History of Medicine

It is sobering to realise that as recently as the year in which On the Origin of Species was published, learned opinion was that diseases such as typhus and cholera were spread by a 'miasma', and suggestions that doctors should wash their hands before examining patients were greeted with mockery by the profession. The Cambridge Library Collection reissues milestone publications in the history of Western medicine as well as studies of other medical traditions. Its coverage ranges from Galen on anatomical procedures to Florence Nightingale's common-sense advice to nurses, and includes early research into genetics and mental health, colonial reports on tropical diseases, documents on public health and military medicine, and publications on spa culture and medicinal plants.

Domestic Medicine

Taking the view that medicine is as much the art of avoiding ill health as it is the cure of disease, physician William Buchan (1729–1805) published this home health guide in 1769. The first part is devoted to preventing ailments through proper diet and exercise, while the second part helps families diagnose and treat maladies ranging from coughs and hiccups to jaundice and gout. Buchan showed particular concern for the health of women and children, whom he believed were often misunderstood and neglected. He condemned corsets and restrictive infant swaddling, discouraged 'high living' and indolence, and blamed the high child-mortality rate on upper-class ignorance of child-rearing wisdom. His book became the most popular health guide prior to the twentieth century, with over a hundred editions by 1871. This reissue is of the first edition. Its diagnoses of physical (and cultural) ailments will illuminate eighteenth-century concerns for modern readers.

Cambridge University Press has long been a pioneer in the reissuing of out-of-print titles from its own backlist, producing digital reprints of books that are still sought after by scholars and students but could not be reprinted economically using traditional technology. The Cambridge Library Collection extends this activity to a wider range of books which are still of importance to researchers and professionals, either for the source material they contain, or as landmarks in the history of their academic discipline.

Drawing from the world-renowned collections in the Cambridge University Library and other partner libraries, and guided by the advice of experts in each subject area, Cambridge University Press is using state-of-the-art scanning machines in its own Printing House to capture the content of each book selected for inclusion. The files are processed to give a consistently clear, crisp image, and the books finished to the high quality standard for which the Press is recognised around the world. The latest print-on-demand technology ensures that the books will remain available indefinitely, and that orders for single or multiple copies can quickly be supplied.

The Cambridge Library Collection brings back to life books of enduring scholarly value (including out-of-copyright works originally issued by other publishers) across a wide range of disciplines in the humanities and social sciences and in science and technology.

Domestic Medicine

Or, the Family Physician

William Buchan

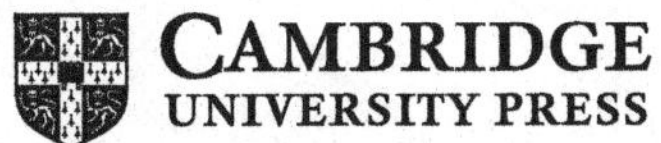

CAMBRIDGE
UNIVERSITY PRESS

University Printing House, Cambridge, CB2 8BS, United Kingdom

Published in the United States of America by Cambridge University Press, New York

Cambridge University Press is part of the University of Cambridge.
It furthers the University's mission by disseminating knowledge in the pursuit of education, learning and research at the highest international levels of excellence.

www.cambridge.org
Information on this title: www.cambridge.org/9781108066259

This edition first published 1769
This digitally printed version 2014

ISBN 978-1-108-06625-9 Paperback

DOMESTIC MEDICINE;

OR THE

FAMILY PHYSICIAN:

BEING AN ATTEMPT

To render the MEDICAL ART more generally uſeful, by ſhewing people what is in their own power both with reſpect to the PREVENTION and CURE of Diſeaſes.

CHIEFLY

Calculated to recommend a proper attention to REGIMEN and SIMPLE MEDICINES.

BY

WILLIAM BUCHAN, M.D.

Sed valitudo ſuſtentatur notitia ſui corporis; et obſervatione, quae res aut prodeſſe ſoleant, aut obeſſe; et continentia in victu omni atque cultu, corporis tuendi cauſa; et praetermittendis voluptatibus; poſtremo, arte eorum quorum ad ſcientiam haec pertinent. CIC. DE OFFIC.

EDINBURGH:
Printed by BALFOUR, AULD, and SMELLIE.

M,DCC,LXIX.

THE

CONTENTS.

PART I. Of PREVENTING DISEASES.

PART

PART II. Of DISEASES.

Of

Of

ADVERTISEMENT.

IT is aſtoniſhing, after medicine has been ſo long cultivated as a liberal art, that philoſophers and men of ſenſe ſhould ſtill queſtion whether it be more beneficial or hurtful to mankind. This doubt could never take its riſe from the nature of medicine, but from the manner in which it has been conducted.

ALL ages and nations have agreed in thinking that the ſick ought to be treated in a manner different from thoſe in health. Indeed the very appetites of the ſick ſhew the neceſſity of, at leaſt, a different regimen. So far medicine is evidently founded in nature, and is quite conſiſtent with reaſon and common ſenſe.

HAD phyſicians been more attentive to *regimen*, and leſs ſollicitous in hunting after wonderful medicines, and concealing their pretended virtues from the reſt of mankind, the medical art would never have become an object of ridicule. The affectation of myſtery may, for a while, draw the admiration of the multitude, but will never ſecure the eſteem of men of ſenſe; and it will always occaſion ſuſpicions in the minds of the more enlightened part of mankind.

EVERY attempt therefore to monopolize or conceal any thing that relates to the preſervation

tion of health or the cure of diseases, must not only be injurious to the interests of society, but likewise detrimental to the medical art. If medicine be a rational science, and founded in nature, it will never lose its reputation by being exposed to public view If it be not able to bear the light, it is high time that it were exploded.

SECRECY in any art lays a foundation for imposition. Had physicians never affected mystery, quacks and quackery could never have existed. Now that they have over-run all Europe, and disgraced both human nature and the medical profession, there is no other method of discrediting them with the people, but a total reverse of behaviour in the Faculty. Let us therefore act with candor, openness, and ingenuity, and mankind will soon learn to dread every thing in medicine that has the smallest appearance of secrecy or disguise.

THE affectation of mystery not only renders the medical art more liable to be abused, but likewise retards its progress. No art ever arrived at any considerable degree of improvement so long as it was kept in the hands of a few who practiced it as a trade. The interested views of a trade will always obstruct the progress of a science. Other arts have been diffused among the people, have become the objects of general attention, and have been improven accordingly. Medicine still continues a mystery. Even the philosopher is not ashamed to own that he is ignorant of the causes and cure of diseases.

diseases. Hence it is, that while other branches of science have arrived at a high degree of perfection, the healing art is still involved in doubt and uncertainty.

Those who follow the beaten tract of a teacher seldom make any useful discoveries. Accordingly we find that most of the real improvements in medicine have either been the effect of chance, or have been made by persons not bred to physic. Men who think and reason for themselves, who are not fettered by theories nor warpt by hypotheses, bid the fairest for improving any art.

As all men are liable to disease, and equally interested in every thing relating to health, it is certainly the duty of physicians to shew them what is in their own power both with respect to the cure of the one, and the preservation of the other. Did men take every method to avoid diseases, they would seldom need the physician; and would they do what is in their own power when sick, there would be little occasion for medicine. It is hard to say if more lives are not lost by people trusting to medicine, and neglecting their own endeavours, than all that are saved by the help of physic.

We do not mean that all men are to be made physicians. This, according to the present acceptation of the word, would be an attempt as ridiculous as it is impossible. We only mean that they should be taught the importance of due *care* for the preservation of health, and of a proper *regimen* in diseases. These they are certainly capable of understanding, and all the rest are of small account.

We are happy to find that some of the most eminent physicians now begin to entertain more liberal ideas with regard to physic. Van Swieten *, Rosen †, Tissot, and some others, have written with a view of diffusing some knowledge of medicine among the people. Their performances have met with that applause from the public, which it is always ready to bestow upon works of real utility. Had Tissot's plan been more extensive, the following pages would probably never have been made public. He confines himself solely to the acute diseases. We have likewise treated the chronic; both because they are very frequent in this country, and because the cure of them chiefly depends on a proper regimen.

Dr Tissot has also treated the prophylaxis, or preventive part of medicine, less minutely than seems necessary. A very slight inquiry into the causes of popular maladies is sufficient to shew that many of them might, by due care, be prevented. For this reason a considerable number of the following pages are employed in pointing out the most common causes of popular

* Physician to their Imperial Majesties.

† First physician of the kingdom of Sweden.

popular diseases, and the means of avoiding them.

THE first part of the prophylaxis is calculated to shew the importance of proper nursing *. The observations were made in a situation where the author had the greatest opportunities of seeing the effects both of the right and wrong management of children, and of being fully convinced that the latter is the principal cause of their great mortality.

PECULIAR attention is paid to the diseases of mechanics. That useful set of people, upon whom the riches and prosperity of Britain depend, can never be too much regarded. Their valuable lives are frequently lost for want of due attention to circumstances which both to themselves and others may often appear trifling.

WE have likewise endeavoured to point out the bad effects of luxury, indolence, &c. All men acknowledge health to be the chief blessing of life; but few shew a proper concern for the preservation of it. There is hardly any pleasure or profit for which people will not hazard their health; and it is often bartered for the most sordid enjoyments. Few things however are more in our own power. Most men may

* Most of the observations contained in the first chapter were made in the Foundling Hospital at Ackworth, and communicated to the public several years ago, in a pamphlet addressed to the governours of that hospital.

may enjoy health if they will. Even thoſe who have had the misfortune to be naturally of a weak conſtitution, have often, by proper care, arrived at an extreme old age, and enjoyed good health to the very laſt; while ſuch as were naturally robuſt, by truſting too much to their ſtrength of conſtitution, and deſpiſing care, have either died young, or dragged out a life of pain and miſery.

In the treatment of diſeaſes we have been chiefly attentive to diet, drink, air, and the other parts of regimen. Regimen ſeems to have been the chief, if not the only medicine of the more early ages, and, to ſay the truth, it is the moſt valuable part of medicine ſtill. But regimen and domeſtic medicines are deſpiſed, while foreign regions are ranſacked for things of leſs value, and every ore which the earth affords is tortured to extract poiſons, and arm the daring empiric for the deſtruction of his fellow men.

We have indeed ventured to recommend ſome ſimple medicines in almoſt every diſeaſe; but even theſe ſhould only be adminiſtred by people of better underſtanding. We would have the ignorant omit them altogether, and atten ſolely to the directions relating to diet and the other parts of regimen.

The laudable diſpoſition which ſo univerſally prevails among the better ſort of people in the country, of aſſiſting their poor neighbours in diſtreſs, ſuggeſted the firſt hint of this attempt. It never was, and, in all probability, never will be be in the power of one half of mankind to obtain the aſſiſtance of phyſicians. What muſt they do? To truſt themſelves in the hands of quacks, or blunder on in the track which their rude forefather's pointed out, are perhaps equally dangerous. The ignorant ruſtic puts little confidence in any endeavours of his own. All his hopes of a cure are placed in ſomething which he does not underſtand, ſomething myſterious and quite above his capacity, as herbs gathered under the influence of ſome planet, charms, the noſtrums of quacks and conjurers, &c. Such are the ridiculous and deſtructive prejudices which prevail among the inhabitants of this country, even in this enlightened age, and ſuch is their entire ignorance of medicine, that they become the eaſy dupes of every pretender to it.

We make no doubt but the ladies, gentlemen, and clergy who reſide in the country will readily concur with us, in endeavouring to root out ſuch pernicious and deſtructive prejudices. Their example will have great weight with their dependents and inferiors; and their advice will be often liſtened to with more attention than that of a phyſician. They will teach the poor the importance of a proper regimen both in health and ſickneſs; the danger of truſting their lives in the hands of quacks and conjurers, and the folly of their own ſuperſtitious notions. By this means they may prevent much evil, do ſome good, and prove real bleſſings to thoſe among whom they reſide.

Nothing

NOTHING is farther from the deſign of the following pages, than to induce ignorant perſons to tamper with dangerous medicines, or truſt to their own ſkill, where better aſſiſtance can be obtained. But where ſomething muſt be done, and no medical aſſiſtance can be had, it is certainly better to direct people what they ought to do than to leave them to blunder on in the dark.

THERE is no doubt but the more mercenary part of the Faculty, whoſe ideas of medicine never riſe above the ſordid views of a trade, will do all in their power to diſcredit every attempt of this kind with the public. With ſuch as are able to ſee through the diſguiſe, their cenſure will paſs for applauſe; and with the leſs enlightened, it will be very little regarded. With us it can have no weight, ſo long as we are conſcious that we have the good of mankind at heart; and that, however imperfect the execution may be, the deſign has been approven by many whoſe names do honour to the medical profeſſion.

As

As people who live in the country cannot always obtain medicines, upon any ſudden emergency, even though they knew how to uſe them, we have here added a liſt of ſuch ſimple druggs and medicines as ought to be kept, at leaſt n every gentleman's family, in order to be in readineſs upon all occaſions.

Rhubarb
Jalap
Senna
Manna
Glaubers ſalts
Cream of tartar
Salt of tartar
Tamarinds
Ipecacuanha
Jeſuits bark
Nitre, or ſalt peter
Sal prunell
Sal. ammoniac
Flowers of ſulphur
Magneſia alba
Crabs claws prepared
Snake root
Liquorice root
Seneka root
Wild Valerian root
Gentian root
Gum arabic
—— camphor
—— ammoniac
—— aſaſœtida
Burgundy pitch
Agaric of the oak
Aſh coloured ground Liver-wort
Cinnamon water
Penny-royal water
Pepper mint water
Syrup of poppies
—— of oranges
—— of lemons
Spirits of wine
—— of hartſhorn
Sweet ſpirits of nitre
—— —— of vitriol
Liquid laudanum
Elixir of vitriol
Vinegar of ſquills
Oil of almonds.
Olive oil
Adheſive plaſter
Bliſtering plaſter
Wax plaſter
Yellow baſilicum ointment
White ointment
Turner's cerate

PART I.

OF PREVENTING DISEASES.

CHAP. I.

OF CHILDREN.

TO avoid diſeaſes, it is neceſſary we ſhould know their cauſes. Theſe indeed are numerous; but we ſhall endeavour to point out ſuch only as have the moſt general influence, as too great minuteneſs in this reſpect would tend rather to perplex than inſtruct the generality of readers.

THE better to trace diſeaſes from their original cauſes, we ſhall take a view of the common treatment of mankind in the ſtate of infancy. In this period of our lives, the foundations of a good or bad conſtitution are generally laid; it is therefore of importance, that parents be well acquainted with the various cauſes which may produce diſeaſes in their offspring. It muſt be owing either to the ignorance or careleſſneſs of parents, that ſo many of the human ſpecies perifh in infancy. This, we prefume, will appear from the following obfervations.

THE annual regifters of the dead fhew, that at leaft one half of the children born in Great Britain die under twelve years of age. To thofe who do not reflect, this appears to be a natural evil, and therefore they think it their duty to fubmit to it. But whoever accurately examines the matter, will find that it is an evil of our own making, and, in a great meafure, owing to mifmanagement Were the death of infants a natural evil, other animals fhould be as liable to die young as man; but that we fee is not the cafe.

IT may feem ftrange that man, notwithftanding his fuperior reafon, fhould fall fo far fhort of other animals in the management of his young: But our furprife will foon ceafe, if we confider that brutes, guided by inftinct, never err in this refpect; while man, trufting folely to art, is feldom right. Were a catalogue of thofe children who perifh annually by art alone exhibited to public view, it would aftonifh moft people.

WHEN parents are above taking care of their children, others muft be employed for that purpofe: Thefe will always endeavour to recommend themfelves by the appearance of extraordinary fkill and addrefs. By this means fo many unneceffary and deftructive articles have been introduced into the diet, cloathing, &c. of children,

dren, that it is no wonder ſo many of them periſh.

NOTHING can be more prepoſterous than for a mother to think it below her to take care of her own child, or to be ſo ignorant as not to know what is proper to be done for it. If we ſearch nature throughout, we cannot find a parallel to this. Every other creature is the nurſe of its own young, and they thrive accordingly. Were the brutes to bring up their young by proxy, they would ſhare the ſame fate with thoſe of the human ſpecies.

WE mean not to impoſe it as a taſk upon every mother to ſuckle her own child. This, whatever ſpeculative writers may ſay to the contrary, is in many caſes impracticable, and would inevitably prove deſtructive both to the mother and child. Women of delicate conſtitutions, ſubject to low ſpirits, hyſteric fits, or other nervous diſorders, make very bad nurſes: But theſe complaints are now ſo common, that it is rare to find a woman of faſhion free from them; for which cauſe few women of better ſtation, ſuppoſe them willing, are really able to ſuckle their own children.

DID mankind live as nature directs, almoſt every mother would be in a condition to give ſuck: But, whoever conſiders how far we have deviated from her dictates, will not be ſurpriſed to find many of them unable to perform that neceſſary office. Mothers, who do not eat enough of ſolid food, nor enjoy the benefit of

free

free air and exercise, can neither have wholesome humours themselves, nor afford proper nourishment to an infant. Children who are suckled by delicate women, either die young, or are weak and sickly all their lives. Nor is this at all to be wondered at. If children suck in nervous diseases with their mother's milk, What have we to expect?

When we say, that every mother is not able to suckle her own child, we would not be understood as discouraging that practice. Every mother who can, ought certainly to perform that tender office. But suppose it to be out of her power, she may, nevertheless, be of great service to her child. The business of nursing is by no means confined to giving suck. To a woman who abounds with milk, that is the easiest part of it. Numberless other offices are necessary for a child, which the mother at least ought to see done. A mother, who abandons the fruit of her womb, as soon as it is born, to the sole care of an hireling, hardly deserves that name. A child, by being brought up under the mother's eye, not only secures her affection, but may reap all the advantages of a mother's care, though it be suckled by another. How can a mother be better employed, than in superintending the nursery? This is at once the most delightful and important office! yet the most trivial business or insipid amusements are often preferred to it. A strong proof both of the bad

bad taſte and wrong education of modern females.

It is much to be regretted, that more pains is not beſtowed in teaching the proper management of children to thoſe whom nature has deſigned for mothers. This, inſtead of being made the principal, is ſeldom conſidered as any part of female education. Is it any wonder, when females, ſo educated, come to be mothers, that they ſhould be quite ignorant of the duties belonging to that ſtation? However ſtrange it may ſeem, it is certainly true, that many mothers, and thoſe of faſhion too, are as ignorant, when they have brought a child into the world, of what is proper to be done for it, as the infant itſelf. Indeed, the moſt ignorant part of the ſex are generally reckoned moſt knowing in the buſineſs of nurſing. Hence, ſenſible people become the dupes of ignorance and ſuperſtition; and the nurſing of children, inſtead of being conducted by reaſon, is the reſult of whim and caprice.

One great deſign of females, no doubt, is to propagate the ſpecies. But to bring forth a child, is the leaſt part of that important buſineſs. Were the care of a parent to ſtop here, the whole human race would ſoon be extinct. Nature has made it neceſſary, that a child ſhould depend on its parents during the ſtate of infancy; and thoſe parents who neglect the proper care of their offspring, not only violate one of the firſt and ſtrongeſt principles of nature,

ture, but actually endeavour to extinguiſh the human race. An infant may be as certainly murdered by neglect, as by any act of violence whatever; and, for one child that loſes its life by the latter, a thouſand periſh by the former, without being regarded.

WERE the time that is generally ſpent by females in acquiring uſeleſs knowledge, employed in learning how to bring up their children; how to dreſs them ſo as not to hurt, cramp, or confine their motions; how to feed them with wholeſome and nouriſhing food; how to exerciſe their tender bodies, ſo as beſt to promote their growth and ſtrength: Were theſe the objects of female inſtruction, mankind would derive the greateſt advantages from it. But, while the education of females implies little more than what relates to dreſs and public ſhow, we have nothing to expect from them but ignorance, even in the moſt important concerns. But ignorance can be no excuſe, where people have it in their power to be better informed; and, if children periſh by the negligence of mothers, they muſt be accountable.

DID mothers know their importance, and lay it to heart, they would embrace every opportunity of informing themſelves of the duties which they owe to their infant-offspring. It is theirs, not only to form the body, but alſo to give the mind its moſt early caſt. They have it very much in their power to make men healthy

healthy or valetudinary, uſeful in life, or the bane of ſociety.

But the mother is not the only perſon concerned in the management of children. The father has an equal intereſt in their welfare, and ought to aſſiſt in every thing that reſpects either the improvement of the body or mind.

It is pity that men pay ſo little regard to this matter. Their neglect is one reaſon why females know ſo little of it. Women will ever be deſirous to excel in ſuch accompliſhments as recommend them to the other ſex. But men generally keep at ſuch a diſtance from even the ſmalleſt acquaintance with the affairs of the nurſery, that many would eſteem it an affront, were they ſuppoſed to know any thing of it. Not ſo, however, with the kennel or the ſtables: A gentleman of the firſt rank is not aſhamed to give directions concerning the management of his dogs or horſes; but would bluſh were he to be ſurpriſed in performing the ſame office for that being, who derived its exiſtence from himſelf, who is the heir of his fortunes, and the future hope of his country. Few fathers indeed run any hazard of being ſurpriſed in this ſituation; yet, certain it is, that man needs culture more than any other creature, and that both his body and mind are capable of the greateſt improvement. Nature has left ſo much in the power of parents, that children are, in a great meaſure, what they pleaſe to make them.

Physicians

PHYSICIANS themſelves have not been ſufficiently attentive to the management of children: That has been generally conſidered as the ſole province of old women, while men of the firſt rank in phyſic have even refuſed to viſit infants when ſick. Such conduct in the faculty has not only cauſed this branch of medicine to be neglected, but has alſo encouraged the other ſex to aſſume an abſolute title to preſcribe for children in the moſt dangerous diſeaſes. The conſequence is, that a phyſician is ſeldom called till the good women have exhauſted all their ſkill; when his attendance can only ſerve to divide the blame and appeaſe the diſconſolate parents.

WE would have nurſes do all in their power to prevent diſeaſes; but, when a child is taken ill, ſome perſon of ſkill ſhould immediately be conſulted. The diſeaſes of children are generally acute, and the leaſt delay is dangerous.

WERE phyſicians more attentive to the diſeaſes of children, they would not only be better qualified to treat them properly when ſick, but likewiſe to give uſeful directions for their management when well. The diſeaſes of children is by no means ſuch a difficult ſtudy as many imagine. It is true, children cannot tell their complaints; but the cauſes of them may be pretty certainly diſcovered, by putting proper queſtions to the nurſes and ſuch as are about them. Beſides, the diſeaſes of infants, being

ing leſs complicated, are eaſier cured than thoſe of adults.

It is really aſtoniſhing, that ſo little attention ſhould in general be paid to the preſervation of infant lives! What labour and expence are daily beſtowed to prop an old rotten carcaſe for a few years, while thouſands of thoſe, who might be uſeful in life, periſh without being regarded, and prove no better than an untimely birth! Mankind are apt to value things not according to their future but their preſent utility. This is of all others the moſt erroneous method of eſtimation; yet, upon no other principle is it poſſible to account for the general indifference with reſpect to the death of infants.

Of DISEASED PARENTS.

Diseased parents cannot beget healthy children. It would be as reaſonable to expect a rich crop from a barren ſoil, as that ſtrong and healthy children ſhould be born of delicate parents, worn out with intemperance or diſeaſe.

An ingenious writer obſerves *, that on the conſtitution of mothers depends originally that of their offſpring. No one who believes this will be ſurpriſed, on a view of the female world, to find diſeaſes and death ſo frequent

* Rouſſeau.

among children. A delicate female brought up within doors, an utter ſtranger to exerciſe and open air, who lives on tea and other ſlops, may bring a child into the world, but it will hardly be fit to live. The firſt blaſt of a diſeaſe will nip the tender plant in the bud: Or, ſhould it ſtruggle through a few years exiſtence, its feeble frame, ſhook with convulſions from every trivial cauſe, would be unable to ſuſtain the common functions of life, and prove a burden to ſociety.

If, to the delicacy of mothers, we add the irregular lives of fathers, we ſhall ſee further cauſe to believe that children are often hurt by the conſtitution of their parents. A ſickly frame may be originally induced by hardſhips or intemperance, but chiefly by the latter. It is impoſſible that a courſe of vice ſhould not ſpoil the beſt conſtitution: And did the evil terminate here, it would be a juſt puniſhment for the folly of the ſufferer; but when once a diſtemper is contracted and rivetted in the habit, it is entailed on all poſterity. What a dreadful inheritance is the gout, the ſcurvy, or the kings-evil, to tranſmit to our offspring! How happy had it been for the heir of many a great eſtate had he been born a beggar, rather than to inherit his father's fortunes at the expence of likewiſe inheriting his diſeaſes!

No perſon who labours under any incurable malady ought to marry, as he thereby both ſhortens his own life and tranſmits miſery to others:

others: But when both parties are deeply tainted with the ſcrophula, the ſcurvy, or the like, the effects muſt be ſtill worſe. Such will either have no iſſue at all, or thoſe whom they have muſt be miſerable indeed. Want of attention to theſe things, in forming connections for life, has rooted out more families than the plague, famine, or the ſword; and while theſe connections are formed from mercenary views, that muſt be the caſe.

In our matrimonial contracts, it is amazing ſo little regard is had to the health and form of the object. Our ſportſmen know, that the generous courſer cannot be bred out of the foundered jade, nor the ſagacious ſpaniel out of the ſnarling cur. This is ſettled upon immutable laws. The man who marries a woman of a ſickly conſtitution, and deſcended of unhealthy parents, whatever his views may be, cannot be ſaid to act a prudent part. A puny ſcrophulous woman may prove fertile; ſhould this be the caſe, the family muſt become an infirmary: What proſpect of happineſs the father of ſuch a family has, we ſhall leave any one to judge.

The Jews, by the poſitive direction of the Almighty, were forbid to have any manner of commerce with the diſeaſed; and indeed to this, all wiſe legiſlators ought to have a ſpecial regard. In ſome ſtates, the marriage of morbid people has actually been prohibited. This is an evil of a complicated kind, a natural deformity

deformity, and political miſchief; and therefore requires a public conſideration.

Such children as have the misfortune to be born of diſeaſed parents, will require to be nurſed with greater care than others. This is the only way to make amends for the defects of conſtitution; and it will often go a great length. A healthy nurſe, wholeſome air, and enough of exerciſe, will do wonders. But, when theſe are neglected, little is to be expected from any other quarter. The defects of conſtitution cannot be ſupplied by medicine.

Those who inherit any family-diſeaſe, ought to be very circumſpect in their manner of living. They ſhould conſider well the nature of ſuch diſeaſe, and guard againſt it by a proper regimen. It is certain, that family-diſeaſes have often, by proper care, been kept off for one generation; and there is great reaſon to believe, that, by perſiſting in the ſame courſe, ſuch diſeaſes might at length be wholely eradicated. This is a ſubject very little regarded, though of the laſt importance. Family-conſtitutions are as capable of improvement, as family-eſtates; and the libertine, who impairs the one, does greater injury to his poſterity, than the prodigal who ſquanders away the other.

Of

Of the CLOATHING of CHILDREN.

THE cloathing of an infant is ſo ſimple a matter, that it is ſurpriſing, how any perſon ſhould err in it; yet many children loſe their lives and others are deformed, by errors of this kind.

NATURE knows no other uſe of cloaths to an infant, but to keep it warm. All that is neceſſary for this purpoſe, is to wrap it in a ſoft, looſe covering. Were a mother left to the dictates of nature and reaſon, this is certainly the method that ſhe would follow. But the buſineſs of dreſſing an infant has long been out of the hands of mothers, and has at laſt become a ſecret, which none but adepts pretend to underſtand.

FROM the moſt early ages it has been thought neceſſary, that a woman in labour ſhould have ſome perſon to attend her. This in time became a buſineſs; and, like all others, thoſe who were employed in it, ſtrove to outdo one another in the different branches of their profeſſion. The dreſſing of a child came of courſe to be conſidered as the midwife's province, who no doubt imagined, that the more dexterity ſhe could ſhow in this article, the more her ſkill would be admired. Her attempts might be ſeconded by the vanity of parents, who wanting to make a ſhow of the infant as ſoon as it was born,

born, were ambitious to have as much finery heaped upon it as poſſible. Thus, it came to be thought as neceſſary for a midwife to excel in bracing and dreſſing an infant, as for a ſurgeon to be expert in applying bandages to a broken limb; and the poor child, as ſoon as it came into the world, had as many rollers and wrappers applied to its body, as if every bone had been fractured in the birth; while theſe were often ſo tight, as not only to gall and wound its tender frame, but even to obſtruct the motion of the heart, lungs, and other organs neceſſary for life.

In ſeveral parts of Britain, the practice of rolling children with ſo many bandages is now in ſome meaſure, laid aſide; but it would ſtill be a difficult taſk to perſuade the generality of women, that the ſhape of a child does not intirely depend on the midwife's care. So far however, are all their endeavours to mend the ſhape of children from being ſucceſsful, that they conſtantly operate the contrary way, and mankind become deformed juſt in proportion to the means uſed to prevent deformity. How little deformity of body is to be found among uncivilized nations? So little indeed, that it is vulgarly believed they put all their deformed children to death. The truth is, they hardly know ſuch a thing as a deformed child. Neither ſhould we, if we followed their example. Savage nations never think of manacling their children. They allow them the full uſe of every

very organ, carry them abroad in the open air, waſh their bodies daily in cold water, *&c.* By this management, their children become ſo ſtrong and hardy, that, by the time our puny infants get out of the nurſe's arms theirs are able to ſhift for themſelves.

Among brute animals, no art is neceſſary to procure a fine ſhape. Though many of them be extremely delicate when they come into the world, yet we never find them grow crooked for want of ſwaddling-bands. Is nature leſs generous to the human kind? No: But we take the buſineſs out of nature's hands.

Not only the analogy of other animals, but the very feelings of infants tell us, that they ought to be kept eaſy and free from all preſſure. They cannot indeed ſpeak their complaints; but they can ſhew ſigns of pain; and this they never fail to do by crying, when pinched by their cloaths. No ſooner are they freed from their bracings, than they ſeem pleaſed and happy; yet, ſtrange infatuation! The moment they hold their peace, they are again committed to their chains.

If we conſider the body of an infant as a bundle of ſoft pipes, repleniſhed with fluids in continual motion, the danger of preſſure will appear in the ſtrongeſt light. Nature, in order to make way for the growth of children, has formed their bodies ſoft and flexible; and, leſt they ſhould receive any injury from preſſure in the womb, has ſurrounded the *fœtus* every

way

way with fluids. This ſhews the care which nature takes to prevent all unequal preſſure on the bodies of infants, and to defend them againſt every thing that might in the leaſt cramp or confine their motions.

Even the bones of an infant are ſo ſoft and cartilaginous, that they readily yield to the ſlighteſt preſſure, and eaſily take on a bad ſhape, which can never after be remedied. Hence it is, that ſo many people appear with high ſhoulders, crooked ſpines, and flat breaſts, who were born with as good a ſhape as others, but had the misfortune to be ſqueezed into monſters by the application of ſtays and bandages.

Pressure, by obſtructing the circulation, prevents the equal diſtribution of nouriſhment to the different parts of the body, by which means the growth becomes unequal. One part of the body grows two large, while another remains too ſmall, and thus in time the whole frame becomes diſproportioned and misſhapen. To this we muſt add, that when a child is cramped in its cloaths, it naturally ſhrinks from the parts affected, and by putting its body into unnatural poſtures, it becomes deformed by habit.

Deformity of body may proceed from weakneſs or diſeaſes; but, in general, it is the effect of improper cloathing. Nine tenths, at leaſt, of the deformity amongſt mankind muſt be imputed to this cauſe. A deformed body is not only diſagreeable to the eye, but injurious

to

to the health. By a bad figure both the animal and vital functions muſt be impeded, and of courſe health impaired. Hence, few people remarkably misſhapen are ſtrong or healthy.

THE new motions which commence at the birth, as the circulation of the blood through the lungs, reſpiration, the periſtaltic motion, *&c.* afford another ſtrong argument for keeping the body of an infant free from all preſſure. Theſe organs, not having been accuſtomed to move, are eaſily ſtopped; but when that happens, death muſt enſue. Hardly any method could be deviſed more effectually to ſtop theſe motions, than bracing the body too tight with * rollers, *&c.* Were theſe to be applied in the ſame manner to the body of an adult, for an equal length of time, they could hardly fail to hurt the digeſtion and make him ſick. How much more hurtful they muſt be to tender infants, we ſhall leave any one to judge.

WHOEVER conſiders theſe things will not be ſurpriſed, that ſo many children die of convulſions ſoon after the birth. Theſe fits are generally attributed to ſome inward cauſe; but, in fact, they oftener proceed from our own imprudent conduct. I have known a child ſeized with convulſion-fits, ſoon after the midwife had done ſwaddling it; but, upon taking off the rollers and bandages, it was immediately relieved,

and

* This is by no means enveighing againſt a thing that does not happen. In many parts of Britain at this day a roller, five or ſix feet in length, is applied round the child's body as ſoon as it is born.

and never had any convulſion-fits afterwards. Numerous examples of this ſort might be brought, were they neceſſary.

It would be ſafer to fix on the cloaths of an infant with ſtrings than pins, as theſe often gall and irritate their tender ſkins, and occaſion convulſions. Inſtances have been known, where pins were found ſticking above half an inch into the body of a child after it had died of convulſion-fits, which, in all probability proceeded from that cauſe.

Children are not only hurt by the tightneſs of their cloaths, but alſo by the quantity. Every child has ſome degree of fever after the birth; and, if it be loaded with too many cloaths, the fever muſt be increaſed. But that is not all; the child is generally laid in bed with the mother, who is likewiſe feveriſh; to which we may add the heat of the lying-in bed-chamber, and the wines, and other heating things too often given to children immediately after the birth. When all theſe are combined, which does not ſeldom happen, they muſt increaſe the fever to ſuch a degree as will endanger the life of the infant.

The danger of keeping infants too hot, will further appear, if we conſider, that, after being for ſome time in the ſituation mentioned above, they are often ſent into the country to be nurſed in a cold houſe *. Is it any wonder, if a child, from ſuch a tranſition, catches a mortal cold, or contracts ſome other fatal diſeaſe? When

* Cadogan.

When an infant is kept too hot, its lungs not being sufficiently expanded, are apt to remain weak and flaccid for life; from whence proceed coughs, consumptions, and other diseases of the breast.

It would answer little purpose to specify the particular pieces of dress proper for an infant. These ever will vary in different places according to custom and the humour of parents. The great rule to be observed is, *That a child have no more cloaths than are necessary to keep it warm, and that they be quite easy for its body.*

Stays are the very bane of children. A volume would not suffice to point out all the ill effects of this useless piece of dress. The madness in favour of stays seems, however, to have been at a height; and it is to be hoped the world will, in time, become wise enough to know, that the human shape does not solely depend upon whale-bone and bend leather *

We shall only add, with respect to the cloaths of children, that they ought to be kept very clean. Children persoire more than adults; and, if their cloaths be not frequently changed, they become very hurtful. Dirty cloaths not only gall and fret the tender skins of infants, but likewise occasion ill smells; and, what is worse tend to produce vermin and cutaneous diseases.

CLEANLINESS

* Stays made of bend leather are worn by all the women of lower station in many parts of England.

Cleanliness is not only agreeable to the eye, but tends greatly to preſerve the health of children. It promotes the perſpiration; and, by that means, frees the body from ſuperfluous humours, which, if retained, could not fail to occaſion diſeaſes. A nurſe can have no excuſe for allowing a child to be dirty. Poverty may oblige her to give it coarſe cloaths; but, if ſhe does not keep them clean, it muſt be her own fault.

Of the FOOD of CHILDREN.

Nature, not only points out the food proper for an infant, but actually prepares it. This however, is not ſufficient to prevent ſome who think themſelves wiſer than nature, from attempting to bring up their children without her proviſion. Nothing can ſhow the diſpoſition which mankind have to depart from nature more than their endeavouring to bring up children without the breaſt. The mother's milk, or that of a healthy nurſe, is unqueſtionably the beſt food for an infant. Neither art nor nature can afford a proper ſubſtitute for it. A child may ſeem to thrive for a few months without the breaſt; but, when teething, the ſmall-pox, and other diſeaſes incident to childhood come on, they generally fall a victim. An evident proof, that their food is unwholeſome, and their humours bad.

A child ſoon after the birth ſhows an inclination to ſuck; and there ſeems to be no reaſon why it ſhould not be gratified. It is true the mother's milk does not always come immediately after the birth; but is not this the way to bring it? The firſt milk that the child can ſqueeze out of the breaſt, anſwers the purpoſe of cleanſing better than all the drugs in the apothecary's ſhop, and at the ſame time prevents inflammations of the breaſt, fevers, and other diſeaſes incident to mothers.

It is ſtrange how people came to think that the firſt thing given to a child ſhould be drugs. This is beginning with medicine by times, and no wonder that they generally end with it. It ſometimes happens, that a child does not paſs the *meconium* ſo ſoon as could be wiſhed. This has induced phyſicians in ſuch caſes to give ſomething of an opening nature to cleanſe the firſt paſſages. Midwives have improved upon this hint, and never fail to give ſyrups, oils, &c. whether they be neceſſary or not. Cramming an infant with ſuch indigeſtible ſtuff as ſoon as it is born, can hardly fail to make it ſick, and is more likely to occaſion diſeaſes, than prevent them. Children are ſeldom long after the birth without having paſſage both by ſtool and urine; though theſe evacuations may be wanting for ſome time without any danger.

Were a child permitted to ſuck its mother as ſoon as it ſhows an inclination for the breaſt, it would need no other phyſic; but, if it muſt have

have ſomething before it be allowed the breaſt, let it be a little ſimple water-pap, to which may be added an equal quantity of new milk. If this be given without any wines, ſugars, or ſpiceries, it will neither heat the blood, load the ſtomach, nor occaſion gripes.

Upon the firſt ſight of an infant, almoſt every perſon is ſtruck with the idea of its being weak, feeble, and wanting ſupport. This naturally ſuggeſts the need of cordials. Accordingly, we find wines univerſally mixed with the firſt food of children. Nothing can be more fallacious than this way of reaſoning, or more hurtful to infants than the conduct founded upon it. Children need very little food for ſome time after the birth; and what they receive ſhould be thin, weak, light, and of a cooling quality. A very ſmall quantity of wine, or even ſugar, is ſufficient to heat and inflame the blood of an infant; but every perſon, converſant in theſe matters, muſt know, that moſt of the diſeaſes of infants proceed from the heat of their humours, as the thruſh, &c.

If the mother or nurſe has enough of milk, the child will need little or no other food before the third or fourth month. It will then be proper to give it, once or twice a-day, a little of ſome food that is eaſy of digeſtion; as water-pap milk-pottage, weak broth with bread in it, or the like. This will eaſe the mother; it will accuſtom the child by degrees to take food, and render the weaning both leſs difficult and dangerous,

ous. All great and ſudden tranſitions are to be avoided in nurſing. For this purpoſe, the food of children ought to be ſimple, as near as poſſible reſembling the properties of milk. Indeed milk itſelf ſhould make a principal part of their food, not only before they be weaned, but for a long time after.

NEXT to milk, we would recommend good light bread. Bread may be given to a child as ſoon as it ſhows an inclination to chew, and it may at all times be allowed as much as it pleaſes. The very chewing of bread will help to cut the teeth and promote the diſcharge of *ſaliva*, while by mixing with the nurſe's milk in the ſtomach, it will afford an excellent nouriſhment. Children ſhow an early inclination to chew whatever is put into their hands. Parents obſerve the inclination, but generally miſtake the object. Inſtead of giving the child ſomething which may at once exerciſe its gums and afford it nouriſhment, they commonly put into its hand a piece of hard metal or impenetrable coral. A cruſt of bread is the beſt gum-ſtick. It not only anſwers the purpoſe better than any thing elſe, but has the additional properties mentioned above, of nouriſhing the child and carrying the *ſaliva* down to the ſtomach, which is too valuable a liquor to be loſt.

BREAD, beſides being uſed dry, may be many ways prepared into food for children. One of the beſt methods of preparing it, is to boil it in

water,

water, afterwards pouring the water off, and mixing with the bread a proper quantity of new milk unboiled: Milk is both more wholeſome and nouriſhing this way than boiled, and is leſs apt to occaſion coſtiveneſs. For a child farther advanced, bread may be mixed in veal or chicken broth, made into puddings, or the like. Bread is a proper food for children at all times, provided it be plain, made of wholeſome grain, and well fermented; but when enriched with fruits, ſugars, or ſuch things, it becomes very unwholeſome.

It is ſoon enough to allow children animal food when they have got teeth to eat it. They ſhould never taſte it till after they are weaned, and even then they ought to uſe it very ſparingly. Indeed, when children live wholely on vegetable food, it is apt to ſour on their ſtomachs; on the other hand, too much fleſh heats the blood and occaſions fevers and other inflammatory diſeaſes. This plainly points out a proper mixture of animal and vegetable food as moſt fit for children.

Few things are more hurtful to children, than the common method of ſweetening their food. It not only makes them grow fat and bloated, but entices them to take more food than they ought to do. It is pretty certain, if childrens food were quite plain, that they would never take more than enough. Thus the exceſſes of children are entirely owing to nurſes. If a child be gorged with food at all hours, and

enticed

enticed to take it, by making it ſweet and agreeable to the palate, is it any wonder if ſuch a child comes in time to crave more food than it ought to have?

CHILDREN may be hurt by too little as well as too much food. After a child is weaned, it ought to be fed four or five times a-day; but ſhould never be accuſtomed to eat in the night; neither ſhould it have too much at one time. Some lay it down as a rule, that no child ought to be fed above three times in twenty-four hours; whereas moſt adults eat four times in the ſame ſpace. The food of children is generally lighter than that of adults; their digeſtion is likewiſe more quickly performed: If to theſe we add the power of habit, we will be inclined to think, that children ſhould be fed oftener than up-grown perſons. If a child, who has been accuſtomed to ſuck its nurſe at all hours, be ſuddenly deprived of that, and reſtricted to three meals a-day, bad conſequences muſt follow. I have often ſeen the ſcheme of bringing children to live on three regular meals a day tried, but never knew it ſucceed. Children thrive much better with ſmall quantities of food frequently given. This neither overcharges the ſtomach, nor hurts the digeſtion, and is certainly moſt agreeable to nature.

WRITERS on nurſing have inveighed with ſuch vehemence againſt too much food, that one would be apt to imagine two thirds of thoſe who die in infancy were actually crammed to death. This has induced many parents to ruin the conſtitutions of their children, by running into the other extreme. The error of pinching children in their food, is more hurtful than its oppoſite. Nature has many ways of relieving herſelf when overcharged; but a child who is pinched with hunger will never become a ſtrong or healthy man That errors are frequently committed on both ſides, we are ready to acknowledge; but where one child is hurt by the quantity of its food, ten ſuffer from the quality. That is the principal evil, and claims our ſtricteſt attention.

MANY people imagine, that food which they love themſelves cannot be bad for their children: But this notion is very abſurd. In the more advanced periods of life we often acquire an inclination for food which when children we could not bear to taſte. There are many things that may agree very well with the ſtomach of an up-grown perſon, which would be very hurtful to a child; as high-ſeaſoned, ſalted, and ſmoke-dried proviſions, &c. It would alſo be improper to feed children with fat meat, ſtrong broths, rich ſoups, gravies, or the like.

ALL ſtrong liquors are hurtful to children. Some parents teach their children to guzzle ale, and other ſtrong liquors at every meal; but ſuch a practice cannot fail to do miſchief. Theſe children ſeldom eſcape the violence of the ſmall-pox, meaſles, hooping cough, or ſome other feveriſh diſorder. Milk, water, butter-

milk.

milk, or whey, make the moſt proper drink for children. It they have any thing ſtronger, it may be fine ſmall beer, or a little wine mixed with water. The ſtomachs of children can digeſt well enough without the aſſiſtance of warm ſtimulants. Young people are naturally hot, and conſequently are eaſily hurt by every thing of a heating quality: Their blood has a conſtant tendency to inflammation, which all ſtrong liquors muſt increaſe.

Few things are more hurtful to children than unripe fruits. Theſe not only ſour the ſtomach, but relax it, and weaken the digeſtion; by which means it becomes a proper neſt fo worms of all kinds. Children indeed ſhow the greateſt inclination for fruit, and I am apt to believe, that if good ripe fruit were allowed them in proper quantity, it would have no bad effects. We ſeldom find a natural inclination wrong, if directed to its proper objects. Fruits are generally of a cooling nature, and correct the heat and acrimony of the humours. This is what moſt children want; only care ſhould be taken leſt they exceed. Indeed the beſt way to prevent children from going to exceſs in the uſe of fruit, or eating that which is bad, is to allow them a proper quantity of what is good.

Roots which contain a crude viſeid juice ſhould be ſparingly given to children. They fill the body with groſs humours, and tend to produce eruptive diſeaſes. This caution is peculiarly neceſſary for the poor; being glad to

get

get what will fill their childrens bellies for a little money, they ſtuff them two or three times a-day with potatoes and the like. Children had better eat a ſmall quantity of ſuch food as would yield a wholeſome nouriſhment, than be crammed with what their digeſtive powers are unable properly to aſſimulate.

BUTTER ought likewiſe to be ſparingly given to children. It both relaxes the ſtomach, and produces groſs humours. Indeed moſt things that are fat or oily, have the ſame effect. Butter, when ſalted, becomes ſtill more hurtful. Inſtead of butter, ſo plentifully eat by children in moſt parts of Britain, we would recommend honey. Honey is not only more wholeſome than butter, but likewiſe cheaper. It is cooling, cleanſing, and tends to ſweeten the humours; whereas butter is juſt the reverſe. Children who eat honey are ſeldom troubled with worms. They are alſo leſs ſubject to the common cutateous diſeaſes, as itch, ſcabbed head, &c.

MANY people err in thinking the diet of children ſhould be always moiſt. When children live entirely upon ſlops, it relaxes their ſolids, renders them weak, and prediſpoſes them to rickets, ſcrophulas, and other glandular diſorders. Relaxation is one of the moſt general cauſes of the diſeaſes of children. Every thing therefore which tends to unbrace their bodies ought to be carefully avoided.

WE would not be underſtood as confining children to any particular kind of food. Their diet

diet may be frequently varied, provided regard be had to ſimplicity. Whatever food we are moſt accuſtomed to in youth, we generally love during life. For this reaſon children ſhould have a little of any kind of food that is plain and wholeſome, leſt they ſhould contract an averſion from it, and afterwards be under a neceſſity of uſing it.

Of the EXERCISE of CHILDREN.

Of all the cauſes which conſpire to render the lives of children ſhort and miſerable, none has greater influence than the want of proper exercise. Healthy parents, wholeſome food, and proper cloathing, will avail little where it is neglected. Enough of exerciſe will make up for ſeveral other defects; but nothing can ſupply the want of it. It is abſolutely neceſſary to the health, the growth, and the ſtrength of children.

The deſire of exerciſe is almoſt coeval with life itſelf. Were this principle attended to, many diſeaſes might be prevented. But while indolence and ſedentary employments keep two thirds of mankind from either taking exerciſe themſelves, or giving it to their children, what have we to expect but diſeaſes and deformity among their offspring? The rickets, ſo deſtructive to children, never appeared in Britain till manufactures began to flouriſh, and people, attracted

tracted by the love of gain, left the country to follow ſedentary employments in great towns. It is amongſt theſe people that this diſeaſe chiefly prevails, and not only deforms, but kills many of their offspring.

THE analogy of other animals ſhews that children require exerciſe. Every creature endeavours to make uſe of its organs as ſoon as it can, and many of them, even when under no neceſſity of moving in queſt of food, cannot be reſtrained without force. This is evidently the caſe with the calf, the lamb, and many other young animals. If theſe creatures were not permitted to friſk about, and take exerciſe, they would ſoon die. The ſame inclination appears very early in the human ſpecies; but as they are not able to take exerciſe themſelves, it is the buſineſs of their parents or nurſes to aſſiſt them.

CHILDREN may be exerciſed various ways. The beſt method, while light, is to carry them about in the nurſe's arms. This gives the nurſe an opportunity of talking to the child, and of pointing out every thing that may pleaſe and delight its fancy. It is much ſafer than ſwinging an infant in a machine, or leaving it to the care of ſuch as are not fit to take care of themſelves. Nothing can be more fooliſh than to ſet one child to keep another; that has proved fatal to many infants, and has rendered others lame for life.

WHEN children begin to walk, the ſafeſt and beſt

beſt method of leading them about is by the hands. The common way of ſwinging children by ſtrings fixed to their backs, has many bad conſequences. It makes them throw their bodies foreward, and preſs with their whole weight upon the breaſt: by that means the breathing is obſtructed, the breaſt flattened, and the bowels compreſſed. This hurts the digeſtion, and occaſions conſumptions of the lungs, and other diſeaſes.

IT is a common notion, that if children be ſet upon their feet too ſoon, their legs will become crooked. There is reaſon to believe, that the very reverſe of this is true. Every member acquires ſtrength in proportion as it is exerciſed. The limbs of children are weak indeed, but their bodies are proportionably light; and had they ſkill to direct themſelves, they would ſoon be able to ſupport their own weight. Who ever heard of any other animal that became crooked by uſing its legs too ſoon? Indeed if a child be not permitted to make uſe of its legs till a conſiderable time after the birth, and be then ſet upon them with its whole weight at once, there may be ſome danger of hurting it; but this proceeds intirely from the child's not having been accuſtomed to uſe its legs from the beginning.

MOTHERS of the poorer ſort think they gain a great deal by making their children lie or ſit while they work. In this they are greatly miſtaken. By neglecting to give their children exerciſe, they are obliged to keep them a long time

time before they can do any thing for themſelves, and to ſpend more on medicine than would have paid for proper care, while it can never ſupply its place. To take care of their children, is the moſt profitable buſineſs in which even the poor can employ themſelves: But alas! it is not always in their power. Poverty often obliges them to neglect their offspring, in order to procure the neceſſaries of life. When that is the caſe, it becomes the intereſt as well as the duty of the public to aſſiſt them. Ten thouſand times more benefit would accrue to the State, by enabling the poor to bring up their own children, than from all the * hoſpitals that ever can be erected for that purpoſe.

WHOEVER conſiders the ſtructure of the human body, will ſoon be convinced of the neceſſity of exerciſe for the health of children. The body is compoſed of an infinite number of veſſels, whoſe contents cannot be puſhed on without the action and preſſure of the muſcles. But if the fluids remain inactive, obſtructions muſt happen, and the humours

* If we make it the intereſt of the poor to keep their offſpring alive, we ſhall loſe very few of them. This I have had many opportunities of obſerving. A ſmall premium given to the poor annually for every child they have alive, would ſave more infant-lives than if the whole revenues of the nation were expended on hoſpitals for that purpoſe. This would make the poor eſteem fertility a bleſſing; whereas many of them think it the greateſt curſe that can befal them; and in place of wiſhing their children to live, ſo far does poverty get the better of natural affection, that they are very happy when they die.

mours will of courſe be vitiated, which cannot fail to occaſion diſeaſes. Nature has furniſhed both the veſſels which carry the blood and lymph with numerous valves, in order that the action of every muſcle might puſh forward their contents; but without action, this admirable contrivance can have no effect. The final cauſe of this part of the animal œconomy proves the neceſſity of exerciſe for the preſervation of health.

ARGUMENTS to ſhew the importance of exerciſe might be drawn from every part of the animal œconomy: Without exerciſe the circulation of the blood cannot be properly carried on, nor the different ſecretions duly performed; without exerciſe the humours cannot be properly prepared, nor the ſolids rendered ſtrong or firm. The action of the heart, the motion of the lungs, and all the vital functions are greatly aſſiſted by exerciſe. But to point out the manner in which theſe effects are produced, would lead us farther into the œconomy of the human body, than moſt of thoſe for whom this treatiſe is intended would be able to follow. We ſhall therefore only add, that where exerciſe is neglected, none of the animal functions can be duly performed; and when that is the caſe, the whole conſtitution muſt go to wreck.

CERTAINLY our firſt object in the management of children ought to be a good conſtitution. This lays a foundation for their being uſeful and happy in life; and whoever neglects it, not only fails in his duty to his offspring, but to ſociety.

One very common error of parents, by which they hurt the conſtitutions of their children, is ſending them too young to ſchool. This is often done ſolely to prevent trouble. When the child is at ſchool, he needs no keeper. Thus the ſchoolmaſter is made the nurſe; and the poor child is nailed to a ſeat ſeven or eight hours a-day, which ought to be ſpent in exerciſe and diverſions. Sitting ſo long cannot fail to produce the worſt effects upon the body; nor is the mind leſs injured. Larly application weakens the faculties, and often fixes in the mind ſuch an averſion from books as can never be removed.

But ſuppoſe this were the way to make children ſcholars, that ought not to be done at the expence of their conſtitutions. Our anceſtors, who ſeldom went to ſchool before they were men, were not leſs learned than we. But we imagine the boy's education will be quite loſt unleſs he be carried to ſchool in his nurſe's arms. No wonder if ſuch hot-bed plants ſeldom become either ſcholars or men!

Not only the confinement in public ſchools, but the number often proves extremely hurtful. Children are much injured by being kept in crowds within doors; their breathing not only renders the place unwholeſome; but if any one of them happens to be diſeaſed, the reſt catch the infection. A ſingle child has been often

often known to communicate the bloody-flux, the hooping-cough, the itch, or other diſeaſes, to almoſt every individual in a numerous ſchool.

But if faſhion will prevail, and infants muſt be ſent to ſchool, we would earneſtly recommend to teachers, as they value the intereſts of ſociety, not to confine them too long at a time; but to permit them to run about and play at ſuch active diverſions as may promote their growth and improve their conſtitutions. Were boys, inſtead of being whipped for ſtealing an hour to run, ride, ſwim, or the like, encouraged to employ their time in theſe manly and uſeful exerciſes, it would have many excellent effects.

It would likewiſe be of great ſervice to boys, if at a proper age, they were all taught the military exerciſe. This would improve their ſtrength, courage, and agility; and, when their country called for their aſſiſtance, it would enable them to act in her defence, without being obliged to undergo a tedious and troubleſome courſe of inſtructions, at a time when they are leſs fit to learn new motions, geſtures, *&c.*

An effeminate education will infallibly ſpoil the beſt natural conſtitution; and, if boys are brought up in a more delicate manner than even girls ought to be, they never will be men.

But the common education of girls is no leſs hurtful to the conſtitution than that of boys. Miſs is ſet down to her frame, before ſhe

ſhe can put on her cloaths; and is taught to believe, that to excell at the needle is the only thing that can intitle her to general eſteem. It is unneceſſary here to inſiſt upon the dangerous conſequences of obliging girls to ſit too much. They are pretty well known, and are too often felt at a certain time of life. But ſuppoſe this critical period to be got over, greater dangers ſtill await them when they come to be mothers. Women who have been early accuſtomed to a ſedentary life, generally run great hazard in childbed; while thoſe who have been uſed to romp about, and take enough of exerciſe, are ſeldom in any danger.

One hardly meets with a girl who can, at the ſame time, boaſt of early performances by the needle, and a good conſtitution. Cloſe and early confinement generally occaſions indigeſtions, headachs, pale complexions, pain of the ſtomach, loſs of appetite, coughs, conſumptions of the lungs, and deformity of body. The latter indeed is not to be wondered at, conſidering the aukward poſtures in which girls ſit at many kinds of needle-work, and the delicate flexible ſtate of their bodies in the early periods of life.

Would mothers, inſtead of having their daughters inſtructed in many uſeleſs accompliſhments, teach them plain work and houſewifery, allowing them enough of time to run about, they would both make them better mothers, and more uſeful members of ſociety. I am no enemy my to genteel accomplishments, but would have them only considered as secondary, and always disregarded when they impair health.

MANY people imagine it a great advantage for children to be early taught to gain their bread. This opinion is certainly right, provided they be so employed as not to hurt their health or growth; but, when these suffer, society, in place of being gainers, are real losers by their labour. There are few employments, except sedentary ones, by which children can earn a livelihood; and, if they be set to those too soon, it ruins their constitutions. Thus, by gaining a few years from childhood, we generally lose twice as many in the other periods of life, and even render the person less valuable while he does live.

IN order to be satisfied of the truth of this observation, one needs only look into the great manufacturing towns, where he will find a puny degenerate race of people, weak and sickly all their lives, seldom exceeding the middle period of life; or, if they do, being unfit for business, they become a burden to society. Thus, arts and manufactures, though they may increase the riches of a country, are by no means favourable to the health of its inhabitants. Good policy would therefore require, that such people as labour during life, should not be set too early to work. Every person conversant in the breeding of horses, or other work-animals, knows, that, if they be set to hard labour

too

too ſoon, they never will turn out to advantage. This is equally true with reſpect to the human ſpecies.

THERE are nevertheleſs various ways of employing young people, without hurting their health. The eaſier parts of gardening, huſbandry, or any buſineſs carried on without doors, are moſt proper. Theſe are employments that moſt young people are fond of, and ſome parts of them may always be adapted to their age, taſte, and ſtrength.

SUCH parents, however, as are under the neceſſity of employing their children within doors, ought to allow them enough of time for active diverſions. This would both encourage them to do more work, and prevent their conſtitutions from being hurt.

SOME imagine, that exerciſe within doors is ſufficient; but they are greatly miſtaken. One hour ſpent in running, or any other exerciſe without doors, is worth ten within. When children cannot go abroad, they ought indeed to be exerciſed at home. The beſt method of doing this is to make them run about in a long room, or dance. This laſt kind of exerciſe, if not carried to exceſs, is of excellent ſervice to young people. It cheers the ſpirits, promotes perſpiration, ſtrengthens the limbs, *&c.* An eminent phyſician uſed to ſay, that he made his children dance inſtead of giving them phyſic. It were well if more people followed his example.

As

As many of the chronic diseases of children might be prevented by the prudent use of the Cold Bath, we shall point out some of those mistakes which commonly prevent its having the desired effect.

The Cold Bath may be considered as an aid to exercise. By it the body is braced and strengthened, the circulation and secretions promoted, and, were it conducted with prudence, many diseases, as the rickets, scrophula, &c. might thereby be prevented. The ancients, who took every method to render children hardy and robust, were no strangers to the use of the cold bath; and, if we may judge from the great number of consecrated wells in this island, many of which possess no other virtues but those of cold water, yet are said to have been famous for curing the diseases of children, we will see cause to believe, that the practice of immersing children in cold water must have been very common amongst our ancestors.

So far as I have been able to observe, the cold bath does as much mischief as good; but that is owing to the want of due care in using it. Children born of delicate parents are not suddenly to be plunged over the head in cold water. They must be gradually brought to it by using tepid water at first, and making it a little cooler every time they are bathed, till by degrees they be able to bear it quite cold. Children afflicted with internal diseases, as inflammations or obstructions of the breast, bowels, &c. ought not to be bathed in cold water.

No

No child ſhould be put into the cold bath when its body is hot, nor immediately after a meal.

It is next to impoſſible to bring nurſes to make a proper uſe of the cold bath: Their prejudices are ſo ſtrong and deep-rooted, that no reaſoning is able to bring them off their own way. I have known ſome of them who would not dry a child's ſkin after bathing it, leſt it ſhould deſtroy the effect of the water. Others will even put cloaths dipt in the water upon the child, and either put it to bed, or ſuffer it to go about in that condition. Some nurſes believe, that the whole virtue of the water depends upon its being dedicated to ſome particular ſaint. Theſe will carry a child 40, 50, or 100 miles to have it once dipt in a certain well; and this is to cure it of whatever diſeaſe it labours under. Others place their confidence in a certain number of dips, as three, ſeven, nine, or the like, and the world could not perſuade them, if theſe do not ſucceed, to try it a little longer.

Thus, by the whims and caprice of nurſes, a valuable medicine is loſt, and the phyſician is often diſappointed in his hopes by their miſconduct. When the cold bath is uſed as a medicine, it ought always to be by the advice of a phyſician, and the nurſe ſhould adhere ſtrictly to his directions. I have ſeen wonderful cures in the moſt obſtinate ſcrophulous caſes performed by the cold bath. The ſalt water in this caſe is always to be preferred. That will

ſucceed

ſucceed where all other medicines have failed.

EVERY child, when in health, ought to have its extremities at leaſt waſhed with cold water daily. This is a partial uſe of the cold bath, and is better than none. In winter this may ſuffice; but in the warm ſeaſon, if a child be relaxed, or ſeem to have a tendency to the rickets or ſcrophula, its whole body ought to be daily immerſed in cold water. Care however muſt be taken not to do this when the body is hot, or the ſtomach full. The child ſhould be dipt only once at a time, ſhould be taken out immediately, and have its ſkin well rubbed with a dry cloth.

Of the bad EFFECTS of unwholſome AIR upon Children.

FEW things are more deſtructive to children than confined or unwholeſome air. This is one reaſon why ſo few of thoſe infants live who are put into hoſpitals, or pariſh-workhouſes. Theſe places are generally crowded with old, ſickly, and infirm people; by that means the air is rendered ſo extremely pernicious, that it becomes a poiſon to infants.

WANT of wholeſome air is likewiſe deſtructive to many of the children born in great towns. There the poorer ſort of inhabitants live in low, dirty, confined houſes, where the fresh air has no access. Tho' up-grown people, who are hardy and robust, may live for a number of years in such situations, yet they generally prove fatal to their offspring, few of whom arrive at maturity, and those who do are weak and deformed. Such people, not being able to carry their children abroad into the open air, we must lay our account with losing the greater part of their progeny. But the rich have not that excuse. It is their business to see that their children be daily carried abroad, and that they be kept in the open air for a sufficient time. This will succeed better if the mother goes along with them. Servants are often negligent in these matters, and allow a child to sit or lie on the damp ground, in place of leading or carrying it about. The mother surely needs air as well as her children; and how can she be better employed than in attending them? Some may think this office below their dignity; but I know no situation in which a mother appears to such advantage, as when surrounded by a circle of healthy children.

A very bad custom prevails of making children sleep in small appartments, or crowding two or three beds into one chamber. In place of that, the nursery ought always to be the largest and best aired room in the house. When children are confined in small appartments, the air is not only unwholesome, but such places being generally too hot, their bodies are relaxed, and this

this diſpoſes them to catch cold when they go abroad, and has many other bad effects.

CHILDREN who are kept within doors all day, and ſleep all night in warm cloſe appartments, may, with great propriety, be compared to plants nurſed in a hot houſe, in place of the open air. Tho' ſuch plants, by extraordinary care, may be kept alive for ſome time; yet they never will arrive at that degree of ſtrength, vigor, and magnitude, which they would have done in the open air, nor would they be able to bear it afterwards ſhould they be expoſed to it.

CHILDREN brought up in the country, who have been accuſtomed to freſh open air, ſhould not be too early ſent to great towns, where the air is confined and unwholeſome. This is frequently done with a view to forward their education, but proves very hurtful to health. Thoſe who are grown up do not ſuffer near ſo much from bad air as young perſons. All ſchools and ſeminaries of learning ought to be ſo ſituated as to have freſh, dry, wholeſome air, and ſhould never be too much crowded.

WITHOUT entering into a detail of the particular advantages of wholeſome air to children, we ſhall only obſerve, that when they enjoy that bleſſing, they generally ſleep well, eat well, and thrive accordingly. It braces and ſtrengthens their bodies, enlivens their ſpirits, and every way promotes their growth and health.

Of

Of NURSES.

NURSES are guilty of many faults, which prove fatal to infants. It is therefore the duty of parents to watch over their conduct with the greatest care, and to be extremely cautious in the choice of them.

ONE of the most common faults of nurses is to dose children with stupifactives, or such things as lull them asleep. An indolent nurse, who does not give a child enough of exercise in the open air to make it sleep, and does not chuse to be disturbed by it in the night, will seldom fail to procure for it a dose of laudanum, diacodium, saffron, or, what answers the same end, a dram of spirits, or other strong liquors. These, tho' they be certain poison to children, are every day administered by many who bear the character of very good nurses.

A nurse who has not enough of milk is apt to imagine, that she can supply that defect by giving the child wines, cordial waters, or other strong liquors. This is an egregious mistake. The only thing that has any chance to supply the place of the nurse's milk, must be somewhat nearly of the same quality, as cow's milk, ass's milk, or the like, with good bread. It never can be done by the help of strong liquors. These, in place of nourishing an infant, never fail to produce the contrary effect.

CHILDREN

Children are often hurt by nurſes permitting them to cry long and vehemently. This ſtrains their tender bodies, and frequently occaſions ruptures, inflammations of the throat, lungs, &c. The nurſe who can hear an infant cry till it has almoſt exhauſted itſelf, without endeavouring to pleaſe it, muſt be cruel indeed, and is unworthy to be truſted with the care of a human creature.

Nurses who deal much in medicine, are always to be ſuſpected. They truſt to it, and neglect their duty. I never knew a good nurſe who had her Godefroy's cordials, Daffy's elixirs, &c. at hand. Such generally imagine, that a doſe of theſe will make up for all defects in food, air, exerciſe, cleanlineſs, &c.

A very pernicious cuſtom of indolent nurſes is the allowing of children to continue long wet. This is not only diſgreeable, but it galls and frets the infant, and by relaxing the ſolids, occaſions ſcrophulas, rickets, and other fatal diſeaſes.

Nature often attempts to free the bodies of children from bad humours, by throwing them out upon the ſkin: By that means fevers, and other diſeaſes are prevented. Nurſes are apt to miſtake ſuch critical eruptions for an itch, or ſome other infectious diſorder. Accordingly they take every method to drive them in. In this way many children loſe their lives; and no wonder, as nature is oppoſed in the very method that ſhe took to relieve them. It ought to be a rule which

every

every nurſe ſhould obſerve, never to ſtop any eruption without proper advice, or being well aſſured, that it is not of a critical nature. At any rate, it is never to be done without previous evacuations.

Loose ſtools is another method by which nature often prevents the diſeaſes of infants. If theſe proceed too far, no doubt they ought to be checked; but this is never to be done without the greateſt caution. Nurſes, upon the firſt appearance of looſe ſtools, frequently fly to the uſe of aſtringents, or ſuch things as bind the belly. Thus inflammations, fevers, and other fatal diſeaſes are brought on. A doſe of rhubarb, a gentle vomit, or ſome other evacuation, ſhould always precede the uſe of aſtringent medicines.

One of the greateſt faults of nurſes is concealing the diſeaſes of children from their parents. This they are extremely ready to do, eſpecially when the diſeaſe is the effect of their own negligence. Every perſon muſt have ſeen inſtances of people who were lame for life by a fall out of the nurſe's arms, while ſhe, through fear, concealed the misfortune till it was paſt cure. Every parent who intruſts a nurſe with the care of a child, ought to give her the ſtricteſt charge not to conceal the moſt trifling diſorder or misfortune that may befal it. Parents, inſtead of being angry when a nurſe informs them of ſuch accidents, ought to reward her for her honeſty; this would encourage her to do the

the ſame upon other occaſions. We can ſee no reaſon why a nurſe ſhould not be puniſhed who conceals any diſorder or misfortune that happens to a child under her care, till it loſes its life. A few examples of this would ſave many infant lives; but as there is little reaſon to expect that it ever will be the caſe, we would earneſtly recommend it to all parents to look carefully after their children, and not to truſt ſo valuable a treaſure entirely in the hands of an hireling.

THESE, and many other faults, being daily committed by thoſe who have the care of children, it ought ſurely to rouſe the attention of all parents who have any regard for their offſpring, and to make them very circumſpect in the choice of thoſe into whoſe hands they commit them. They ought at leaſt to take care that a nurſe be ſober, cleanly, honeſt, healthy, not too young, nor the contrary; that ſhe have the neceſſaries of life, and a comfortable habitation, *&c.*

WERE it practicable to have all children nurſed and educated in the country, we ſhould loſe very few of them. One ſeldom ſees a country-farmer without a numerous offſpring, moſt of whom arrive at maturity. Many things conſpire to that end. The children of theſe people are generally nurſed by their mothers, they eat plain wholeſome food, enjoy the benefit of freſh air, and have enough of proper exerciſe; they have rural ſports and paſtimes ſuited to their

age,

age, and as they grow up, find employments adapted to their ſtrength, agreeable to their inclinations, and conducive to their health: They learn induſtry and ſobriety from their parents, and ſeldom fail to practiſe theſe virtues for life. In fine, we cannot help joining with the learned Mr Locke *, in recommending the example of theſe people as a model to all in the management of their children.

As many people can underſtand the meaning of a ſhort rule, who are not able to attend to a chain of reaſoning, we ſhall reduce the leading principles of nurſing under the following general heads.

1. EVERY mother ought to ſuckle her own child, if ſhe can do it with ſafety.

2. A weak, conſumptive, nervous, or hyſteric mother ought not to give ſuck, where a healthy nurſe can be had.

3. No child ſhould be brought up without the breaſt, if it be poſſible to obtain a proper nurſe.

4. The cloaths of an infant ſhould be ſoft, light, looſe, and eaſy for its body. They ought to be faſtened on with ſtrings rather than pins.

5. THE cloaths of children ought to be kept very clean.

6. A new born infant ſhould not be kept too hot.

* On education.

7. AN

7. An infant ſhould be permitted to ſuck as ſoon as it ſhows an inclination for the breaſt.

8. An infant ſhould neither be crammed with food nor phyſic as ſoon as it is born; but permitted to lie quiet for ſome time, in order to recover the fatigue of the birth, *&c.*

9. If an infant muſt have food before it ſucks, let it be water-pap mixed with new milk, free of all wines, ſugars, ſpiceries, or the like.

10. While the child ſucks, it ſeldom needs much of any other food. It will however be right, about the third or fourth month, to begin to give it once or twice a-day a little of ſome food that is light and eaſy of digeſtion. This will make the weaning both leſs troubleſome and dangerous.

11. A child ſhould not be weaned all at once but by degrees; as all ſudden changes in the diet of children are dangerous.

12. The food of children ought at all times to be ſimple, but nouriſhing. It ſhould conſiſt of a proper mixture of animal and vegetable ſubſtances.

13. Children ſhould not be permitted to eat too much fruit, or roots of any kind; but all ſorts of green traſh ought to be kept from them with the greateſt care.

14. Children ought not to be pinched in their food. They require to eat oftener than adults.----If their food be ſimple, and they know that they can have it when hungry, they will ſeldom or never eat more than enough.

15. As ſoon as children can take exerciſe, they ought to be allowed as much as they pleaſe; till then it is the buſineſs of the nurſe to carry and toſs them about.

16. A nurſe ought not only to carry an infant about, but to divert and amuſe it ſo as to keep it in good humour.

17. An infant ſhould never be ſuffered to cry long and vehemently.

18. Eruptions, or looſeneſs in children ought not to be ſtopt, but with the greateſt caution.

19. Nurses ſhould uſe no means to force children to ſleep; but they may always be permitted to take as much as they pleaſe.

20. Children ought never to have medicine unleſs they are diſeaſed.

21. Children ſhould neither be too early ſet to ſchool, nor confined to any mechanical employment within doors.

22. Schoolmasters, and all who have the care of youth, ſhould allow them plenty of time for exerciſe and diverſions.

23. All children ſhould be nurſed and educated in the country, if poſſible. When that cannot be done, they ought to be carried abroad every day, and kept for a ſufficient time in the open air.

24. The children of delicate and diſeaſed parents muſt be managed with more care than thoſe of the hardy and robuſt.

25. A mother ſhould never abandon her child ſolely to the care of a mercenary nurſe.

LET no one imagine theſe matters unworthy of his attention. On the proper management of children depend not only their health and uſefulneſs in life, but likewiſe the ſafety and proſperity of the ſtate to which they belong. Effeminacy ever muſt prove the ruin of any kingdom; and when its foundations are laid in infancy, it can never afterwards be wholely eradicated. We would therefore recommend to all who wiſh well to their country, to ſtudy every method to render their offspring ſtrong and healthy.

——————————By arts like theſe
Laconia nurs'd of old her hardy ſons;
And Rome's unconquer'd legions urg'd their way,
Unhurt, thro' every toil in every clime *.

* *Armſtrong on health.*

CHAP.

CHAP. II.

Of ADULTS.

HAVING endeavoured to point out ſome of the ſources from which the diſeaſes and mortality of infants proceed, we ſhall next take a view of the more general cauſes of diſeaſes, or ſuch things as endanger the health of mankind in the more advanced periods of life.

No man, however careful, can at all times avoid diſeaſes; yet nothing is more certain than that many of them, and thoſe too of the moſt dangerous nature, are often owing to the want of care. The ſmalleſt cauſes, when neglected, generally produce the greateſt effects. This is ſtrictly true with reſpect to diſeaſes. A little care would often prevent what no medicine can cure.

The moſt common cauſe of diſeaſes in this iſland is an obſtructed perſpiration, or what commonly goes by the name of CATCHING COLD. The perſpiration is by far the moſt conſiderable diſcharge from the body; and ſo long as it goes on properly, we have ſeldom any complaints; but when it is obſtructed, the health muſt ſuffer. Men being leſs ſenſible of this than of the other evacuations, are conſequently not ſo attentive to the various cauſes which obſtruct it: We ſhall therefore point out ſome of the moſt

most considerable of them, in order to put people upon their guard.

Common CAUSES of catching COLD.

COLDS are often occasioned by sudden changes in the atmosphere. There is no country where such changes happen more frequently than in Britain. The degrees of heat and cold are not only various in the different seasons of the year, but often change from the one extreme to the other in a few days, and sometimes even in the course of one day: As these changes cannot fail to increase or diminish the perspiration, they must of course affect the health.

THE best method of fortifying the body against the changes of the weather, is to be abroad every day. Those who keep much within doors, are most liable to catch cold. Such people feel even the slightest changes in the atmosphere, and by their coughs, pains, and oppressions of the breast, &c. become a kind of living barometers.

THE frequent changes of the weather ought to make us cautious in changing our apparel. All persons, but especially the valetudinary, should be careful not to put off their winter-garments too soon, nor to wear their summer ones too long. The commencement of our warm season is so uncertain, that a few hot days in April or May often make us believe summer is arrived;

arrived; when all of a ſudden, the weather ſets in more intenſely cold than at Chriſtmas. The like ſudden changes frequently happen in September or October; and where no care is taken to guard againſt their influence, the gout, rheumatiſms, fluxes, and fevers, often enſue.

Labourers frequently ſuffer by not attending to the changes of the weather. They ſtrip to work while it is warm, but neglect to put on their cloaths when it grows cold; ſome are even thoughtleſs enough to diſregard being wet; ſuch however, in the end, generally find cauſe to repent their fool-hardineſs.

Nothing more certainly obſtructs the perſpiration than wet cloaths. Nor is the moſt robuſt conſtitution proof againſt their effects. The perſpiration is not only obſtructed by wet cloaths, but the moiſture is likewiſe abſorbed, which greatly encreaſes the danger.

It is impoſſible for people who go abroad, always to avoid being wet. But the danger might generally be leſſened, if not wholely prevented, by changing their cloaths ſoon; when that cannot be done, they ſhould keep in motion till they dry. So far are many from obſerving this rule, that they will ſit, or even lie down in the fields with their cloaths wet, and frequently ſleep whole nights in that condition. Every perſon muſt have known inſtances of fevers, rheumatiſms, and even conſumptions, brought on in this way. Though theſe happen daily, yet they

they are not ſufficient to deter others from the like conduct.

EVEN wet feet often occaſion fatal diſeaſes. Coughs, inflammations of the breaſt, and ulcers in the lungs, frequently proceed from that cauſe. The cholic, a fit of the gout, the iliac paſſion, and *cholera morbus*, are likewiſe often occaſioned by wet feet. Habit will, no doubt, render this leſs dangerous; but it ought, as far as poſſible, to be avoided. The delicate, and thoſe who are not accuſtomed to have their cloaths or feet wet, ſhould be peculiarly careful in this reſpect.

THE perſpiration is often obſtructed by NIGHT-AIR; the abſence of the ſun renders it damp and foggy. Even in ſummer, the night-air ought to be avoided. The dews which fall plentifully after the hotteſt day make the night more dangerous than when the weather is cool. Hence, in warm countries, the dews are more hurtful than where the climate is more temperate.

IT is very agreeable indeed, after a warm day, to be abroad in the cool evening; but this is a pleaſure to be avoided by all who value their health. The effects of evening-dews are gradual and almoſt imperceptible; but they are not the leſs to be dreaded: We would therefore adviſe travellers, labourers, and all who are much heated by day, carefully to avoid them. When the perſpiration has been great, theſe become dangerous in proportion: By not attending to this, in flat marſhy countries, where the exhalations and dews are copious, labourers often catch intermitting fevers, quinſies, and the like.

DAMP

Damp beds seldom fail to obstruct the perspiration. Beds become damp, either from want of use, standing in damp houses, or in rooms without fire. Nothing is more to be dreaded by travellers than damp beds, which are very common in all places where feuel is scarce. When a traveller cold and wet arrives at an inn, he may by means of a good fire, and a dry bed, have the perspiration restored; but if he be put into a cold room, and laid on a damp bed, it will be more obstructed, and the worst consequences must ensue. Travellers should avoid inns which are noted for damp beds, as they would a house infected with the plague; as no man, however robust, is proof against the danger arising from them.

But inns are not the only places where damp beds are to be met with. Beds kept in private families for the reception of strangers, are no less dangerous. All kinds of linen and bedding, when not frequently used, become damp. How then is it possible, that beds which are not slept in above two or three times a-year, should be otherwise? Nothing is more common than to hear of people having caught cold by changing their bed. The reason is obvious: Were they careful never to sleep on a bed but what was frequently used, they would seldom find any ill consequences from a change.

Nothing is more to be dreaded by a delicate person when on a visit, than being laid in the guest-chamber. That ill-judged piece of com-

complaisance becomes a real injury. All the bad consequences from this quarter might be easily prevented in private families, by causing their servants to sleep in the spare beds, and to resign them to strangers when they come. This is the custom of many families in London, and we would earnestly recommend it to all who value the health of their friends. In inns where the beds are used almost every night, nothing else is necessary than to keep the rooms well seasoned by frequent fires, and the linen dry.

DAMP HOUSES frequently produce the like ill consequences; for this reason those who build should be careful to chuse a dry situation. A house which stands on a damp marshy soil must be hurtful to the health of the inhabitants. Not only a marshy soil, but being situated in the neighbourhood of large woods, lakes, or standing water, must make a house damp. Large woods both prevent the free current of air, and send forth great quantities of moist exhalations, which render all places near them unwholesome. This is one reason why new discovered countries commonly prove unhealthy, till they be cleared of their woods. Even in England, at this day, there is greatly more planting in several parts than is either conducive to the fertility of the soil, or the health of its inhabitants. This taste, instead of being any improvement, is the way to reduce the country back to its original ſtate, and to render the climate leſs healthy than it otherwiſe would be.

COLD is not near ſo hurtful to the health as moiſture. Cold, in a moderate degree, braces and ſtrengthens the body; but moiſture relaxes and pre-diſpoſes it to diſeaſes. That is the reaſon why intermittents and other fevers are ſo frequent in low damp marſhy countries abounding with woods and ſtanding water. This likewiſe ſhews the danger of inhabiting new houſes before they be thoroughly dry. Nothing is more common than for people, merely to avoid ſome trifling inconveniency, to hazard their lives, by inhabiting a houſe almoſt as ſoon as the maſons, plaiſterers, &c. have done with it: Such houſes are not only dangerous from their dampneſs, but likewiſe from the ſmell of lime, paints, &c. The aſthma's, conſumptions, and other diſeaſes of the lungs, ſo common to people who work in theſe articles, are a plain proof of their being unwholeſome.

HOUSES are often rendered damp by an unſeaſonable piece of cleanlineſs; I mean the ridiculous cuſtom of waſhing rooms immediately before company is put into them. Many people are ſure to catch cold, if they ſit but a ſhort while in a room that has been lately waſhed; the delicate ought carefully to avoid ſuch a ſituation, and even the robuſt would run leſs hazard by ſitting without doors. People who are accuſtomed to live in dry houſes, ought, as far as poſſible,

ſible, to ſhun damp ones, and by all means not to continue long in rooms that have been lately waſhed.

All houſes, unleſs where the ground is extremely dry, ſhould have the firſt floor a little raiſed. Such ſervants, as are obliged to live for the moſt part in cellars and ſunk ſtories, ſeldom continue long in health; and ſurely maſters ought to pay ſome regard to the health of their ſervants as well as to their own.

Even houſes which are built for the poor ought to be dry. Theſe people generally live on the ground-floor, and if it be damp, they muſt ſuffer. This is one cauſe of the aches, cramps, and rheumatic pains, which poor people are ſo ſubject to in the decline of life.

But nothing ſo frequently obſtructs the perſpiration as SUDDEN TRANSITIONS from heat to cold. Colds are ſeldom caught unleſs when people have been too much heated. Heat rarifies the blood, quickens the circulation, and increaſes the perſpiration; but when theſe are ſuddenly checked, the conſequences muſt be bad. It is indeed impoſſible for labourers not to be too hot upon certain occaſions; but it is generally in their power to put on their cloaths when they leave off work, to make choice of a dry place to reſt themſelves in, and to avoid falling aſleep in the fields. Theſe eaſy rules, if obſerved, would ſave many uſeful lives.

Nothing is more common than for people when

when hot, to drink freely of cold ſmall liquors. This conduct is extremely dangerous. Thirſt indeed is hard to bear, and the inclination to gratify that appetite frequently gets the better of reaſon, and makes us do what our judgment diſapproves. Every peaſant knows if his horſe be permitted to drink his belly full of cold water after violent exerciſe, and be immediately put into the ſtable, or ſuffered to remain at reſt, that it will kill him. This they take the utmoſt care to prevent. It were well if they were equally attentive to their own ſafety.

THIRST may be quenched many ways without ſwallowing large quantities of cold liquor. The fields afford variety of acid fruits and plants, the very chewing of which would abate thirſt. Water kept in the mouth for ſome time, and ſpit out again, if frequently repeated, will have the ſame effect. If a bit of bread be eat along with a few mouthfuls of water, it will both quench thirſt more effectually, and make the danger leſs. When a perſon is extremely hot, a mouthful of brandy, or other ſpirits, ought to be preferred to any thing elſe, if it can be obtained. But if any one has been ſo fooliſh, when hot, as to drink freely of cold liquor, he ought to continue his exerciſe at leaſt, till what he drank be thoroughly warmed upon his ſtomach.

IT would be tedious to enumerate all the bad effects which flow from drinking cold thin liquors

quors when the body is hot. Sometimes this has occaſioned immediate death. Hoarſeneſs, quinſeys, and fevers of various kinds, are its common conſequences. Neither is it ſafe when warm to eat freely of raw fruits, ſallads, or the like. Theſe indeed have not ſo ſudden an effect on the body as cold liquors, but they are notwithſtanding dangerous, and ought to be avoided.

SITTING in a warm room, and drinking hot liquors till the pores are quite open, and immediately going into the cold air, is extremely dangerous. Colds, coughs, and inflammations of the breaſt, are the uſual effects of this conduct: Yet how common is it? Many people, after having drank warm liquors for ſeveral hours, walk or ride a number of miles in the coldeſt night; while others ſit up at their bottle all night, or ramble about in the ſtreets. Such conduct is one cauſe why coughs and colds are ſo common in the winter-ſeaſon.

PEOPLE are very apt when a room is hot, to throw open a window, and to ſit near it. This is a moſt ready way to catch cold. A delicate perſon had better ſit without doors than in ſuch a ſituation, as the current of air is directed againſt one particular part of the body. Inflammatory fevers and conſumptions have often been occaſioned by ſitting or ſtanding thinly cloathed near an open window. Nor is ſleeping with open windows leſs to be dreaded. That

ought

ought never to be done even in the hotteſt ſeaſon. I have known mechanics frequently contract fatal diſeaſes, by working ſtript at an open window, and would adviſe all of them to beware of ſuch a practice.

Nothing expoſes people more to catch cold than keeping their own houſes too warm; ſuch perſons may be ſaid to live in a ſort of hot-houſes; they can hardly ſtir abroad to viſit a neighbour, but at the hazard of their lives. Were there no other reaſon for keeping houſes in a moderate degree of warmth, that alone is ſufficient: But no houſe that is too hot can be wholeſome; heat deſtroys the ſpring and elaſticity of the air, and renders it leſs fit for expanding the lungs, and other purpoſes of reſpiration. Hence it is, that conſumptions and other diſeaſes of the lungs prove ſo fatal to people who work in forges, glaſs-houſes, and the like.

Some are even ſo fool-hardy, as to bathe themſelves when hot in cold water. Not only fevers, but madneſs itſelf has frequently been the effect of this conduct. Indeed it looks too like the action of a madman to deſerve a ſerious conſideration.

We ſhall conclude theſe obſervations on the common cauſes of catching cold, by recommending it to every one to avoid, with the utmoſt attention, all ſudden tranſitions from heat to cold, and to keep the body in as uniform a temperature as poſſible; or, where that cannot be done, to take care to cool gradually.

It

It may be thought that too ſtrict an attention to theſe things would tend to render people delicate. So far however is this from being our deſign, that the firſt rule laid down for preventing colds, is to harden the body, by enuring it daily to bear the open air.

It is a true ſaying, that colds kill more than plagues. On examining patients, one finds moſt of them impute their diſeaſes either to violent colds, or to ſlight ones which had been neglected. This ſhows the importance of guarding againſt every thing that may obſtruct the perſpiration, and likewiſe of uſing proper means immediately to remove ſuch obſtruction when it does happen. The want of due attention to theſe coſts Britain annually ſome thouſands of uſeful lives.

UNWHOLESOME FOOD.

As our bodies conſiſt of what we eat and drink, unwholeſome food muſt be dangerous. There is no queſtion but the whole conſtitution of body may be changed by diet. This is often done more quickly than people would imagine. A diet conſiſting too much of alkaline ſubſtances, will ſoon render the humours putrid. On the other hand, if acids be uſed too freely, they will receive a taint of an oppoſite nature. The ſolids may be relaxed or weakened

ened by the uſe of oily or watery ſubſtances, or they may be too much conſtricted by eating ſpiceries, auſtere vegetables, &c.

It is not eaſy to aſcertain the exact quantity and quality of food proper for every age, ſex, and conſtitution: But a ſcrupulous nicety here is by no means neceſſary. The beſt rule is to avoid all extremes. Mankind were never intended to weigh and meaſure their food. Nature teaches every creature when it has enough of food, and a very ſmall degree of reaſon is ſufficient for the choice of it. Men ſeldom err in this reſpect through ignorance. The moſt knowing are generally the moſt guilty.

Tho' *moderation* be the only rule neceſſary with reſpect to the quantity of food, yet the quality of it merits further attention. Many people, if they can ſatisfy the appetites of hunger and thirſt, are very indifferent what they eat or drink. The following obſervations will ſhow the danger of ſuch conduct.

Provisions may be rendered unwholeſome various ways. Bad ſeaſons may either prevent the ripening of grain, or damage it afterwards. Wet and cold ſummers ſeldom bring the fruits of the earth to maturity; and if the harveſt likewiſe prove rainy, they are often ſo damaged as to be very hurtful. Theſe indeed are acts of Providence; it is therefore our duty to ſubmit to them: But ſurely no puniſhment can be too ſevere for thoſe who ſuffer proviſions to be ſpoilt, by hoarding them on purpoſe to enhance the price.

price. The soundest grain, if kept too long, must become unfit for use.

The poor are generally the first who suffer by unsound provisions: But the lives of the labouring poor are of the greatest importance to the state. Besides, diseases occasioned by unwholesome food often prove infectious, and by that means reach people in every station. The poor judge ill in buying low-priced and coarse provisions. They had better have a smaller quantity of what is sound and good; as that would both afford more nourishment, and be attended with less danger.

Animal as well as vegetable food becomes unwholesome when kept too long. All animal substances have a constant tendency to putrefaction, and when that has proceeded too far, they not only become offensive to the senses, but hurtful to health. Diseased animals, and such as die of themselves, ought not to be eaten. It is common enough in grasing countries for servants and poor people to eat such animals as die of any disease in the spring or winter, or are killed by accident. I have been frequently told by people who live in places where this is done, that when much flesh of that kind is eaten, it never fails to occasion fevers.

The injunctions given to the Jews, not to eat any creature which died of itself, seem to have a strict regard to health, and ought to be observed by Christians as well as Jews. Animals never die of themselves without some previous diſeaſe; but how a diſeaſed animal ſhould be wholeſome food is inconceivable: Even thoſe which die by accident muſt be hurtful, as their blood is mixed with the fleſh, and ſoon turns putrid.

Animals which feed groſs, as tame ducks, ſwine, *&c.* are neither eaſily digeſted, nor afford wholeſome nouriſhment. No animal can be wholeſome food which does not take ſufficient exercíſe. Moſt of our ſtalled cattle, hogs, &c. are crammed with groſs food, but not allowed exerciſe nor free air; by which means they indeed grow fat, but their humours not being properly prepared or aſſimulated, they muſt remain crude. The fleſh of an animal which has not properly digeſted its own food, can never be eaſily digeſted by another: Yet ſuch are the delicacies of modern luxury, and ſuch the animals daily devoured even by the weak and valetudinary. Is it any wonder that ſuch ſhould complain of crudities, indigeſtions, and oppreſſion of the ſpirits? Let them eat the ſame quantity of an animal which runs wild, and they will not feel any load on their ſtomach, or difficulty of digeſtion. We would not have people live on carrion; but ſurely the oppoſite extreme of eating animals which are gorged with groſs food till they are unfit to live, muſt be as pernicious.

Animals may likewiſe be rendered unwholeſome by being over-heated. Heat cauſes a fever, exhalts the ſalts of the animal, and mixes the

the blood ſo intimately with the fleſh, that it cannot be ſeparated. For this reaſon people ought not to eat freely of ſuch animals as are hunted down, their fleſh being apt to occaſion putrid fevers. Butchers ſhould alſo be careful not to over-drive their cattle. No perſon would chuſe to eat the fleſh of an animal which had died in a high fever; yet that is the caſe with all over-drove cattle; and the fever is often raiſed even to the degree of madneſs.

No people in the world eat ſuch quantities of animal food as the Engliſh; that is one reaſon why they are ſo generally tainted with the ſcurvy, and its numerous train of conſequences, as indigeſtion, low ſpirits, hypochondriaciſm, &c. Animal food was ſurely deſigned for man, and with a proper mixture of vegetables, it will be found the moſt wholeſome; but to gorge beef, mutton, pork, fiſh, and fowl, twice or thrice a-day, is certainly too much. All who value health ought to be contented with making one fleſh-meal in the twenty-four hours, and this ought to conſiſt of one kind only.

The moſt obſtinate ſcurvy has often been cured by a vegetable diet; nay, milk alone will frequently do more in that diſeaſe than any medicine. From hence it is evident, that if vegetables and milk were more uſed in diet, we ſhould have leſs ſcurvy, and likewiſe fewer putrid and inflammatory fevers.

Our aliment ought neither to be too moiſt, nor too dry. Moiſt aliment relaxes the ſolids,

and

and renders the body feeble. Thus we ſee females who live much on tea and other watery diet generally become weak, and unable to digeſt ſolid food; from whence proceed hyſterics, and all their dreadful conſequences. On the other hand, food that is too dry, renders the ſolids in a manner rigid, and the humours viſcid, which prediſpoſes the body to inflammatory fevers, ſcurvies, and the like.

THE arts of cookery render many things unwholeſome, which are not ſo in their own nature. By jumbling together a number of different ingredients, in order to make a poignant ſauce, or rich ſoup, the compoſition proves almoſt a poiſon. All high ſeaſoning, pickles, &c. are only incentives to luxury, and never fail to hurt the ſtomach. It were well for mankind if cookery, as an art, were intirely prohibited. Plain roaſting or boiling is all that nature points out, and all that the ſtomach requires. Theſe alone are ſufficient for people in health, and the ſick have ſtill leſs need of a cook.

THE liquid part of our aliment likewiſe claims our attention. Water is not only the baſis of moſt liquors, but alſo compoſes a great part of our ſolid food. Good water muſt therefore be of the greateſt importance in diet. The beſt water is that which is moſt pure, and free from any mixture of foreign bodies. Water takes up parts of every body with which it comes in contact; by which means it is often impregnated

ted with metals or minerals of a hurtful or poisonous nature.

The inhabitants of ſome hilly countries have peculiar diſeaſes, which in all probability proceed from the water. Thus the people who live near the Alps in Switzerland, and the inhabitants of the Peak of Derby in England, have large tumors or wains on their necks. This diſeaſe is generally imputed to the ſnow-water; but there is more reaſon to believe it is owing to the minerals in the mountains thro' which the waters paſs. Were it owing to the ſnow-water, it ſhould happen to the inhabitants of all mountainous countries, where ſnow lies long; but there are many parts of Britain where the ſnow lies much longer than in the Peak of Derby; yet the inhabitants have no ſuch diſeaſe. The Peak of Derby is well known to be a bed of minerals of different kinds; and, as far as what is called the mineral country extends, theſe tumors are common, and generally go by the name of *Derbyſhire-necks*.

When water is impregnated with foreign bodies, it generally appears by its weight, colour, taſte, ſmell, heat, or ſome other ſenſible quality. Our buſineſs therefore is to chuſe ſuch water, for common uſe, as is lighteſt, and without any particular colour, taſte, or ſmell. In moſt places of Britain the inhabitants have it in their power to make choice of their water, and few things would contribute more to health than a due attention to this article. But mere indolence often induces

duces people to make uſe of the water that is neareſt them, without conſidering its qualities.

BEFORE water be brought into great towns, the ſtricteſt attention ought to be paid to its qualities, as epidemic diſtempers are often occaſioned by bad water; and when it has been procured at a great expence, we are unwilling to give it up.

THE common methods of rendering water clear by filtration, or ſoft by expoſing it to the ſun and air, &c. are ſo generally known, that it is unneceſſary to ſpend time in explaining them. We ſhall only in general adviſe all to avoid waters which ſtagnate long in ſmall lakes, ponds, or the like; ſuch waters often become putrid with inſects and other vermine, which breed and die in them. Even cattle frequently ſuffer by drinking, in dry ſeaſons, water which has ſtood long in ſmall reſervoirs, without being ſupplied by ſprings, or freſhened with ſhowers. All wells ought to be kept clean, and to have a free communication with the air. When either animal or vegetable ſubſtances are ſuffered to lie at the bottom of wells, they corrupt and taint the water. Even the air itſelf when confined in wells becomes poiſonous, and muſt of courſe render the water unwholeſome.

MUCH noiſe has been made about the uſe of fermented liquors; they notwithſtanding ſtill continue to be the common drink of almoſt every perſon who can afford them. As this

this is, and in all probability will be the caſe, we ſhall rather endeavour to aſſiſt people in their choice of theſe liquors, than pretend to condemn what cuſtom has eſtabliſhed. It is not the moderate uſe of ſound fermented liquors which hurts mankind; it is exceſs, or the abuſe of them, and uſing ſuch as are ill-prepared or vitiated.

FERMENTED liquors which are too ſtrong, hurt digeſtion inſtead of aſſiſting it, by which means their intention is loſt, and the body, in place of being ſtrengthened by them, is weakened and relaxed. Many imagine, that hard labour could not be ſupported without drinking ſtrong liquors: This, tho' a common, is a very erroneous notion. Men who never taſte ſtrong liquors are not only able to endure more fatigue, but alſo live much longer than thoſe who uſe them daily. But ſuppoſe ſtrong liquors did enable a man to do more work, they muſt nevertheleſs waſte the powers of life, and of courſe occaſion premature old age. They keep up a conſtant fever, which waſtes the ſpirits, heats and inflames the blood, and prediſpoſes the body to numberleſs diſeaſes.

BUT fermented liquors may be too weak as well as too ſtrong: When that is the caſe, they muſt either be drank new, or they become ſour and dead; when ſuch liquors are drank new, the fermentation not being over, they generate air in the bowels, and occaſion flatulencies; and when kept till ſtale, they ſour on the

the ſtomach, and greatly hurt digeſtion. For this reaſon all malt-liquor, cyder, &c. ought to be of ſuch ſtrength as will make them keep till they be ripe, and then they ſhould be uſed. When ſuch liquors are kept too long, tho' they ſhould not become ſour, yet they generally contract a hardneſs, which renders them unwholeſome. Hence it is, that bottled ale hurts the ſtomach, occaſions the gravel, &c.

ALL families, who can, ought to prepare their own liquors. Since preparing and vending of liquors became one of the moſt general branches of buſineſs, every method has been tried to adulterate them. The great object both of the makers and venders of liquor is, to render it intoxicating. But it is well known that this may be done by other ingredients than thoſe which ought to be uſed for that purpoſe. It would be imprudent even to name thoſe things which are daily made uſe of to render liquors heady. It is ſufficient to obſerve, that the practice is very common, and all the ingredients uſed for that purpoſe are of an opiate or ſtupifactive nature. But as all opiates are of a poiſonous quality, it is eaſy to ſee what muſt be the conſequence of their general uſe. Tho' they do not kill ſuddenly; yet they hurt the nerves, relax and weaken the ſtomach, and of courſe ſpoil the digeſtion.

WERE fermented liquors faithfully prepared, not too ſtrong, nor too weak, kept to a proper age, and uſed in moderation, they would prove real

real bleſſings to mankind. But while they are ill prepared, various ways adulterated, and taken to exceſs, they muſt have many bad conſequences. Theſe however we ſhall not mention at preſent, as they will be pointed out under another article.

To ſpecify the different kinds of aliment, to explain their nature and properties, and to point out their effects in different conſtitutions, would far exceed the limits of our deſign. Inſtead of a detail of this kind, which in all probability would be very little attended to, and would not be generally underſtood, we ſhall only mention the following eaſy rules with reſpect to the choice of aliment.

Those whoſe ſolids are weak and relaxed, ought to avoid all viſcid food, or ſuch things as are hard of digeſtion; and to take plenty of exerciſe in a dry open air.

Such as abound with blood ſhould be ſparing in the uſe of every thing that is highly nouriſhing, as fat meat, rich wines, ſtrong ale, &c. Their food ſhould conſiſt moſtly of bread and other vegetable ſubſtances; and their drink ought to be milk, whey, and the like.

Fat people ſhould not eat freely of oily nouriſhing diet. They ought frequently to uſe raddiſh, garlic, ſpices, or ſuch things as are heating and promote perſpiration and urine. Their drink ſhould be water, coffee, tea, or the like; and they ought to take much exerciſe and little ſleep.

THOSE who are too lean muſt follow an oppoſite courſe.

SUCH as abound with acidities, or whoſe food is apt to ſour on their ſtomach, ſhould live much on fleſh-meats; and thoſe who are troubled with alkaline eructations, or heat of the ſtomach, ought to uſe a diet conſiſting chiefly of acid vegetables.

PEOPLE who are affected with the gout, low ſpirits, hypochondriac, or hyſteric diſorders, ought to avoid all flatulent food, every thing that is viſcid, or hard of digeſtion, all ſalted or ſmoke-dried proviſions, and whatever is auſtere, acid, or apt to ſour on the ſtomach. Their food ſhould be light, ſpare, cool, and of an opening quality.

THE diet ought not only to be ſuited to the age and conſtitution, but alſo to the manner of life. A ſedentary or ſtudious perſon ſhould live more ſparingly than one who labours hard without doors. Food will nouriſh a peaſant very well, which would be almoſt indigeſtible to a citizen; and the latter will live upon a diet on which the former would ſtarve.

DIET ought not to be too uniform. The conſtant uſe of one kind of food might have bad effects. Nature points out this by the great variety of aliments which ſhe has provided for man, and likewiſe by giving him an appetite for different kinds of food.

THOSE who labour under any particular diſeaſe, ought to avoid ſuch aliments as have a tendency

tendency to increaſe it: For example, a gouty perſon ſhould not uſe rich wines, ſtrong ſoups, or gravies, and ſhould avoid all acids. One who is troubled with the gravel, ought to ſhun all auſtere and aſtringent aliments; and thoſe who are ſcorbutic, ſhould not indulge in animal food, &c.

In the firſt period of life our food ought to be light, nouriſhing, and of a diluting nature, but frequently uſed. Food that is ſolid, with a ſufficient degree of tenacity, is moſt proper for the ſtate of manhood. The diet ſuited to the laſt period of life, when nature is upon the decline, approaches near to that of the firſt. It ſhould be lighter, and more diluting than that of vigorous age, and likewiſe more frequently taken.

Irregularities in DIET, SLEEP, &c.

It is not only neceſſary for health, that our diet be wholeſome, but alſo that it be taken at regular periods. Some imagine, that long faſting will attone for exceſs; but that, inſtead of mending the matter, never fails to make it worſe. When the ſtomach and inteſtines are over diſtended with food, they loſe their proper tone, and by long faſting they become weak, and inflated with wind. Thus either gluttony or faſting deſtroys the powers of digeſtion.

The frequent repetition of aliment is not only

ly neceſſary for repairing the continual waſte of our bodies, but likewiſe to keep the humours ſound and ſweet. Our humours, even in the moſt healthy ſtate, have a conſtant tendency to become putrid, which can only be prevented by frequent ſupplies of freſh nouriſhment: When that is wanting too long, the putrefaction often proceeds ſo far, as to occaſion very dangerous fevers. From hence we may learn the neceſſity of regular meals. No perſon can enjoy a good ſtate of health, whoſe veſſels are either frequently overcharged, or the humours long deprived of freſh ſupplies of chyle.

Long faſting is extremely hurtful to young people; it vitiates their humours, and prevents their growth and ſtrength: Nor is it leſs injurious to the aged. Many in the decline of life are afflicted with wind: That complaint is not only increaſed, but even rendered dangerous, and often fatal, by long faſting. Old people, when their ſtomachs are empty, are frequently ſeized with giddineſs, headachs, and faintneſs. Theſe complaints may generally be removed by a bit of bread and a glaſs of wine, or taking any other ſolid food; which plainly points out the method of preventing them. It is more than probable, that many of the ſudden deaths which happen in the advanced periods of life, are occaſioned by faſting too long, as it exhauſts the ſpirits, and fills the bowels with wind; we would therefore adviſe people, in the decline of life, never

never to allow their ſtomachs to be too long empty. Many take nothing but a few cups of tea and a bit of bread, from nine o'clock at night till two or three next afternoon. Such may be ſaid to faſt almoſt three fourths of their time. This can hardly fail to ruin the appetite, vitiate the humours, and fill the bowels with wind; All which might be prevented by a ſolid breakfaſt. That would tend more to ſtrengthen the nerves, and expel wind, than all the cordial or carminative medicines which can be adminiſtred.

THE ſtrong and healthy do not indeed ſuffer ſo much from faſting as the weak and delicate; but they run great hazard from its oppoſite, *viz.* repletion. Many diſeaſes, eſpecially fevers, are the effect of a plethora, or too great fulneſs of the veſſels. Strong people in high health, have generally a great quantity of blood and other humours. When theſe are ſuddenly increaſed by an overcharge of rich and nouriſhing diet, the veſſels become diſtended, and being unable to contract themſelves, obſtructions and inflammations enſue. Hence ſo many people are ſeized with inflammatory and eruptive fevers, after a feaſt or debauch. This ſhows the danger of all ſudden tranſitions from a ſpare to a full and luxurious diet.

EXCESS in diet is not peculiar to the rich and opulent; the poor are often guilty of it, and frequently feel its bad effects. The poor ſeldom loſe an opportunity of gorging themſelves either

ther with meat or drink, when they can obtain it; and the leſs they are accuſtomed to it, the danger is the greater.

WHEN we recommend regularity in diet, we would not be underſtood as condemning every ſmall deviation from it. It is next to impoſſible for people at all times to avoid ſome degree of exceſs, and living too much by rule might make even the ſmalleſt deviation dangerous. It may therefore be prudent to vary a little, ſometimes taking more, ſometimes leſs than the uſual quantity of meat and drink, provided always that regard be had to moderation.

SLEEP as well as diet ought to be duly regulated. Too little ſleep exhauſts the ſpirits, weakens the nerves, and occaſions diſeaſes; and too much renders the mind dull, the body groſs, and diſpoſes it to apoplexies, lethargies, &c. A medium therefore ought to be obſerved; but that is not eaſy to fix. The young require more ſleep than thoſe who are grown, the laborious than the idle, and ſuch as eat and drink freely than thoſe who live abſtemiouſly. Beſides, the real quantity of ſleep cannot be meaſured by time; as one perſon will be more refreſhed by five or ſix hours of ſleep than another by eight or ten. The beſt way to make ſleep ſound and refreſhing is to riſe by times. The indolent cuſtom of lolling a-bed for nine or ten hours relaxes the body, unbraces the nerves, and greatly hurts the conſtitution.

CHILDREN may be allowed as much ſleep as they chuſe; but for adults ſix or ſeven hours is is certainly enough, and none ought to exceed eight. Thoſe who lie more than eight hours a-bed may ſlumber, but they can hardly be ſaid to ſleep; ſuch generally toſs and dream away the fore-part of the night, ſink to reſt towards morning, and doſe till noon. Inſtead of encouraging a habit of this kind, riſing early would make them fall into a ſound ſleep as ſoon as they went to bed, and they would ſeldom wake till morning, when they would find themſelves ſufficiently refreſhed.

NATURE points out night as the proper time for ſleep. Thoſe who think it too vulgar to ſleep in that ſeaſon, ſeldom enjoy health. Nothing more certainly deſtroys the conſtitution than night-watching. It is great pity that a practice ſo deſtructive to health ſhould be ſo much in faſhion. How quickly the want of reſt in due ſeaſon will blaſt the moſt blooming complexion, or ruin the beſt conſtitution, is evident from the ghaſtly countenances of thoſe who, as the phraſe is, turn day into night, and night into day.

To make ſleep refreſhing, the following things are neceſſary. Firſt, that we take enough of exerciſe in the open air, through the day; next, to eat a light ſupper; and laſtly, to lie down with a mind chearful and ſerene.

IT is certain, that too much fatigue will prevent ſleep, as well as too little. We ſeldom however hear the active and laborious complain of reſtleſs nights. It is the indolent and ſlothful who

who generally have theſe complaints. Is it any wonder that a bed of down ſhould not be refreſhing to a perſon who lolls all day in an eaſy chair? A great part of the pleaſure of life conſiſts in alternate reſt and motion; but they who neglect the latter can never reliſh the former. The labourer enjoys more true luxury in plain food and ſound ſleep, than is to be found in ſumptuous tables and downy pillows, where exerciſe is wanting.

THAT light ſuppers cauſe ſound ſleep, is true even to a proverb. Many, if they exceed the leaſt at that meal, are ſure to have uneaſy nights; and if they drop aſleep, the load and oppreſſion on their ſtomach and ſpirits occaſion frightful dreams, broken and diſturbed repoſe, with night-mares, &c. Were the ſame perſons to go to bed with a light ſupper, or ſit up till what they eat were pretty well digeſted, they might enjoy ſound ſleep, and riſe refreſhed and chearful.

NOTHING more certainly diſturbs our repoſe than anxiety. When the mind is not at eaſe, we ſeldom enjoy ſound ſleep. That greateſt of human bleſſings often flies the wretch who needs it moſt, and viſits the happy, the chearful, and the gay. This is a good reaſon why every man ſhould endeavour to be as eaſy in his mind as poſſible, when he goes to reſt. Many, by neglecting this rule, and by indulging grief and anxious thoughts, have baniſhed ſleep

ſo

ſo long, that they could never afterwards enjoy it.

Few things contribute more to health than keeping the belly regular. When the fœces lie too long in the bowels, they become acrid, and ſpoil the humours; and when they are diſcharged too ſoon, the body is not properly nouriſhed. Regular ſtools depend greatly upon regularity in eating and drinking, and proper exerciſe; people have reaſon to ſuſpect a fault in one or other of theſe, whenever the belly is not regular.

To prevent coſtiveneſs, one good rule is, to riſe betimes and go abroad in the open air. Not only the poſture in bed is unfavourable to regular ſtools, but likewiſe the warmth. This, by promoting the perſpiration, cannot fail to leſſen all the other diſcharges. Mr Locke's advice, to ſollicite nature by going regularly to ſtool every morning, is a very good one, and has more effect than moſt people would imagine. Any habit will in time become natural. It is always more ſafe to keep the belly regular by proper diet, exerciſe, &c. than by the uſe of drugs. Thoſe who have frequent recourſe to medicine for that purpoſe, ſeldom fail to ruin their conſtitutions. But if opening medicines muſt be uſed, the ſafeſt is fine rhubarb, which may either be taken in ſmall doſes in powder, or a little of it chewed daily. Cuſtom will render this ſufficiently agreeable.

Such as are troubled with habitual looſeneſs,

ought to suit their food to the nature of their complaint. Looseness may often be removed by a change of diet: For example, boiled milk may be used in place of raw, wheat bread instead of that which is mixed, red wine or brandy and water may be drank in place of malt-liquor, white broths may be eat instead of flesh, and rice or sago greuels, with light flour puddings, in place of barley or oat meal. An habitual looseness is often occasioned by an obstructed perspiration. In that case a flannel vest and thick shoes are the best medicines.

BAD AIR.

BAD air is a very common cause of diseases. Few are aware of the danger arising from it; people generally pay some attention to what they eat and drink, but seldom regard what goes into the lungs, tho' the one often proves fatal as well as the other.

PERHAPS no air is perfectly pure; that however which has fewest noxious particles in it, is no doubt the best. Air as well as water takes up parts of most bodies with which it comes into contact, and is often so replenished with those of a noxious quality, as to occasion immediate death. But such violent effects seldom happen, as people are generally on their guard against them. The less perceptible influences of bad air prove more hurt-

hurtful to mankind ; we ſhall therefore endeavour to point out ſome of theſe, and to ſhow wherein the danger conſiſts.

Air may become noxious many ways. Whatever deſtroys its ſpring or elaſticity, renders it unfit for reſpiration: Wherever therefore great numbers of people are crowded into one place, if the air has not a free current, it ſoon becomes unwholeſome. Hence it is that delicate perſons are ſo apt to faint or be ſick, in crowded churches, aſſemblies, or any place where the air is exhauſted by breathing, fires, candles, or the like.

In great cities ſo many things tend to pollute the air, that it is no wonder it proves ſo fatal to the inhabitants. The air in cities is not only breathed over and over by thouſands, but is likewiſe exhauſted by fires, loaded with ſulphur, ſmoke, and other exhalations, beſides the vapours continually ariſing from innumerable putrid ſubſtances. All poſſible care ſhould be taken to keep the ſtreets of large towns open and wide, that the air may have a free current. They ought likewiſe to be kept very clean. Nothing tends more to pollute and contaminate the air than dirty ſtreets, dunghills, ſlaughter-houſes, &c.

It is very common in this country to have church-yards in the middle of populous cities. Whether that be the effect of ancient ſuperſtition, or owing to the increaſe of ſuch towns, is a matter of no conſequence. Whatever gave riſe

to

to the cuſtom, it is a bad one. It is habit alone which reconciles us to theſe things; by means of it the moſt ridiculous, nay, pernicious cuſtoms, often become ſacred. Certain it is, that thouſands of putrid carcaſes, ſo near the ſurface of the earth, in a place where the air ſtagnates, cannot fail to taint it; and that ſuch air being breathed into the lungs, and mixed with the blood, muſt occaſion diſeaſes *.

WHEREVER air ſtagnates long, it becomes unwholeſome. Hence the unhappy inmates of jails not only contract malignant fevers themſelves, but often communicate them to others. Nor are many of the holes, for we cannot call them houſes, poſſeſſed by the poor in great towns, much better than jails. Theſe low dirty habitations are the very lurking places of bad air and contagious diſeaſes. Such as live in them ſeldom enjoy good health; and their children commonly die young. In the choice of a houſe, the greateſt attention ought always to be paid to free air.

THE various methods which luxury has invented to make houſes cloſe and warm, contribute not a little to render them unwholeſome. No houſe can be wholeſome unleſs the air has a free paſſage through it. For which reaſon houſes ought daily to be ventilated by opening oppoſite

* In moſt eaſtern countries it is cuſtomary to bury the dead at ſome diſtance from any town. It were to be wiſhed the inhabitants of Europe would follow this example.

posite windows, and admitting a current of fresh air into every room. This would expel any noxious vapour, and could not fail to promote the health of the inhabitants. In hospitals, jails, ships, &c. where that cannot be conveniently done, ventilators should be used. The method of expelling foul, and introducing fresh air, by means of ventilators, is a most salutary invention, and is indeed the most useful of all our modern medical improvements. We wish, for the benefit of mankind, it were more generally regarded. It is capable of universal application, and fraught with numerous advantages, both to those in health and sickness.

Air not only loses its spring, and becomes unwholesome from heat and stagnation, but likewise from moisture. Thus, in low marshy countries, the air is generally bad, as also in countries over run with wood, or any thing that sends forth moist exhalations.

Air that stagnates in mines, wells, cellars, &c. must be noxious. That kind of air is to be avoided as the most deadly poison. It often kills almost as quick as lightening. For this reason people should be very cautious in opening cellars that have been long shut, or going down into deep wells, especially if they have been close covered.

Many people who have splendid houses, chuse to sleep in small appartments. This conduct is very imprudent. A bed-chamber ought always to be well aired; as it is generally occupied in the

the night only, when all doors and windows are ſhut. If a fire be kept in it, the danger becomes ſtill greater. Many have been ſtiffled when aſleep by a fire in a ſmall appartment. Some are even ſo inconſiderate as to make fires in bed-chambers which have no chimneys, and imagine by uſing that kind of coal which has little or no ſmoke, that they are ſafe; whereas the danger becomes thereby the greater, ſuch coal generally abounding with ſulphur. The moſt fatal conſequences are always to be dreaded from every attempt of this nature.

Those who are obliged, on account of buſineſs, to ſpend the day in cloſe towns, ought, if poſſible, to ſleep in the country. Breathing good air in the night will, in ſome meaſure, make up for the want of it through the day. This practice would have a greater effect in preſerving the health of citizens than is commonly imagined.

Care ſhould be taken to admit a conſtant ſtream of freſh air into all crowded places, as churches, aſſembly-rooms, colleges, courts of juſtice, &c. The neglect of this has had ſo many fatal conſequences, that it is ſufficient only to mention it.

It was neceſſary in former times, for ſafety, to ſurround cities, colleges, and even ſingle houſes, with high walls. Theſe, by obſtructing the current of air, never fail to render ſuch places damp and unwholeſome. As ſuch walls are now, generally ſpeaking, become uſeleſs, they ought to be be thrown down, and every method taken to admit a free paſſage to the air. Were proper attention paid to AIR and CLEANLINESS, it would tend more to preſerve the health of the inhabitants of great towns than all the endeavours of the Faculty.

IF freſh air be neceſſary for thoſe in health, it is ſtill more ſo for the ſick, who often loſe their lives for the want of it. The notion that ſick people muſt be kept very hot, is ſo common, that one can hardly enter the chamber where a patient lies without being ready to faint, by reaſon of the hot ſuffocating ſmell. How this muſt affect the ſick, any one may judge. No medicine is ſo beneficial to the ſick as freſh air. It is the moſt reviving of all cordials, if it be adminiſtred with prudence. We are not however to throw open doors and windows at random upon the ſick. Freſh air is to be let into the chamber gradually, and, if poſſible, by opening the windows of ſome other appartment.

THE air of a ſick perſon's chamber may be greatly freſhened, and the patient much revived, by ſprinkling the floor, bed, &c. frequently with vinegar, juice of lemon, or any other ſtrong vegetable acid.

IN places where numbers of ſick are crowded into the ſame houſe, or, which is often the caſe, into the ſame appartment, freſh air becomes abſolutely neceſſary. Infirmaries, hoſpitals, &c. often become ſo noxious for want of proper ventilation, that the ſick run more hazard

zard from them than from the diſeaſe; this is particularly the caſe when dyſenteries, putrid fevers, or other infectious diſeaſes prevail.

PHYSICIANS, ſurgeons, and others who attend hoſpitals, ought, for their own ſake, to take care that they be properly ventilated. They are obliged to ſpend much of their time amongſt the ſick, and run great hazard of being themſelves infected when the air is bad. All hoſpitals, and places for the ſick, ought to have an open ſituation, at ſome diſtance from any great town.

Want of CLEANLINESS.

THE want of cleanlineſs is a fault which admits of no excuſe. Where water can be had for nothing, it is ſurely in the power of every perſon to be clean. The continual diſcharge from our bodies by perſpiration renders frequent changes of apparel neceſſary. Change of apparel greatly promotes the ſecretion from the ſkin, ſo neceſſary for health. When that matter which ought to be carried off by perſpiration, is either retained in the body, or re-abſorbed from dirty cloaths, it is apt to occaſion fevers and other diſeaſes.

MOST diſeaſes of the ſkin proceed from want of cleanlineſs. Theſe indeed may be caught by infection; but they will ſeldom continue long where cleanlineſs prevails. To the ſame cauſe muſt

must we impute the various kinds of vermin which infest the human body, houses, &c. These may generally be banished by cleanliness alone. Perhaps the intention of nature in permitting such vermin to annoy mankind, is to induce them to the practice of this virtue.

One common cause of putrid and malignant fevers is the want of cleanliness. These fevers commonly begin among the inhabitants of close, dirty houses, who breathe bad air, take little exercise, use unwholesome food, and wear dirty cloaths. There the infection is generally hatched, which often spreads far and wide, to the destruction of many. Hence cleanliness may be considered as an object of public attention. It is not sufficient that I be clean myself, while the want of it in my neighbour affects my health as well as his own. If dirty people cannot be removed as a common nuisance, they ought at least to be avoided as infectious. All who regard their health should keep at a distance even from their habitations.

In places where great numbers of people are collected, cleanliness becomes of the utmost importance. It is well known, that infectious diseases are communicated by tainted air. Every thing therefore which tends to pollute the air, or spread the infection, ought, with the utmost care, to be avoided. For this reason in great towns no filth, of any kind, should be permitted to lie upon the streets. Nothing is more apt to convey infection than the excrements of the

 diseased.

diſeaſed. Theſe, in many caſes, are known to be highly infectious. The ſtreets in many great towns are little better than dunghills, being frequently covered with aſhes and naſtineſs of every kind. How eaſily might this be prevented by active magiſtrates, who have it always in their power to make proper laws relative to things of this nature, and to enforce the obſervance of them?

WE are ſorry to ſay, that the importance of general cleanlineſs does by no means ſeem to be ſufficiently underſtood. It were well if the inhabitants of Britain would imitate their neighbours the Dutch in the cleanneſs of their ſtreets, houſes, &c. Water indeed is eaſily obtained in Holland; but the ſituation of moſt towns in Britain is more favourable to cleanlineſs. Nothing can be more agreeable to the ſenſes, more to the honour of the inhabitants, or conducive to their health, than a clean town; nor does any thing impreſs a ſtranger ſooner with a diſreſpectful idea of any people than its oppoſite.

THE peaſants in moſt countries ſeem to hold cleanlineſs in a ſort of contempt. Were it not for the open ſituation of their houſes, they would often feel the bad effects of this diſpoſition. One ſeldom ſees a farm-houſe without a dunghill before the door, and frequently the cattle and their maſters lodge under the ſame roof. Peaſants are likewiſe extremely careleſs with reſpect to change of apparel, keeping their ſkins

ſkins clean, &c. Theſe are merely the effects of indolence and a dirty diſpoſition. Habit may indeed render them leſs diſagreeable; but no habit can ever make it ſalutary to wear dirty cloaths, or breathe unwholeſome air.

In camps the ſtricteſt regard ſhould be paid to cleanlineſs. By negligence in this matter infectious diſeaſes are often ſpread amongſt a whole army; and frequently more die of theſe than by the ſword. The Jews, during their encampments in the wilderneſs, received particular inſtructions with reſpect to cleanlineſs *. The rules enjoined them ought to be obſerved by all in the like ſituation. Indeed the whole ſyſtem of laws delivered to that people, has a manifeſt tendency to promote cleanlineſs. Whoever conſiders the nature of their climate, and the diſeaſes to which they were liable, will ſee the propriety of ſuch laws.

It is remarkable, that in moſt eaſtern countries cleanlineſs makes a great part of their religion. The Mahometan, as well as the Jewiſh religion, enjoins various bathings, waſhings, and purifications. No doubt theſe were deſigned to repreſent inward purity; but they are at the ſame time calculated for the preſervation of health. However

* Thou ſhalt have a place alſo without the camp, whither thou ſhalt go forth abroad; and thou ſhalt have a paddle upon thy weapon: and it ſhall be when thou ſhalt eaſe thyſelf abroad, thou ſhalt dig therewith, and ſhalt turn back, and cover that which cometh from thee, &c.

Deuter. chap. xxiii. ver. 12. 13.

However whimsical these washings may appear to some, few things ould tend more to prevent diseases than a proper attention to many of them. Were every person, for example, after handling a dead body, visiting the sick, &c. to wash before he went into company, or sat down to meat, he would run less hazard either of catching the infection himself, or communicating it to others.

FREQUENT washing not only removes the filth and sordes which adhere to the skin, but likewise promotes the perspiration, braces the body, and enlivens the spirits. Even washing the feet tends greatly to preserve health. The sweat and dirt with which these parts are frequently covered, cannot fail to obstruct the perspiration. This piece of cleanliness would often prevent colds and fevers. Were people careful to bathe their feet and hands in warm water at night, after being exposed to cold or wet through the day, they would seldom experience any of the fatal effects which often proceed from these causes.

A proper attention to cleanliness is no where more necessary than on shipboard. If epidemical distempers break out there, no one can be safe. The best way to prevent them is to take care that the whole company be cleanly in their cloaths, diet, &c. When infectious diseases do break out, cleanliness is the most likely means to prevent their spreading. Above all things, the cloaths, bedding, &c. of the sick ought to be carefully washed, and fumigated with brimstone, or the

the like. Infection will lodge a long time in dirty cloaths, and will afterwards break out in the most terrible manner.

In places where great numbers of sick people are kept, cleanliness ought most religiously to be observed. The very smell in such places is often sufficient to make one sick. It is easy to imagine what effect that is likely to have upon the diseased. A person in perfect health has a greater chance to become sick, than a sick person has to get well, in an hospital or infirmary, where cleanliness is neglected.

The brutes themselves set us an example of cleanliness. Most of them seem uneasy, and thrive ill, if they be not kept clean. A horse that is kept thoroughly clean will thrive better on a smaller quantity of food, than with a greater where cleanliness is neglected. Even our own feelings are a sufficient proof of the necessity of cleanliness. How refreshed, how chearful, and agreeable does one feel on being shaved, washed, and dressed; especially when these offices have been long neglected? Most people esteem cleanliness; and even those who do not practice it themselves often admire it in others. Superior cleanliness sooner attracts our regard than even finery itself, and often gains esteem where the other fails.

To point out the numerous advantages arising from cleanliness of person, houses, streets, &c. would be a very useful and agreeable task; but as our plan only permits us to name things,

we

we muſt conclude this article by recommending the practice of that virtue to people of all ſtations and conditions in life. We do not indeed pretend to rank cleanlineſs amongſt the *cardinal virtues;* but we would recommend it as neceſſary for ſupporting the dignity of human nature, as uſeful and agreeable to ſociety, and as highly conducive to health.

INTEMPERANCE.

A modern author * obſerves, that temperance and exerciſe are the two beſt phyſicians in the world. He might have added, that if theſe were duly regarded, there would be little occaſion for any other. Temperance may juſtly be called the parent of health; but numbers of mankind act as if they thought diſeaſes and death too ſlow in their progreſs, and by intemperance and debauch ſeem, as it were, to ſollicit their approach.

The danger of intemperance appears from the very conſtruction of the human body. Health depends on that ſtate of the ſolids and fluids which fits them for the due performance of the vital functions; and ſo long as theſe go regularly on, we are ſound and well; but whatever diſturbs them, neceſſarily impairs health. Intemperance never fails to diſorder the whole animal œconomy:

* Rouſſeau.

œconomy; it ſpoils the digeſtion, relaxes the nerves, renders the different ſecretions irregular, vitiates the humours, and of courſe occaſions diſeaſes.

THE analogy between the nouriſhment of plants and animals affords a ſtrong proof of the danger of intemperance. Moiſture and manure greatly promote vegetation; but an over-quantity of either will entirely prevent it. The beſt things become hurtful, nay deſtructive, when carried to exceſs. From hence we learn, that the greateſt pitch of human wiſdom conſiſts in regulating our appetites and paſſions ſo as to avoid all extremes. 'Tis that alone which entitles us to the character of rational beings. The ſlave of appetite will ever be the diſgrace of human nature.

THE Author of nature hath endued us with various paſſions, for the propagation of the ſpecies, the preſervation of the individual, &c. Intemperance is the abuſe of theſe paſſions; and in the proper regulation of them moderation conſiſts. Men, not content with ſatisfying the ſimple calls of nature, create artificial wants, and are perpetually in ſearch after ſomething that may gratify them; but imaginary wants can never be gratified. Nature is content with a little; but luxury knows no bounds. The epicure, the drunkard, and the debauchee ſeldom ſtop in their carreer till caſh or conſtitution fails: Then indeed they generally ſee their error when too late.

IT

It is impoſſible to lay down determined rules of temperance, on account of the different conſtitutions of mankind. The moſt ignorant perſon however certainly knows what is meant by exceſs; and it is in the power of every man to avoid it if he chuſes. The great rule in regulating our diet, is to ſtudy ſimplicity. Nature delights in the moſt plain and ſimple food, and every animal, except man, follows her dictates. Man alone riots at large, and ranſacts the whole creation in queſt of luxuries, to his own deſtruction. An elegant writer * of the laſt age ſpeaks thus of intemperance: "For my part, when I behold a faſhionable table ſet out in all its magnificence, I fancy that I ſee gouts and dropſies, fevers and lethargies, with other innumerable diſtempers, lying in ambuſcade among the diſhes."

Intemperance does not hurt its votaries alone; the innocent too often feel the direful effects of it. How many wretched orphans are to be ſeen embracing dunghills, whoſe parents, regardleſs of the future, ſpent in riot and debauch what might have ſerved decently to feed and cloath their offspring? How often do we behold the miſerable mother, with her helpleſs infants, pining in want, while the cruel father is indulging even at the expence of their lives!

Families are not only reduced to miſery, but extirpated by means of intemperance. Nothing tends ſo much to prevent propagation, and to ſhorten

* Addiſon.

ſhorten the lives of children. The poor man who labours all day, and at night lies down contented with his humble fare, can boaſt a numerous offspring, while his pampered lord, ſunk in eaſe and luxury, has neither ſon nor nephew. Even ſtates and empires feel the influence of intemperance, and riſe or fall as it prevails.

INSTEAD of mentioning the different kinds of intemperance, and pointing out their influence upon health, we ſhall confine our obſervations to one particular ſpecies of that vice, *viz.* the abuſe of intoxicating liquors.

EVERY act of intoxication puts nature to the expence of a fever in order to diſcharge the ſuperfluous load; but when that is repeated almoſt every day, it is eaſy to foreſee the conſequences. That conſtitution muſt be ſtrong indeed which is able long to hold out under a daily fever! But fevers occaſioned by drinking do not always go off in a day; they frequently end in an inflammation of the breaſt, liver, or brain, and produce fatal effects.

THO' the drunkard ſhould not fall by an acute diſeaſe, he ſeldom eſcapes thoſe of a chronic nature. Intoxicating liquors, when uſed to exceſs, weaken the bowels and ſpoil the digeſtion; they deſtroy the power of the nerves, and occaſion paralytic and convulſive diſorders; they heat and inflame the blood, deſtroy its balſamic quality, render it unfit for circulation, and the nouriſhment of the parts, *&c.* Hence obſtructions, atrophies, dropſies, and conſumptions of the lungs. Theſe are the common ways in which drunkards make their exit. Diſeaſes of this kind, when brought on by hard drinking, ſeldom admit of a cure.

MANY people injure their health by drinking, who ſeldom get drunk. The continual habit of ſoaking, as it is called, though its effects be not ſo violent, is no leſs pernicious. When the veſſels are kept conſtantly full and upon the ſtretch, the different digeſtions can neither be duly performed, nor the humours properly prepared. Hence moſt people of this character are afflicted with the gout, the gravel, ulcerous ſores in the legs, &c.; if theſe diſorders do not appear, they are ſeized with low ſpirits, hypochondriacal diſorders, and other ſymptoms of indigeſtion.

ALL intoxicating liquors may be conſidered as poiſons. However diſguiſed, that is their real character, and ſooner or later they will have their effect. Conſumptions are now ſo common, that it is thought one tenth of the inhabitants of great towns die of that diſeaſe. Drunkenneſs is one of the cauſes to which we muſt impute the increaſe of conſumptions. The great quantities of viſcid malt-liquor drank by the common people of England, cannot fail to render the blood ſizy and unfit for circulation; from whence proceed obſtructions and inflammations of the lungs. There are few great ale-drinkers who are not phthiſical; nor is that to be wondered at, conſidering the glutinous and almoſt indigeſtible

indigeſtible nature of ſtrong ale. Thoſe who drink ardent ſpirits or ſtrong wines do not run leſs hazard; theſe liquors heat and inflame the blood, and tear the tender veſſels of the lungs in pieces.

The habit of drinking proceeds frequently from misfortunes in life. The miſerable fly to it for relief. It affords them indeed a temporary eaſe. But alas, this ſolace is ſhort-lived, and when it is over the ſpirits ſink as much below their natural pitch as they had before been raiſed above it. Hence a repetition of the doſe becomes neceſſary, and every freſh doſe makes way for another, till the unhappy wretch becomes a ſlave to the bottle, and at length falls a ſacrifice to what nature intended only as a medicine. No man is ſo dejected as the drunkard when his debauch is gone off. Hence it is, that thoſe who have the greateſt flow of ſpirits while the glaſs circulates freely, are of all others the moſt melancholy when ſober, and often put an end to their own miſerable exiſtence in a fit of ſpleen or ill humour.

Drunkenness not only proves deſtructive to health, but likewiſe to the faculties of the mind. It is ſtrange that creatures who value themſelves on account of a ſuperior degree of reaſon to that of the brutes, ſhould take pleaſure in ſinking ſo far below them. Were ſuch as voluntarily deprive themſelves of the uſe of reaſon, to continue ever after in that condition, it would ſeem but a juſt puniſhment. Though that be not the conſequence

consequence of one act of drunkenness, it seldom fails to succeed a course of intoxication. By a habit of drinking, the greatest genius is often reduced to a mere dunce.

INACTIVITY.

MANY look upon the necessity man is under of earning his bread by labour as a curse. Be that as it may, it is evident from the structure of the body, that exercise is not less necessary for the preservation of health, than food. Those whom poverty obliges to labour for daily bread, are not only the most healthy, but generally the most happy. Industry seldom fails to place such above want, and activity serves them instead of physic. This is peculiarly the case with those who live by the culture of the ground. The great increase of inhabitants in infant-colonies, and the common longevity of such as follow agriculture every where, evidently prove it to be the most healthful as well as the most useful employment.

THE love of activity shows itself very early in man. So strong is this principle, that a healthy youth cannot be restrained from exercise, even by the fear of punishment. Our love of motion is surely a strong proof of its utility. Nature implants no disposition in vain. Some imagine, that the love of motion was implanted ed in man, becauſe without it he could not obtain the neceſſaries of life; but ſuppoſe the neceſſaries of life could be univerſally obtained without motion, it would nevertheleſs be indiſpenſable. It ſeems to be a catholic law throughout the whole animal creation, that no creature, without exerciſe, can enjoy health. Every creature, except man, takes as much exerciſe as is neceſſary. He alone, and ſuch animals as are under his direction, deviate from this original law, and they ſuffer accordingly.

INACTIVITY never fails to bring on univerſal relaxation of the ſolids, which occaſions innumerable diſeaſes. When the ſolids are relaxed, neither the digeſtion, nor any of the ſecretions, can be duly performed. In this caſe, the worſt conſequences muſt enſue. How can thoſe who loll all day in eaſy chairs, and ſleep all night on beds of down, fail to be relaxed? Nor do ſuch greatly mend the matter, who never ſtir abroad but in a coach, or ſedan, &c. Theſe elegant pieces of luxury are become ſo common, that the inhabitants of great towns ſeem to be in ſome danger of loſing the uſe of their limbs altogether. 'Tis now below any one to walk who can afford to be carried. How ridiculous would it ſeem to a perſon unacquainted with modern luxury, to behold the young and healthy ſwinging along on the ſhoulders of their fellow-creatures! or to ſee a fat carcaſe, over-run with diſeaſes occaſioned by inactivity, dragged thro' the ſtreets by half a dozen horſes.

GLAN-

Glandular obstructions generally proceed from inactivity. These are the most obstinate of all maladies. So long as the liver, kidnies, and other glands, duly perform their functions, health is seldom impaired; but when they fail, nothing can preserve it. Exercise is almost the only cure we know for glandular obstructions; indeed it does not always succeed; but there is reason to believe that it would seldom fail to prevent these complaints. One thing is certain, that amongst those who take enough of exercise, glandular diseases are very little known; whereas the indolent and inactive are seldom free from them.

Weak nerves are the constant companions of inactivity. Nothing but exercise and open air can brace and strengthen the nerves, or prevent the endless train of diseases which proceed from a relaxed state of these organs. We seldom hear the active or laborious complain of nervous diseases; these are reserved for the sons of ease and affluence. Many have been compleatly cured of nervous disorders by being reduced from a state of opulence to labour for their daily bread. This plainly points out the sources from whence such diseases flow, and the means by which they may be prevented.

It is absolutely impossible to enjoy health without a free perspiration; but that necessary discharge never goes properly on where exercise is wanting. When the matter which ought to be thrown off by perspiration is retained in the body,

body, it cannot fail to vitiate the humours. Hence proceed the gout, fevers, rheumatism, &c. In a word, none of the vital or animal functions can be duly performed when exercise is neglected. It alone would prevent many diseases which cannot be cured, and would remove others where medicine proves ineffectual.

A late author *, in his excellent treatise on health, says, that the weak and valetudinary ought to make exercise a part of their religion. We would recommend this, not only to the weak and valetudinary, but to all whose business does not oblige them to take sufficient exercise, as sedentary artificers, shop-keepers, studious people, &c. Such ought to take exercise as regularly as they take food. This, were people careful to husband their time well, might be done without any interruption to business or study.

No piece of indolence hurts the health more than the modern custom of lolling a-bed too long in a morning. This is universally the case in great towns. The inhabitants of cities seldom do much business before breakfast; but that is the best time for exercise, while the stomach is empty, and the body refreshed with sleep. Rising early would not only give those who cannot leave their business through the day, an opportunity of taking exercise, but it would prevent the bad effects of loitering in bed too long. The morning-air braces and strengthens the nerves,

* Cheyne.

nerves, and, in ſome meaſure, anſwers the purpoſe of a cold bath. Let any one who has been accuſtomed to lie a-bed till eight or nine o'clock, riſe by ſix or ſeven, ſpend a couple of hours in walking, riding, or any active diverſion without doors, and he will find his ſpirits chearful and ſerene through the day, his appetite keen, and his body braced and ſtrengthened. Cuſtom ſoon renders early riſing agreeable, and nothing contributes more to the preſervation of health.

Exercise, if poſſible, ought always to be taken in the open air. When that cannot be done, various methods may be contrived for exerciſing the body within doors, as dancing, fencing, the dumb bell, playing at tennis, &c. It is not neceſſary to adhere ſtrictly to any particular kind of exerciſe. The beſt way is to take them by turns, and to uſe that longeſt which is moſt ſuitable to the ſtrength and conſtitution. Theſe kinds of exerciſe which give action to moſt of the bodily organs, are always to be preferred, as riding, walking, running, digging, ſwiming, and ſuch like.

It is much to be regreted, that active and manly diverſions are now ſo little regarded. Diverſions make people take more exerciſe than they otherwiſe would do, and are of the greateſt ſervice to ſuch as are not under the neceſſity of labouring for their bread. As active diverſions loſe ground, thoſe of a ſedentary kind ſeem to prevail. Sedentary diverſions are of

no

no other uſe than to conſume the time which might be employed in exerciſe: Inſtead of relieving the mind, they often require more thought than either ſtudy or buſineſs. Every thing that induces people to ſit ſtill, unleſs it be ſome neceſſary employment, ought to be avoided.

THE diverſions which afford the beſt exerciſe are, hunting, ſhooting, playing at cricket, hand-ball, golff *, &c. Theſe exerciſe the limbs, promote perſpiration, and the other ſecretions. They likewiſe ſtrengthen the lungs, and give firmneſs and agility to the whole body.

SUCH as can, ought to ſpend two or three hours a day on horſeback; thoſe who cannot, ſhould employ the ſame time in walking. The beſt time for taking exerciſe is in the morning, or at leaſt before dinner; but it ſhould never be continued too long. Over fatigue prevents the benefit of exerciſe, and weakens inſtead of ſtrengthening the body.

EVERY man ſhould lay himſelf under ſome ſort of neceſſity to take exerciſe. Indolence, like all other vices, when indulged, gains ground, and at length becomes agreeable. Hence many who were fond of exerciſe in the early part of life,

O become

* Golff is a diverſion very common in North Britain. It is well calculated for exerciſing the body, and may always be taken in ſuch moderation, as neither to over heat nor fatigue. It has greatly the preference over cricket, tennis, or any of thoſe games which cannot be played without violence.

become quite averſe from it afterwards. This is the caſe of moſt hypochondriac and gouty people, which renders their diſeaſes in a great meaſure incurable.

In ſome countries laws have been made, obliging every man, of whatever rank, to learn ſome mechanical employment. Whether ſuch laws were deſigned for the preſervation of health, or encouragement of manufacture, is a queſtion of no importance. Certain it is, that if gentlemen were frequently to amuſe and exerciſe themſelves in this way, it might have many good effects. They would at leaſt derive as much honour from a few maſterly ſpecimens of their own workmanſhip, as from the character of having ruined moſt of their companions by gaming, or hard drinking. Beſides, men of leiſure, by applying themſelves to the mechanical arts, might improve them, to the great benefit of ſociety. This would afford a more comfortable reflection at the cloſe of life, than the conſciouſneſs of having lived in the world for no other purpoſe than to eat and drink.

Indolence not only occaſions diſeaſes, and renders men uſeleſs to ſociety, but promotes all manner of vice. To ſay a man is idle, is perhaps, in the ſtrongeſt terms, to call him vicious. The mind, if not engaged in ſome uſeful purſuit, is conſtantly in queſt of ideal pleaſures, or impreſſed with the apprehenſion of ſome imaginary evil. From theſe ſources proceed moſt of the miſeries of mankind. Sure man never was intended

tended to be idle. Inactivity frustrates the very design of his creation. An active life is the best guardian of virtue, and the greatest preservative of health.

INFECTION.

Most diseases are infectious. Every person ought therefore, as far as he can, to avoid all communication with the diseased. The common practice of visiting the sick, though well meant, has many ill consequences. Far be it from us to discourage any act of charity or benevolence, especially towards those in distress; but we cannot help blaming such as endanger their own or neighbours lives by a mistaken friendship, or an impertinent curiosity.

The houses of the sick, especially in the country, are generally crowded from morning till night with idle visitors. It is customary, in such places, for servants and young people to wait upon the sick by turns. It would be a miracle indeed should such always escape. Experience teaches us the danger of this conduct. People often catch fevers in this way, and communicate them to others, till at length they become epidemic.

It would be thought highly improper for one who had not had the small pox, to wait upon a patient in that disease; yet many other fevers

vers are almoſt as infectious as the ſmall pox, and not leſs fatal. Some imagine, that fevers prove more fatal in villages than in great towns, for want of proper medical aſſiſtance. How far that is true, we will not pretend to ſay; but we are inclined to think, that it rather proceeds from the cauſe above mentioned.

WERE a plan to be laid down for communicating infection, it could not be done more effectually than by the common method of viſiting the ſick. Such viſitors not only endanger themſelves and their connections, but likewiſe hurt the ſick. By crowding the houſe, they render the air unwholeſome, and by their private whiſpers and diſmal countenances, diſturb the imagination of the ſick and depreſs his ſpirits. Sick perſons, eſpecially in fevers, ought to be kept as quiet as poſſible. The ſight of ſtrange faces, and every thing that diſturbs the mind, hurts them.

THE common practice in country-places of inviting great numbers of people to funerals, and crowding them into the ſame appartment where the corps lies, is another way of ſpreading infection. The infection by no means dies with the patient. In many caſes it rather grows ſtronger as the body becomes putrid. This is peculiarly the caſe of thoſe who die of malignant fevers, or other putrid diſeaſes. Such ought not to lie long unburied; and people ſhould keep at a diſtance from them. It is very common for people, after attending the funeral of a friend, to be ſeized with the ſame diſ-

caſe

ease of which he died, and to share the same fate.

It would tend greatly to prevent the spreading of infectious diseases, if those in health were kept at a proper distance from the sick. The Jewish Legislator, among many other wise institutions for preserving health, has been peculiarly attentive to the means of preventing infection, or *defilement* as it is called, either from a diseased person or a dead body. In many cases the diseased were to be separated from those in health; and it was deemed a crime even to approach their habitations. If a person only touched a dead body, he was appointed to wash himself in water, and to keep for some time at a distance from society.

Infectious diseases are often communicated by cloaths. It is extremely dangerous to wear apparel which has been worn by the diseased, as infection will lodge in it a long while, and afterwards produce very tragical effects. This shows the danger of buying at random the cloaths which have been used by other people.

Infectious disorders are frequently imported. Commerce, together with the riches of foreign climes, brings us also their diseases. These do often more than counterbalance all the advantages of that trade by means of which they are introduced. It is to be regretted, that so little care is commonly taken, either to prevent the introduction or spreading of infectious diseases. Some attention indeed is generally

rally paid to the plague; but other diſeaſes paſs unregarded.

INFECTION is often ſpread by jails, hoſpitals, &c. Theſe are frequently ſituated in the very middle of cities, or populous towns; and when infectious diſeaſes break out in them, it is impoſſible for the inhabitants to eſcape. Were magiſtrates to pay any regard to the health of the people, this evil might be eaſily remedied.

MANY are the cauſes which tend to diffuſe infection through populous cities. The whole atmoſphere of a large town is one contaminated maſs, abounding with every kind of infection, and muſt be pernicious to health. The beſt advice that we can give to ſuch as live in cities, is, to chuſe an open ſituation; to avoid narrow, dirty, crowded ſtreets; to keep their own houſes and offices clean; to admit the freſh air every day into their appartments; and to be as much abroad as their time will permit.

IT would tend greatly to prevent the ſpreading of infectious diſeaſes, were proper nurſes every where employed to take care of the ſick. This might often ſave a family, or even a whole town, from being infected by one perſon. We do not mean that people ſhould abandon their friends or relations in diſtreſs, but only to put them on their guard againſt being too much in company with thoſe who are afflicted with diſeaſes of an infectious nature.

SUCH as wait upon the ſick in infectious diſeaſes, ought to ſtuff their noſes with tobacco, or ſome

ſome other ſtrong ſmelling herb, as rue, tanſy, or the like. They ought likewiſe frequently to ſprinkle the room where the patient lies with vinegar, or other ſtrong acids; and to avoid the patient's breath as much as they can.

HOWEVER eaſy theſe hints may ſeem; yet a proper attention to them would ſave many lives. A fever, or other infectious diſeaſe, ſeldom breaks out in a family, but it affects the moſt of them, and frequently ſeizes every individual. The ſcenes of calamity and diſtreſs produced by this means, are too often witneſſed by thoſe who attend the ſick.

YOUNG people are peculiarly liable to catch infection; and therefore ought to be kept at the greateſt diſtance from the diſeaſed. Their minds are eaſily affected with ſcenes of diſtreſs, and they often catch diſeaſes even by the force of imagination.

WE would not only recommend it to magiſtrates, to take proper meaſures to prevent the ſpreading of infectious diſeaſes, but alſo to maſters of families. A ſingle ſervant may ſpread a diſeaſe amongſt a whole family, which may prove fatal to many of them. For this reaſon, when a ſervant is ſeized with a fever, or other infectious diſeaſe, he ought to be kept in ſome ſeparate appartment, or rather ſent to an hoſpital or infirmary. Servants would not only be taken better care of in this way, but fatal diſeaſes might be often prevented.

INFECTION is often caught by ſleeping with the

the diseased. Every person knows that this is the case in consumptions of the lungs; but other diseases are infectious as well as consumptions: Nay, we hardly know any disease that is not so in some degree. If a sound person communicates health, surely a diseased one must have the contrary effect. Were this attended to in the choice of companions for life, it would save many from a premature end.

Not only the diseases of the body, but also those of the mind are infectious. For this reason our companions ought to be of a sound mind, as well as a sound body. A melancholy person, for example, diffuses a gloom all around him, and generally taints the minds of his companions with the temper of his own. Those who would be healthy and happy, ought therefore to associate with the young, the chearful, and good humoured.

The PASSIONS.

The passions have great influence both in the cause and cure of diseases. How mind acts upon matter will, in all probability, ever remain a secret. It is sufficient for us to know, that there is established a reciprocal influence betwixt the mental and corporeal parts, and that whatever disorders the one likewise hurts the other.

The

The passion of *anger* ruffles the mind, distorts, the countenance, hurries on the circulation of the blood, and disorders the whole vital and animal functions. It often occasions fevers, with other acute diseases; and sometimes brings on sudden death. This passion is peculiarly hurtful to the delicate, and those of weak nerves. I have known a hysteric woman lose her life by a violent fit of anger; all such ought to guard against the excess of this passion with the utmost care.

It is not always in our power to prevent being angry; but we may surely avoid harbouring resentment in our breast. Resentment preys upon the mind; it occasions the most obstinate chronical disorders, and gradually wastes the constitution. Nothing shows true greatness of mind more than to forgive injuries: It promotes the peace of society, and greatly conduces to our own ease, health, and felicity.

Such as value health should avoid violent gusts of anger, as they would the most deadly infection. They ought never to indulge resentment, but to endeavour at all times to keep their minds calm and serene. Nothing tends so much to the health of the body as a constant tranquility of mind.

The influence of *fear*, both in occasioning and aggravating diseases, is very great. No man ought to be blamed for a decent concern about life; but too great a desire to preserve it, is often the way to lose it. Fear and anxiety, by depreſſing the ſpirits, pre-diſpoſe us to diſeaſes, and often render thoſe fatal which an undaunted mind would overcome.

SUDDEN fear has generally violent effects. Epilectic fits, and other convulſive diſorders, are often occaſioned by it. Hence the danger of that practice, ſo common among young people, of frightening one another. By this many have loſt their lives; and others have been rendered uſeleſs ever after. It is dangerous to tamper with the human paſſions. They may eaſily be thrown into ſuch diſorder as never again to act with regularity.

BUT the gradual effects of fear prove more generally hurtful. The conſtant dread of ſome future evil, by dwelling upon the mind, often occaſions the very evil itſelf. Hence it comes to paſs that ſo many die of theſe diſeaſes of which they long had a dread, or which ſome accident, or fooliſh prediction, had impreſſed on their minds. This often happens to women in child-bed. Many of thoſe who die in that ſituation are impreſſed with the notion of their death a long while before it happens; and there is reaſon to believe, that ſuch impreſſions are often the cauſe of it.

THE methods taken to impreſs the minds of women with apprehenſions of the great danger and peril of child-birth are very hurtful. Few women die in labour, tho' many loſe their lives after it; which may be thus accounted for. A woman after delivery finding herſelf weak and exhauſted, ed, immediately apprehends ſhe is in danger; But fear ſeldom fails to obſtruct the neceſſary evacuations upon which her recovery depends. Thus the ſex often fall a ſacrifice to their own imaginations, when there would be no danger, did they apprehend none.

It ſeldom happens that two or three women who are generally known, die in child-bed, but their death is followed by many others. Every woman of their acquaintance who is with child dreads the ſame fate, and the diſeaſe becomes epidemical by the mere force of imagination. This ſhould induce pregnant women to deſpiſe fear, and by all means to avoid thoſe tattling goſſips who are continually telling them the misfortunes of others. Every thing that may in the leaſt alarm a pregnant, or child-bed woman, ought with the greateſt care to be guarded againſt. Many women have loſt their lives in child-bed by the old ſuperſtitious cuſtom, ſtill kept up in moſt parts of Britain, of tolling the pariſh-bell for every perſon who dies. People who think themſelves in danger are very inquiſitive; and if they come to know that the bell tolls for one who died in the ſame ſituation, what muſt be the conſequence?

But this cuſtom is not pernicious to child-bed women only. It is hurtful in many other caſes. When low fevers, in which it is difficult to ſupport the patient's ſpirits, prevail, what muſt be the effect of a funeral peal ſounding five or ſix times a day in his ears? His imagination will

will no doubt ſuggeſt, that others died of the ſame diſeaſe which he labours under. Nor will the matter be at all mended by endeavouring to perſuade him of the contrary. This will tend rather to confirm than remove his ſuſpicions.

If this childiſh cuſtom cannot be aboliſhed, we ought to keep the ſick as much from hearing it as poſſible, and from every thing elſe that may tend to alarm them. So far is this from being attended to, that many make it their buſineſs to viſit the ſick, on purpoſe to whiſper diſmal ſtories in their ears. Such may paſs for ſympathizing friends, but they ought rather to be reckoned enemies, and ranked amongſt murderers. All who wiſh well to the ſick, ought to keep ſuch perſons at the greateſt diſtance from them.

A cuſtom has long prevailed among phyſicians of prognoſticating, as they call it, the patient's fate, or foretelling the iſſue of the diſeaſe. Vanity no doubt introduced this practice, and ſtill ſupports it, in ſpite of common ſenſe and the ſafety of mankind. I have known a phyſician barbarous enough to boaſt, that he pronounced more *ſentences* than all his Majeſty's judges. Would to God that ſuch ſentences were not often equally fatal! It may be alledged, that the doctor does not declare his opinion before the patient. So much the worſe. A ſenſible patient had better hear what the doctor ſays than learn it from the diſconſolate looks, the watery eyes, and the broken

ken whiſpers of thoſe about him. It ſeldom happens, when the doctor gives an unfavourable opinion, that it can be concealed from the patient. The very embaraſſment which generally appears in diſguiſing what he has ſaid, is ſufficient to diſcover the truth.

We do not ſee what right any man has to announce the death of another, eſpecially if ſuch a declaration has a chance to kill him. Mankind are indeed very fond of prying into future events, and ſeldom fail to importune the phyſician for his opinion. A doubtful anſwer, however, or one that may tend to encourage the hopes of the patient, is ſurely the moſt ſafe. This conduct could neither hurt the patient nor the phyſician. Nothing tends more to deſtroy the credit of phyſic than thoſe bold prognoſticators, who, by the bye, are generally the moſt ignorant. The miſtakes which daily happen in this way are ſo many ſtanding proofs of human vanity, and the weakneſs of ſcience.

The vanity of foretelling the fate of the ſick is not peculiar to the Faculty. Others follow their example, and thoſe who think themſelves wiſer than their neighbours often do much miſchief in this way. Humanity ſurely calls upon every one to comfort the ſick, and not to add to their affliction by alarming their fears. A phyſician may often do more good by a mild and ſimpathizing behaviour than by medicine, and ſhould never neglect to adminiſter that greateſt of all cordials, Hope.

Grief

Grief is the moſt deſtructive of all the paſſions. Its effects are permanent, and when it ſinks deep into the mind, it generally proves fatal. Anger and fear being of a more violent nature, ſeldom laſt long; but grief often changes into a fixed melancholy, which preys upon the ſpirits, and waſtes the conſtitution. We ſhould beware of indulging this paſſion. It may generally be conquered at the beginning; but when it has gained ſtrength, all our attempts become vain.

No perſon can prevent misfortunes; but it ſhows true greatneſs of mind to bear them with ſerenity. Many make a merit of indulging grief, and when misfortunes happen, they obſtinately refuſe all conſolation till the mind, overwhelmed with melancholy, ſinks under the load. Such conduct is not only deſtructive to health, but inconſiſtent with reaſon, religion, and common ſenſe.

Change of ideas is as neceſſary for health as change of poſture. When the mind dwells long upon one object, eſpecially of a diſagreeable nature, it hurts the whole functions of the body. Thus grief indulged ſpoils the digeſtion, and deſtroys the appetite. By that means the ſpirits are depreſſed, the nerves relaxed, the bowels inflated with wind, and the humours, for want of freſh ſupplies of chyle, vitiated. Thus many an excellent conſtitution has been ruined by a family-misfortune, or any thing that occaſioned exceſſive grief.

It

It is utterly impoſſible, that any perſon of a dejected mind ſhould enjoy health. Life may indeed be dragged on for a few years: But whoever would live to a good old age, muſt be good humoured and chearful. This indeed is not altogether in our own power; yet our temper of mind, as well as actions, depends greatly upon ourſelves. We can either think of agreeable or diſagreeable objects, as we chuſe; we can go into chearful or melancholy company; we can mingle in the amuſements and offices of life, or ſit ſtill and brood over our calamities. Theſe, and many ſuch things, are certainly in our power, and from theſe the mind generally takes its caſt.

The variety of ſcenes which preſent themſelves to the ſenſes, were certainly deſigned to prevent our attention from being too long fixed upon any one object. Nature abounds with variety, and the mind, unleſs fixed down by habit, delights in contemplating new objects. This at once points out the method of relieving the mind in diſtreſs. Turn the attention to other objects. Examine them with accuracy. When the mind begins to recoil, ſhift the ſcene. By this means a conſtant ſucceſſion of new ideas may be kept up, till the diſagreeable ones entirely diſappear. Thus travelling, the ſtudy of any art or ſcience, reading or writing on ſuch ſubjects as engage the attention, will ſooner expel grief than the moſt ſprightly amuſements.

It has already been obſerved, that exerciſe is abſolutely neceſſary for the health of the body; but it is no leſs ſo for that of the mind. Indo-

lence

lence nouriſhes grief. When the mind has nothing elſe to think of but calamities, no wonder that it dwells there. Few people who purſue buſineſs with attention are hurt by grief. Inſtead of abſtracting ourſelves from the world or buſineſs, when misfortunes happen, we ought to engage in it with more than uſual attention, to diſcharge with double diligence the functions of our ſtation, and to mix with friends of an eaſy ſocial temper.

INNOCENT amuſements are by no means to be neglected. Theſe, by leading the mind inſenſibly to the contemplation of agreeable objects, help to diſpel the gloom which misfortunes caſt over it. They make time ſeem leſs tedious, and have many other happy effects.

SOME, when overwhelmed with grief, betake themſelves to drinking. This is making the cure worſe than the diſeaſe. It ſeldom fails to end in the ruin of fortune, character, and conſtitution.

THE beſt way to counteract the violence of any paſſion is to encourage its oppoſite. Thus, under the moſt preſſing calamities, HOPE is always to be kept in view. Hope is the very ſupport of life, and abſolutely neceſſary to the happineſs of a rational being.

SHOULD all other means of comfort fail, the Chriſtian religion affords an inexhauſtible ſource of conſolation. It teaches us, that the ſufferings of this life are deſigned to prepare us for a future ſtate of happineſs; and that all who purſue the paths of virtue ſhall at laſt arrive at complete felicity.

CHAP. III.

Of ARTIFICERS, LABOURERS, &c.

THAT men are expoſed to particular diſeaſes from the occupations which they follow, is a fact well known; but to remedy that evil is a difficult matter. People are under a neceſſity of purſuing the employments in which they are bred, whether they be favourable to health or not. Hence all that we can propoſe, under this article, is to point out thoſe diſeaſes to which men are more immediately expoſed from their particular occupations; and to ſhew how far ſuch diſeaſes, by due care, may be avoided.

THE firſt cauſe of the diſeaſes of artificers that we ſhall mention, is the unwholeſome ſmells and noxious exhalations which often proceed from thoſe materials in which they are employed. Thus tallow chandlers, boilers of oil, dreſſers of leather, and all who work upon putrid animal ſubſtances are afflicted with diſeaſes of the ſtomach and lungs. Ill ſmells not only create a nauſea and hurt the digeſtion, but even taint the humours themſelves, and frequently prove the cauſe of fevers, conſumptions, &c.

THESE occupations are not only hurtful to ſuch as are employed in them, but likewiſe to thoſe who live in the neighbourhood of the places where they are carried on; for which reaſon they ought always to be at a proper diſtance from any town.

THE beſt advice that we can give to ſuch as are employed in this way, is, to pay the utmoſt attention to cleanlineſs. They are indeed obliged to wear dirty cloaths while at work; but the moment they leave off, they ought to waſh themſelves, ſtrip off their dirty cloaths, put on clean ones, and remove at a proper diſtance from the ſmell of their work ſhops, &c. No one, who has not made the trial, can imagine how far an attention to theſe, and other pieces of cleanlineſs, will go in preſerving the health of thoſe artificers who are obliged to follow ſuch employments.

CHYMISTS, founders, glaſs-makers, &c. beſides the noxious exhalations from thoſe bodies in which they work, are forced to breathe an air that is in a manner burnt, or at leaſt too much rarified to expand the lungs, or anſwer the important purpoſes of reſpiration. Such people are generally thin, pale, and of a weak conſumptive habit. They are melted down with ſweat, in order to ſupply which evacuation large quantities of liquor become neceſſary. Thus by hard working and faſt living, their conſtitutions are worn out in a few years.

SUCH artiſts ought to work by turns, and ſhould never continue long near the furnace at a time. They ſhould be careful, when they leave off work, to cool gradually, avoiding every thing that may ſuddenly check the perſpiration.

The

The places where theſe occupations are carried on ſhould be properly conſtructed for diſcharging the ſmoke, and other exhalations, and admitting a free current of freſh air; otherwiſe the people who work in them can never enjoy health.

THE exhalation from metals and minerals is not only hurtful to founders, chymiſts, and others who manufacture them for particular purpoſes, but likewiſe to miners, or thoſe who dig them out of the earth. Falloppius obſerves, that ſuch as work in mines of mercury ſeldom live above three or four years. They are generally affected with palſies, vertigos, and other diſeaſes of the nerves, which ſoon put an end to their miſerable lives. Thoſe alſo who work in lead mines are very liable to paralitic diſorders, with gripes, colics, and other complaints of the bowels.

MINERS ſuffer from their ſituation as well as from the metals in which they work. The air in mines being totally excluded from the ſun's rays, by ſtagnation loſes its ſpring, and often becomes damp This kind of air is to be avoided as the moſt deadly poiſon: Beſides, mines are often wet, which renders them ſtill more hurtful. This is one reaſon why miners are very ſubject to aches, cramps, and rheumatic pains, &c.

MINERS ſhould never continue too long under ground at a time; neither ought they at any time to go to work faſting, nor to ſuffer their ſtomachs

ſtomachs to be empty while they continue in the mines. They ought not to live too low; and their liquor ſhould be generous. They ſhould by all means avoid coſtiveneſs, by either taking food of an opening nature, or, when that does not ſucceed, a gentle purge. Oils are found to be a good preſervative againſt gripes from the effluvia of metals. Oils both open the belly, and ſheath the coats of the inteſtines, which prevents their being hurt by the poiſonous particles of the metal.

MINERS ſhould by all means take care that the air have a free current through the mines, and that neither it nor the water be ſuffered to ſtagnate. All who work in mines or metals ought to waſh when they leave off work, and to change their cloaths. Thoſe parts of the metal which adhere either to the ſkin or the cloaths, being continually abſorbed into the body, muſt neceſſarily do hurt. People are too apt to look upon ſuch circumſtances as unworthy of their attention; but theſe ſmall cauſes, by being neglected, never fail to produce the moſt dreadful effects.

PLUMBERS, painters, gilders, and all who work in metals, are ſubject to the ſame diſeaſes as thoſe who dig them. They are afflicted with colics, aſthmas, palſies, &c. and ſhould obſerve the ſame precautions as miners. It is impoſſible for people thus employed, at all times to avoid ſome degree of danger; but it conſiſts with obſervation, that, by due care, they may prolong

prolong their lives to a good old age, with a tolerable ſhare of health. We have ſeldom ſeen a perſon in danger from any of the above cauſes, but it proceeded from his own foolhardineſs or want of care.

As it would greatly exceed our bounds to ſpecify the diſorders peculiar to every occupation, we ſhall therefore conſider mankind under the following general claſſes, *viz. Laborious*, *Sedentary*, and *Studious*.

The LABORIOUS.

Though thoſe who follow laborious employments are in general the moſt healthy, yet the nature of their occupations, and the places where they are carried on, expoſe them to many diſeaſes. Huſbandmen, for example, are expoſed to all the viciſſitudes of the weather, which are often very great and ſudden. They are likewiſe forced to work hard, and often to carry loads above their ſtrength, which, by overſtraining the veſſels, occaſion many diſeaſes, as aſthmas, fevers, ruptures, &c.

Intermittent fevers, or agues, are very common amongſt thoſe who labour without doors. Theſe are occaſioned by the frequent viciſſitudes of heat and cold to which they are expoſed, by the bad water which they are often obliged to drink, by the low marſhy ſituation of of their houſes, and by their frequent expoſure to the evening dews, night-air, &c.

ASTHMAS and inflammations of the breaſt are very incident to the laborious. Theſe are occaſioned by the violent exerciſe and the frequent extremes of heat and cold to which they are expoſed. Thoſe who bear heavy burdens, as porters, &c. are obliged to draw in the air with much greater force, and alſo to keep their lungs diſtended with more violence than is neceſſary for common reſpiration: By this means the tender veſſels of the lungs are over-diſtended, and often burſt, inſomuch that a ſpitting of blood or fever enſues. Hippocrates mentions an inſtance to this purpoſe of a man, who, upon a wager, had carried an aſs. The man, he ſays, was immediately ſeized with a fever, a vomiting of blood, and a rupture.

CARRYING heavy burdens is often the effect of mere indolence, which prompts people to do at once what ſhould be done at twice. It likewiſe proceeds frequently from bravado, or an emulation to outdo others. Hence it is that the ſtrongeſt men are moſt generally hurt by heavy burdens, hard labour, or feats of activity. It is rare to find one who excels in this way, without a hernia, a hæmoptoe, or ſome other diſeaſe, which he enjoys as the fruit of his folly. One would imagine, that the daily inſtances we have of the fatal effects of carrying great weights, running, wreſtling, &c. ſhould be ſufficient to put a ſtop to ſuch practices.

THERE

THERE are indeed ſome employments which neceſſarily require a violent exertion of ſtrength, ſuch as blackſmiths, carpenters, &c. None ought to follow theſe occupations but men of a ſtrong body; and they ſhould never exert their ſtrength to the utmoſt, nor work too long. When the muſcles are violently ſtrained, frequent reſt is neceſſary, in order that they may recover their tone; where that is neglected, the ſtrength and conſtitution will ſoon be worn out, and a premature old age brought on.

THE quinſy and eriſipelas, or St Anthony's fire, are likewiſe diſeaſes very incident to the laborious. Theſe are occaſioned by whatever gives a ſudden check to the perſpiration, as drinking cold liquor when the body is warm, keeping on wet cloaths, ſitting or lying on the cold ground, damp houſes, wet feet, &c. As the great danger of theſe practices has already been pointed out, it is unneceſſary to inſiſt upon them here.

THE laborious are often afflicted with the iliac paſſion, the colic, and other complaints of the bowels. Theſe are often occaſioned by wet feet, or wet cloaths; but they more generally proceed from flatulent and indigeſtable food. Labourers eat unfermented bread made of peas, beans, rye, and other windy ingredients. They alſo eat great quantities of unripe fruits, baked, ſtewed, or raw, with various kinds of roots and herbs, upon which they drink ſour milk, ſtale ſmall beer, &c. Such a compoſition cannot fail

fail to fill the bowels with wind, and occafion difeafes. Accordingly we find thefe people in the decline of life univerfally complaining of flatulencies; a diforder which renders many of them very unhappy, and for which no cure is yet known. The beft advice that we can give them is to avoid windy food as far as poffible.

INFLAMMATIONS, whitloes, and other difeafes of the extremities, are very common amongft thofe who labour without doors. Thefe difeafes are often attributed to venom, or fome kind of poifon; but they generally proceed either from fudden heat after cold, or the contrary. When fuch people come from the fields cold and wet, they run to the fire, and often plunge their hands in warm water, by which means the blood and other humours in thefe parts are fuddenly expanded, and the veffels not yielding fo quickly, a ftrangulation happens, and an inflammation or mortification enfues.

WHEN labourers come home cold, they ought to keep at a diftance from the fire for fome time, to wafh their hands in cold water, and to rub them well with a dry cloth. It fometimes happens that people are fo benumbed with cold, as to lofe the ufe of their limbs altogether. In fuch a cafe the only remedy is to rub the parts affected with fnow, or, failing it, with cold water. If they be held near the fire, or plunged into warm water, a mortification will certainly enfue.

LABOURERS in the hot feafon are apt to ly down

down and ſleep in the ſun. This practice is ſo dangerous, that they often riſe in a high fever. The burning fevers which prove ſo fatal about the end of ſummer, and beginning of autumn, are often occaſioned by this means. When labourers leave off work, which they ought always to do during the heat of the day, they ſhould go home, or, at leaſt, get under ſome cover, where they may repoſe themſelves in ſafety.

The different ſeaſons of the year expoſe thoſe who labour without doors to different diſeaſes. Thus in the ſpring agues are frequent; in ſummer, as has been obſerved, burning fevers abound; and in autumn, dyſenteries and fluxes prevail. The latter proceed not only from the perſpiration being, at that time, obſtructed, but alſo from the green traſh, or unripe fruits, which country-people eat in great quantities. Indeed if fruit be ripe, and eat in moderation, it rather prevents than occaſions dyſenteries; but it is equally certain, that much bad fruit will bring on a flux.

Labourers are often hurt by long faſting. They frequently follow their employments in the fields from morning till night, without eating any thing. This cannot fail to hurt their health. However homely their fare be, they ought to have it at regular times, and the harder they work, the more frequently ſhould they eat.

LABOURERS likewiſe ſuffer from the nature of their food. They are extremely careleſs with reſpect to what they eat or drink, and often, thro' mere indolence, eat unwholeſome food, when they might. for the ſame expence, have that which is wholeſome. The poor often hurt their health for want of a proper method of living, and in the end ſave nothing by it. In many parts of Britain, the peaſants are too careleſs to take the trouble of dreſſing their victuals, though they have feuel for nothing. Such people will live upon one meal a-day in indolence, rather than labour, though it were to procure them the greateſt affluence.

POVERTY is doubtleſs a very general cauſe of diſeaſes among the labouring part of mankind. Few of them have much foreſight; and if they had, it ſeldom is in their power to lay any thing up againſt hard times. They are glad to make a ſhift to live from day to day; and when any diſeaſe renders them unfit for work, their families are ready to ſtarve. Here the God-like virtue ot charity ought ever to exert herſelf. To relieve the induſtrious poor when in diſtreſs, is ſurely the moſt exalted act of religion, and can never loſe its reward. They alone who witneſs thoſe ſcenes of calamity, can form a notion of what numbers periſh in diſeaſes for want of proper aſſiſtance, and even for want of the neceſſaries of life. It were to be wiſhed, for the honour of human nature, as well as for the good

good of society, that these things were more looked into.

FEVERS of a very bad kind are often occasioned by what is called *poor living*. When the body is not sufficiently nourished, the humours become bad, and the spirits sink; from whence the most fatal consequences must ever ensue. *Poor living* is likewise productive of cutaneous diseases. It is remarkable that cattle, when pinched in their food, are generally affected with diseases of the skin. These diseases seldom fail to disappear when they are put upon a good pasture: which shews how much a good state of the humours depends upon a sufficient quantity of proper nourishment.

LABOURERS often suffer from a foolish emulation, which prompts them to vie with one another, till they drop down dead, or over-heat themselves to such a degree as to occasion a fever. As this is the effect of vanity, it ought always to be checked by those who have the superintendence of them. Such as wantonly throw away their lives in this manner, deserve to be looked upon in no better light than self-murderers. It is pity that poor widows and fatherless children should suffer by such childish conduct: Could we speak to the passions of men, we would bid them think of these, and then consider of how great importance their lives are.

THE office of a soldier in time of war, may be ranked amongst laborious employments. Soldiers

Soldiers ſuffer many hardſhips from the inclemency of ſeaſons, long marches, hunger, bad proviſions, &c. Theſe occaſion fevers, fluxes, rheumatiſms, and other fatal diſeaſes. which often do more execution than the ſword, eſpecially when campaigns are continued too late in the ſeaſon. One week of cold rainy weather will kill more men than many months when it is dry and warm.

Every commander ſhould take care that his ſoldiers be well cloathed and well fed. He ought alſo to endeavour to put an end to the campaign in due ſeaſon, and to provide his men with winter quarters that are dry and well-aired. Theſe eaſy rules, with taking care to keep the ſick at a proper diſtance from thoſe in health, will go a great length in preſerving the lives of the ſoldiery.

It is indeed to be regretted, that ſoldiers ſuffer no leſs by indolence and intemperance in time of peace, than from hardſhips in time of war. When men are idle, they will be vicious. It would therefore be of the greateſt importance, could a ſcheme be formed for rendering the military in time of peace leſs vicious, more healthy, and more uſeful to ſociety. All thoſe deſirable objects might certainly be promoted by only employing them five or ſix hours every day, and advancing their pay in proportion. By this means idleneſs, the mother of vice, would not only be prevented, but the price of labour might be lowered. Public works, as harbours,

harbours, canals, turnpike-roads, &c. might be made without hurting manufactures; and ſoldiers might be enabled to marry, and bring up children.

A ſcheme of this kind might be ſo conducted as to raiſe inſtead of depreſſing the martial ſpirit, provided the men were never allowed to work above a certain number of hours, and obliged always to work without doors. No ſoldier ſhould ever be allowed to work too long, nor permitted to follow any ſedentary employment. Sedentary employments render men weak and effeminate, and quite unfit for the hardſhips of war; whereas working a few hours daily without doors would inure them to the weather, brace their nerves, and promote their ſtrength and courage.

SAILORS may alſo be numbered amongſt the laborious. They undergo great hardſhips from change of climate, the violence of weather, hard labour, bad proviſions, &c. Sailors are of ſo great importance both to the trade and ſafety of this kingdom, that too much pains can never be beſtowed in pointing out the proper means of preſerving their lives.

EXCESS is one great ſource of the diſeaſes of ſea-faring people. When they get on ſhore, after being long at ſea, without regard to the climate, or their own conſtitutions, they plunge headlong into all manner of riot, and often perſiſt till a fever puts an end to their lives. Thus intemperance, and not the climate, is is often the cause why so many of our brave sailors die on foreign coasts. We would not have sea-faring people live too low; but they will find temperance the best defence against fevers, and many other maladies.

SAILORS when on duty are often exposed to cold and wet. When that happens, they should change their cloaths as soon as they are relieved, and take every proper method to restore the perspiration. In this case they should not have recourse to spirits, or other strong liquors, but should rather drink such as are weak and diluting, of a proper warmth, and go immediately to bed, where a sound sleep and a gentle sweat will set all to rights.

THE health of sailors suffers most from unwholesome food. The constant use of salted provisions vitiates the whole humours, and occasions the scurvy, and other obstinate maladies. It is no easy mater to prevent this disease in long voyages; yet we cannot help thinking, that much might be done towards effecting so desirable an end, were due pains bestowed for that purpose. For example, various roots, greens, and fruits might be kept a long time at sea, as potatoes, cabbages, lemons, oranges, tamarinds, apples, &c. When fruits cannot be kept, the juices of them either fresh or fermented, may. With these all the drink, and even the food of the ship's company, ought to be acidulated in long voyages. But suppose the vegetable acids should fail, yet the chymical,

cal, as cream of tartar, elixir of vitriol, &c, may be kept for any length of time; and as they are attended with no expence, it is in the power of every ſailor to lay in enough of theſe for the longeſt voyage. Theſe, though not ſo good as the vegetable acids, are ſtill better than none, and ſhould always be uſed when the others fail.

Stale bread and beer likewiſe contribute to vitiate the humours. Meal will keep for a long while on board, of which freſh bread might frequently be made. Malt too might be kept on board, and infuſed with boiling water at any time. This liquor, when drank even in the form of wort, is very wholeſome, and is found to be an excellent antidote againſt the ſcurvy. Small wines and cyder might likewiſe be plentifully laid in, and ſhould they turn ſour, they would ſtill be uſeful, as vinegar. Vinegar is a very great antidote againſt diſeaſes, and ſhould be uſed by all travellers, eſpecially at ſea.

Such animals as can be kept alive ought likewiſe to be carried on board, as hens, ducks, pigs, &c. Freſh broths made of portable ſoup, and puddings made of peas, or other vegetables, ought to be uſed frequently. Many other things will occur to people converſant in theſe matters, which would tend to preſerve the health of that brave and uſeful ſet of men. Pity it is that ſo little attention ſhould be paid to theſe things by ſuch as have it in their power to rectify

tify them; but intereſt blinds the eyes of ſome, while others, totally regardleſs of the future, will make no proviſion againſt diſeaſes till they feel them.

THERE is reaſon to believe, if care were taken with reſpect to the diet, air, cloathing, &c. of ſea-faring people, that they would be the moſt healthy ſet of men in the world; but when theſe are not duly regarded, the very reverſe muſt happen.

PERUVIAN bark is the beſt *medical antidote* that we can recommend to ſailors or ſoldiers on foreign coaſts. This will often prevent fevers, and other fatal diſeaſes. A dram or ſo of it may be chewed every day, or if this ſhould prove diſagreeable, an ounce of bark, with half an ounce of orange-pill, and two drams of ſnake-root coarſely powdered, may be infuſed for two or three days in an Engliſh quart of brandy, and half a wine glaſs of it taken twice or thrice a-day, when the ſtomach is moſt empty. This has been found to be an excellent antidote againſt fluxes, putrid, intermitting, and other fevers, in unhealthy climates. It is not material in what form this medicine be adminiſtred. It may either be infuſed in water, wine, or ſpirits as recommended above, or made into an electuary with ſyrip of lemons, oranges, or the like.

The

The SEDENTARY.

THO' nothing can be more contrary to the nature of man than a ſedentary life, yet the far greater part of the human ſpecies are comprehended under this claſs. Almoſt the whole female world, and, in manufacturing countries, the major part of the males, may be reckoned ſedentary.

AGRICULTURE, the firſt and moſt healthful of all employments, is now followed by few who are able to carry on any other buſineſs. Thoſe who imagine that the culture of the earth is not ſufficient to employ all its inhabitants, are greatly miſtaken. An ancient Roman, we are told, could maintain his family from the produce of one acre of ground. So might a modern Britain, if he could be contented to live like a Roman. This ſhows what an immenſe increaſe of inhabitants Britain might admit of, and all of them live by the culture of the ground. Agriculture is the great ſource of domeſtic riches. It is of all employments the moſt favourable to health and population. When it is neglected, whatever wealth may be imported from abroad, poverty, wretchedneſs, and miſery will abound at home. Such is, and ever will be, the fluctuating nature of manufactures, that ten thouſand people may be in bread to-day, and in beggary to-morrow. This can never happen to thoſe who cultivate the ground. They can eat the fruit of their labour, and can always by induſtry obtain, at leaſt, the neceſſaries of life.

THO' ſedentary employments be neceſſary, yet there ſeems to be no reaſon why any perſon ſhould be confined for life to theſe alone. Were ſuch employments intermixed with the more active and laborious, they would never do hurt. It is conſtant confinement that ruins the health. A man may not be hurt by ſitting four or five hours a-day, who, were he obliged to ſit ten or twelve, would ſoon contract diſeaſes.

BUT it is not want of exerciſe alone which hurts ſedentary people; they often ſuffer from the unwholeſome air which they breathe. It is very common to ſee ten or a dozen taylors, or ſtay-makers, for example, crouded into one ſmall appartment, where there is hardly room for one ſingle perſon to breathe freely. In this ſituation they generally continue for many hours at a time, with often the addition of ſundry candles, which help to waſte the air, and render it leſs fit for reſpiration. Air that is breathed over and over, loſes its ſpring, and becomes unfit for expanding the lungs. This is one cauſe of the phthiſical coughs, and other complaints of the breaſt, ſo incident to ſedentary artificers.

EVEN the perſpiration from a great number of

of bodies pent up together, renders the air unwholesome. The danger from this quarter is greatly increased, if any one of them happens to have bad lungs, or to be otherwise diseased. Those who sit near him, being forced to breathe the same air, can hardly fail to be infected. It would be a rare thing indeed to find a dozen of sedentary people all sound. The danger of crouding them together must therefore be evident to every one.

MANY of those who follow sedentary employments are constantly in a bending posture, as shoemakers, taylors, cutlers, &c. Such a situation is extremely hurtful. A bending posture obstructs all the vital motions, and of course must ruin the health. Accordingly we find such artificers generally complain of indigestions, flutulencies, headaches, pains of the breast, &c. In such people the first concoction is generally bad, and as that fault can never be mended in any of the subsequent ones, it cannot fail to induce a total vitium of the humours, which paves the way to innumerable diseases.

THE aliment in sedentary people, instead of being pushed forewards by an erect posture, the action of the muscles, &c. is in a manner confined in the bowels. Hence costiveness, wind, and other hypochondriacal symptoms, the never failing companions of the sedentary. Indeed none of the excretions can be duly performed where exercise is wanting, and when any one of these is retained

retained too long in the body, it muſt have bad effects, as it is again taken up into the maſs of humours.

A bending poſture is very hurtful to the lungs. When this organ is compreſſed, the air cannot have free acceſs into all its parts, ſo as to expand them properly Hence tubercles, adheſions, &c. are formed, which often end in conſumptions. The proper action of the lungs is likewiſe neceſſary for making good blood. When that organ fails, the humours ſoon become univerſally depraved, and the whole conſtitution goes to wreck. In fine, both the pectoral and abdominal viſcera ought to be kept as free and eaſy as poſſible. Their continual action is abſolutely neceſſary to life, and being of a ſoft texture, their functions are eaſily obſtructed by any ſort of preſſure.

The ſedentary are not only hurt by preſſure on the bowels, but alſo on the inferior extremities, which obſtructs the circulation in theſe parts, and renders them weak and feeble. Thus taylors, ſhoemakers, &c. frequently loſe the uſe of their legs altogether; beſides the blood and other humours, by ſtagnating in theſe parts, are vitiated; from whence proceed the ſcab, ulcerous ſores, foul blotches, and other cutaneous diſeaſes, ſo common among ſedentary artificers.

A bad figure of body is a very common conſequence of cloſe application to ſedentary employments. The ſpine, for example, by being continually bent, puts on a crooked ſhape, and generally

generally remains ſo ever after. But a bad figure of body has already been obſerved to be hurtful to health, as the vital functions, &c. are thereby impeded.

A ſedentary life never fails to occaſion an univerſal relaxation of the ſolids. This is the grand ſource from whence moſt of the diſeaſes of ſedentary people flow. The ſcrofula, conſumption, rickets, and many other maladies which now abound, were very little known in this country before ſedentary artificers became ſo numerous; and they are very little known ſtill among ſuch of our people as follow active employments without doors, tho' in the great manufacturing towns, at leaſt two thirds of the inhabitants are afflicted with them.

It is the more difficult to remedy thoſe evils, becauſe many who have been accuſtomed to a ſedentary life, like rickety children, loſe all inclination for exerciſe; we ſhall however give a few hints with reſpect to the moſt likely means for preſerving the health of this uſeful ſet of people, which ſome of them, we hope, will be wiſe enough to obſerve.

It has been obſerved, that ſedentary artificers are often hurt by their bending poſture. They ought therefore to ſtand or ſit as erect as the nature of their employments will permit. They ſhould likewiſe change poſtures frequently, and ſhould never ſit too long at a time, but leave off work and walk, ride, run, or do any thing that will promote the vital functions.

Seden-

SEDENTARY artificers are allowed too little time for exercife; yet, fhort as it is, they feldom employ it properly. A journeyman taylor or weaver, inftead of walking abroad for exercife and frefh air, at his hours of leifure, chufes often to fpend them in a public houfe, or in purfuing fome fedentary diverfion, at which he generally lofes both his time and money.

THE aukward poftures in which many fedentary artificers work, feem rather to be the effect of cuftom than neceffity. For example, a table might furely be contrived for ten or a dozen taylors to fit round it, with liberty for their legs either to hang down, or reft upon a foot board, as they fhould chufe. A place might be cut out in the table for every perfon to fit in, by which means his work would lie as ready to his hand, as in the prefent mode of fitting crofs-legged.

WE would recommend to all fedentary artificers the moft religious regard to cleanlinefs. Both their fituation and occupations render this highly neceffary. Nothing would contribute more to preferve fendentary artificers in health, than a ftrict attention to this rule; and fuch of them as neglect it, not only run the hazard of lofing their health, but of becoming a nuifance to fociety.

SEDENTARY people fhould live fpare. They ought likewife to avoid food that is windy, or hard of digeftion, and fhould pay the ftricteft regard

gard to ſobriety. A perſon who works hard without doors will ſoon throw off an overcharge of liquor, but one who ſits has by no means an equal chance. Hence it often happens, that ſedentary people are ſeized with fevers after hard drinking. When ſuch people feel their ſpirits low, inſtead of running to the tavern for relief, they ſhould ride, or walk into the fields. This would remove the complaint more effectually than ſtrong liquor, and would never hurt the conſtitution.

INSTEAD of multiplying rules for preſerving the health of the ſedentary, we ſhall recommend the following general plan, viz. That every perſon who follows a ſedentary employment ſhould cultivate a piece of ground with his own hands. This he might dig, plant, ſow, and weed at his leiſure-hours, ſo as to make it both an exerciſe and amuſement, while it produced many of the neceſſaries of life. After working an hour in a garden, a man will return with more keenneſs to his employment within doors, than if he had been all the while idle.

LABOURING the ground is every way conducive to health. It not only gives exerciſe to every part of the body, but the very ſmell of the earth and freſh herbs, revive and chear the ſpirits, whilſt the perpetual proſpect of ſomething coming to maturity, delights and entertains the mind. We are ſo made as to be always pleaſed with ſomewhat in proſpect, however diſtant or however trivial. Hence

Hence the happineſs that moſt men feel in planting, ſowing, building, &c. Theſe ſeem to have been the chief employments of the early ages; and when kings and conquerors cultivated the ground, there is reaſon to believe, that they knew as well wherein true happineſs conſiſted as we do.

It may ſeem romantic to recommend gardening to manufacturers in great towns; but obſervation proves, that the plan is very practicable. In the town of Sheffield, in Yorkſhire, where the great iron manufacture is carried on, there is hardly a journeyman cutler who does not occupy a piece of ground which he cultivates as a garden. This practice has many ſalutary effects. It not only induces theſe people to take exerciſe without doors, but alſo to eat many greens, roots, &c. of their own produce, which they would not think of purchaſing. There ſeems to be no reaſon why manufacturers in any other town in Great Britain ſhould not follow this example.

Mechanics are too much inclined to croud into great towns. This ſituation may have ſome advantages; but it has many diſadvantages. All mechanics who live in the country, have it in their power, and indeed moſt of them do, occupy a piece of ground, which not only gives them exerciſe, but enables them to live more comfortably. So far at leaſt as our obſervation reaches, mechanics who live in the country are far more happy than thoſe in great towns.

towns. They enjoy better health, live in greater affluence, and ſeldom fail to rear a healthy and numerous offspring.

In a word, exerciſe without doors, in one ſhape or other, is abſolutely neceſſary to health. Thoſe who neglect it, though they may for a while drag out life, can hardly be ſaid to enjoy it. Their humours are generally vitiated, their ſolids relaxed and weak, and their ſpirits low and depreſſed.

The STUDIOUS.

Intense thought is ſo deſtructive to health, that few inſtances can be produced of ſtudious perſons who live to an extreme old age. Hard ſtudy always implies a ſedentary life; and when want of exerciſe is joined to intenſe thinking, the conſequences muſt be bad. We have frequently known even a few months intenſe ſtudy ruin an excellent conſtitution, and bring on a train of nervous complaints, which never could be removed. Man is evidently not formed for continual thought more than for perpetual action, and would be as ſoon worn out by the one as by the other.

So great is the power of the mind over the body, that by its influence the whole vital motions may be accelerated or retarded, to almoſt any degree. Chearfulneſs and mirth quicken the circulation, and promote all the ſecretions; whereas ſadneſs and profound thought never fail to retard them. Thus even a degree of thoughtleſsneſs is neceſſary to health. The perpetual thinker ſeldom enjoys either health or ſpirits; while the perſon who can hardly be ſaid to think at all, ſeldom fails to enjoy both. The mind, by a habit of thinking, in ſome meaſure loſes the power of unbending itſelf. This may be called a diſeaſe of the mind, and ſhould be as carefully guarded againſt as any other malady.

PERPETUAL thinkers, as they are called, ſeldom think to much purpoſe. Such people, in a courſe of years, generally become quite ſtupid, and exhibit a melancholy proof how readily the greateſt bleſſings may be abuſed. Thought, like all other things, when carried to extreme, becomes a vice. Hence nothing can afford a greater proof of wiſdom than for a man frequently and ſeaſonably to unbend his mind. This may always be done by chearful company, active diverſions, muſic, or the like.

THE gout is the common companion of the ſtudious. This excrutiating diſeaſe generally proceeds from indigeſtions, and an obſtructed perſpiration. It is impoſſible that the man who ſits all day in a cloſet ſhould either digeſt his food, or have any of the ſecretions in due quantity. When that matter, which ſhould be thrown off by the ſkin, is retained in the body, it cannot

not fail to vitiate the humours, and of course to produce the gout, or some other malady.

THE studious are often afflicted with the stone and gravel. Motion greatly assists the secretion and discharge of urine; consequently a sedentary life must have the contrary effect. Of this any one may be sensible by observing, that he passes much more urine by day than in the night, and also when he walks or rides than when he sits. A free discharge of urine not only prevents the gravel and stone, but many other diseases. When the blood or other humours are disordered, nature generally attempts to free herself of the offending cause, by the urinary passages; but when these become unfit for performing their proper functions, this attempt must fail, and consequently diseases will ensue.

OBSTRUCTIONS of the liver prove often fatal to the studious. Diseases of that organ are very obstinate, and generally complicated. The circulation in the liver being slow, obstructions can hardly fail to be the consequence of inactivity. Hence sedentary people are frequently afflicted with schirrous livers, the jaundice, &c. The proper secretion and discharge of the bile is so necessary a part of the animal œconomy, that where it is not duly performed, the health must needs be impaired. Indigestion, loss of appetite, and a wasting of the whole body, seldom fail to be the consequences of a vitium, or obstructions of the bile.

FEW diseases prove more fatal to the studious than

than consumptions of the lungs. It has already been observed, that this organ cannot be duly expanded in those who do not take proper exercise, and where that is the case, obstructions, adhesions, &c. must ensue. Not only want of exercise, but the posture in which studious people often sit, is very hurtful to the lungs. Those who read or wiite much are apt to contract a habit of bending forwards, and often press with their breast upon a table or bench, &c. It is impossible this posture should fail to hurt the lungs. It ought therefore to be avoided with the utmost care.

THE studious are often afflicted with want of appetite and indigestions. These lay the foundation of numerous diseases. When the digestions fail, the humours must soon be depraved, to which succeed low spirts, weak nerves, with the whole train of hysteric and hypochondriac maladies.

HEADACHES often afflict the studious. These proceed from long and intense thinking, and sometimes they are aggravated by costiveness. The best way to prevent them is never to study too long, and to keep the belly regular either by proper food, or taking frequently a little of some opening medicine.

DISEASES of the eyes often afflict the studious. Such therefore as read or write much should early accustom themselves to use *preserves*. Night-study is most destructive to the sight, and should never be prolonged too late. Indeed late studies

ſtudies are not only hurtful to the eyes, but to the whole body. Nothing more certainly ruins the health, than the practice of ſpending thoſe hours in the cloſet which ſhould be allotted to ſleep. Studious perſons will find their eyes greatly ſtrengthened by bathing them frequently in cold water, or brandy and water mixed.

THE dropſy is another of thoſe diſeaſes which commonly affect the ſtudious, and very often puts an end to their lives. It has already been obſerved, that the ſecretions are generally defective in the ſtudious, and that various diſeaſes, among which is the dropſy, are occaſioned by the retention of theſe humours which ought to be thrown off in that way. Any perſon may obſerve, that ſitting makes his legs ſwell, and that this will go off by exerciſe; which clearly points out the method of prevention to all who can take it. To thoſe who cannot take exerciſe, we would recommend the uſe of the fleſh-bruſh, cold bathing, and ſuch food as is of a bracing and ſtrengthening nature.

FEVERS, eſpecially of the nervous kind, are often the effect of ſtudy. Nothing is ſo deſtructive to the nerves as intenſe thought. It is able, in a manner, to unhinge the whole machine. It not only hurts the vital motions, but diſorders the mind itſelf. Hence a delirium, melancholy, and even madneſs, are often the effect of cloſe application to ſtudy. There is no diſeaſe which can proceed either from a bad ſtate of the humours, a defect of the uſual ſecretions, or a debility

bility of the nervous ſyſtem, which may not be brought on by intenſe thinking.

But the moſt afflicting of all the diſeaſes which attack the ſtudious, are the hypochondriacal. Theſe ſeldom fail to be the companions of deep thought, and may rather be called a complication of maladies than a ſingle one. To what a wretched paſs are the beſt of men often reduced by theſe maladies? Their ſtrength and appetite fail. A perpetual gloom hangs over their minds. They live in the conſtant dread of death, and are continually in ſearch of relief from medicine, where alas! it is not to be found. This diſeaſe far exceeds all deſcription, and thoſe who labour under it, tho' they be often made the ſubject of ridicule, juſtly claim our higheſt ſympathy and compaſſion.

Nothing can be more prepoſterous than for any man to make ſtudy his ſole buſineſs. A mere ſtudent is ſeldom an uſeful member of ſociety. Indeed it rarely happens, that an uſeful invention is the effect of ſtudy. The farther that men dive into profound reſearches, they generally deviate the more from common ſenſe, and too often loſe ſight of it altogether. Hence it is that profound ſpeculations, inſtead of making men wiſer or better, generally render them mere ſceptics, and overwhelm them in doubt and uncertainty. All that is neceſſary for man to know, in order to be happy, is eaſily obtained, and the reſt, like the forbidden tree, ſerves only to increaſe his miſery.

Studious

STUDIOUS people, in order to relieve their minds, muſt not only diſcontinue to read and write, but engage in ſome employment or amuſement, that will ſo far occupy the thought as to make them forget the buſineſs of the cloſet. A ſolitary ride or walk are ſo far from relieving the mind, that they rather encourage thought. Nothing can divert the mind, when it gets into a train of ſerious thinking, but an attention to ſubjects of a more trivial nature. Theſe, when compared with the other, prove a kind of play to the mind, and conſequently relieve it.

THINKING men are apt to contract a contempt for what they call trifling company. They are aſhamed to be ſeen with any but philoſophers. This however is no proof of their being philoſophers themſelves. No man deſerves the name of a philoſopher who is aſhamed to unbend his mind by aſſociating with the cheerful and gay. Even the ſociety of children will relieve the mind, and expel the gloom which application to ſtudy is too apt to occaſion. It is remarkable, that ſuch as have numerous families, whatever hardſhips they may labour under, are generally the moſt cheerful and happy.

As ſtudious people are neceſſarily much within doors, they ſhould make choice of a large and well aired place for ſtudy. That would not only prevent the bad effects which attend confined

fined air, but would cheer the ſpirits, and have a moſt happy influence both on the body and mind. Is is ſaid of Euripides the Tragedian, that he uſed to retire to a dark cave to compoſe his tragedies, and of Demoſthenes the Grecian orator, that he choſe a place for ſtudy where nothing could either be heard or ſeen. With all deference to ſuch venerable names, we cannot help condemning this taſte. A man may ſurely think to as good purpoſe in an elegant appartment as in a cave; and may have as happy ideas where the all-cheering rays of the ſun render the air wholeſome, as in places where they never reach.

THOSE who read or write much ſhould be very attentive to their poſture. They ought to ſit and ſtand by turns, always keeping as near an erect poſture as poſſible. Thoſe who dictate may do it walking. It has an excellent effect frequently to read or ſpeak aloud. This not only exerciſes the lungs, but almoſt the whole body. Hence ſtudious people are greatly benefited by delivering diſcourſes in public, Such indeed ſometimes hurt themſelves by over-acting their part; but that is their own fault. The man who dies a martyr to mere vociferation merits not our ſympathy.

THE morning has by all medical writers been reckoned the beſt time for ſtudy. It is ſo. But it is alſo the moſt proper ſeaſon for exerciſe, while the ſtomach is empty, aud the ſpirits refreſhed with ſleep. Studious people ſhould there-

therefore frequently ſpend the morning in ſome manly diverſion abroad. This would make them return to ſtudy with greater alacrity, and would be of more ſervice than twice the time after their ſpirits are worn out with fatigue. It is not ſufficient to take diverſion only when we can think no longer. Every ſtudious perſon ſhould make it a part of his buſineſs, and ſhould let nothing interrupt his hours of recreation more than thoſe of ſtudy.

Music has a moſt happy effect in relieving the mind. It would be well if every ſtudious perſon were ſo far acquainted with that ſcience as to amuſe himſelf after ſevere thought, by playing ſuch airs as have a tendency to rouſe the ſpirits, aud inſpire cheerfulneſs and good humour.

Studious perſons generally ſpend their mornings in the cloſet, and their evenings in company. It were better to invert this rule. It is the reproach of learning, that ſo many of her ſons, to relieve the mind after ſtudy, betake themſelves to the uſe of ſtrong liquors. This indeed is a remedy; but it is a deſperate one, and always ends in deſtruction. Would ſuch perſons, when their ſpirits are low, get on horſeback, and gallop ten or a dozen miles, they would find it a more effectual remedy than all the ſtrong liquors in the world. A good horſe is the beſt preventive medicine that we can recommend to the ſtudious. This is better than all the nervous antidotes of the ſhops, and will in the end be found much cheaper.

It is really to be regretted that men, while in health, pay ſo little regard to theſe things! How common is it to ſee a wretch, over-run with nervous diſeaſes, bathing, walking, riding, and, in a word, doing every thing for health after it is gone; yet if any one had recommended theſe things by way of prevention, his advice would have been treated with contempt, or at leaſt, with neglect. Such is the weakneſs of human nature, and ſuch the folly and want of foreſight, even of thoſe who ought to be the wiſeſt of mankind!

PART II.

OF DISEASES.

CHAP. IV.

OF DISTINGUISHING DISEASES.

BEFORE we proceed to the particular treatment of diſeaſes, it will be neceſſary to lay down ſome general rules for diſtinguiſhing one diſeaſe from another, as the danger of miſtaking the diſeaſe often deters people from attempting to relieve the ſick.

To diſtinguiſh diſeaſes is the moſt difficult part of the practice of phyſic. So near a reſemblance do the ſymptoms of one diſeaſe often bear to thoſe of another, that they may deceive the moſt ſkilful phyſician. We do not mean in this place to give the diſtinguiſhing marks of every particular diſeaſe, but only to put the reader upon his guard by pointing out a few a few of thoſe diſeaſes which have the neareſt reſemblance to one another, and which the unwary and inattentive may be moſt apt to miſtake.

THE ſmall-pox and meaſles are both preceeded by chilneſs and ſhivering, with heat and cold by turns, a quick pulſe, great thirſt, and other ſymptoms of a fever. In both the eruption appears about the third or fourth day in little ſpots reſembling flea-bites. Thus far the diſeaſe cannot be certainly known; but on the ſecond or third day from the eruption, the ſmall-pox begin to riſe and to fill with matter; which plainly ſhows the nature of the diſeaſe.

THE petechial or ſpotted fever, may be known from the miliary by this mark, that in the former the ſpots never riſe above the ſkin; whereas in the latter the ſkin is rough, and before the eruption appears the patient complains of chilneſs, itching in the ſkin, and oppreſſion of the breaſt.

THO' there be a great ſimilarity in the firſt ſymptoms of all fevers, yet an attentive obſerver may generally diſcover to what claſs they belong. Thus a burning fever may be known by the intenſe heat of the whole body, a dry parched ſkin, a chapt tongue, and unquenchable thirſt. An inflammatory fever generally affects one particular part, as the lungs, the ſtomach, the brain, &c. This kind of fever has a natural tendency to a mortification. Malignant fevers are generally owing to infection. They may be known by the patient's ſudden loſs of ſtrength, perpetual watching, &c. A catarrhal fever

fever is known by a running at the nofe, a hoarfenefs, and a fenfe of fulnefs in the breaft.

The peripneumony and pleurify may be diftinguifhed by this, that in the latter the pain is more acute, and in the former the oppreffion of the breaft, and difficulty of breathing are greater, and the fpittle is generally tinctured with blood.

Intermittent fevers or agues are known by their leaving the patient, and returning at certain periods, as once a day, once in two days, three days, or the like. They are denominated from the fpace between the fits, as quotidian, or every day agues, tertian, or fuch as return every other day, quartan, &c.

A hectic fever may be known by its fupervening to fome other diforder, as the dropfy, confumption, fcurvy, &c. It differs from a flow fever in this, that the pulfe is always quick, but remarkably fo in the morning; whereas the pulfe in a flow fever is more natural in a morning, and before meals, though it be more quick after eating: Befides, in a flow fever the weaknefs is not fo great as in a hectic.

An inflammation of the ftomach may be diftinguifhed from a cardialgia, an inflammation of the liver, &c. by a fenfe of the moft intenfe heat in the ftomach, a fever attended with a quick, unequal, and weak pulfe, and a prodigious uneafinefs upon taking any thing into the ftomach.

An

An inflammation in the concave part of the liver may be diſtinguiſhed from the baſtard pleuriſy, by the fever being leſs violent, the breathing eaſier, and the pain lower down. Beſides, the baſtard pleuriſy generally goes off on the ſeventh day; whereas the inflammation of the liver is a tedious diſeaſe, and often ends in an abſceſs, which occaſions a hectic fever or a dropſy, &c.

A phrenzy, or inflammation of the membranes of the brain, may be diſtinguiſhed from madneſs, a common delirium, the hydrophobia, &c. by the burning fever, the continual watching, and the violent pulſation of the arteries about the head and temples, which always attend it. It differs from a delirium in being more violent, from madneſs in being an acute diſeaſe, and from the hydrophobia in this, that the patient has no averſion from liquids.

A nephritis, or inflammation of the kidneys, may be diſtinguiſhed from a fit of the gravel, by a fixed, dull, preſſing pain in the loins, which continues long; whereas the pain in a fit of the gravel is more violent, leſs fixed, and generally extends downwards.

External inflammations are eaſily diſtinguiſhed. An *eryſipelas*, or St Anthony's fire, only affects the ſkin with redneſs, tumour, and pain; whereas a *phlegmon* reaches to the ſubjacent muſcles, and a *gangrene* penetrates not only the muſcles, but even the tendinous and nervous parts, and is attended with great heat, pain,

pain, and redneſs, which at length change into a livid or black colour.

A ſtone deſcending by the ureters may eaſily be miſtaken for a fit of the colic, as both are attended with violent pain, vomiting, &c. In the former, however, the pain is more fixed in the loins, is attended with ſhiverings, and as the ſtone deſcends, the pain reaches downwards, and occaſions a numbneſs of the thigh on the ſide affected; there is alſo a frequent inclination to paſs water, with ſome degree of ſtrangury; whereas in the colic the pain is chiefly about the navel, and the belly is generally diſtended with wind.

The gout may be diſtinguiſhed from the rheumatiſm by its attacking the extremities chiefly, and being attended with a greater inflammation, and more violent pain. It may likewiſe be diſtinguiſhed from venereal pains, by its being more violent in the day; whereas they are moſt ſevere in the night.

The piles may be miſtaken for a dyſentery, as both tinge the ſtools with blood, tho' the one be a dangerous diſeaſe, and the other in many caſes a ſalutary evacuation. In the piles however the blood flows without pain or gripes; whereas in the dyſentery the ſtools are attended with the moſt violent gripes, ſpaſms, &c.

Coughs may be owing to cold, an ulcer in the lungs, an aſthma, &c. The beſt way to diſtinguiſh them is to examine into the cauſe, to obſerve

obſerve what the patient ſpits, and to mark the continuance of the diſeaſe. A cough occaſioned by catching cold is generally attended with a diſcharge of phlegm, and is ſeldom of long continuance. That which is owing to an ulcer of the lungs is generally attended with an hectic fever, and the ſpittle is mixed with matter. An aſthmatic cough is generally owing to wind or ſpaſms, and ſeldom admits of relief from medicine.

A headach, which proceeds from too great a quantity of blood being forced into the veſſels of the brain, is generally attended with heat, redneſs, and a ſwelling of the face, a great pulſation of the arteries of the neck, &c. That kind of headach, which is the effect of venereal contagion, may be known by its being generally worſt in the night. When the headach is owing to an effuſion of ſerum or blood into the ſinuoſities of the bones of the forehead, the pain is obſtinate, ſharp, and fixed; it is generally ſituated in the bottom of the forehead, and above the eyes. When the head is diſordered from crudities in the ſtomach or wind, it may be known from belching, and the increaſe of the diſorder upon uſing flatulent food, &c.

An apoplexy may be diſtinguiſhed from a ſyncope or fainting fit, by the colour of the face, the breathing, and the pulſe continuing much the ſame as in health; whereas in a ſyncope the pulſe and breathing are imperceptible, the

the face is pale, and the body grows cold. An apoplexy may be diſtinguiſhed from a catalepſy, becauſe the latter comes on ſuddenly, and keeps the member quite rigid, and in the ſame poſture as at the time of the attack.

A proper attention to the age, ſex, conſtitution, temper of mind, &c. of the patient, would greatly aſſiſt us in finding out and diſtinguiſhing diſeaſes. Thus, in children the fibres are lax and ſoft; in adults, rigid and tenſe. In young people the nerves are extremely irritable, and the fluids thin. In old age the nerves become almoſt inſenſible, and many of the veſſels imperviable. Theſe, and numberleſs other peculiarities, render the diſeaſes of the young and thoſe of the aged very different; and of courſe they muſt require different treatment.

NOT only the age, but alſo the ſex of the patient, claims our attention. Females are liable to many peculiar diſeaſes. Their nervous ſyſtem being weak and delicate, they are eaſier affected with ſpaſtic or convulſive diſorders than males. This is the true ſource of moſt of the diſeaſes of the fair ſex, and ought always to be kept in view in the treatment of their diſorders.

WE ought likewiſe to attend to the particular conſtitution. This not only prediſpoſes perſons to peculiar diſeaſes, but likewiſe makes it neceſſary, that their diſeaſes be treated in a very different manner. For example, a de-

X licate

licate perſon with weak nerves, can neither bear bleeding, nor any other evacuation, to the ſame extent as one whoſe conſtitution is hardy and robuſt.

The temper of mind ought likewiſe to be attended to in diſeaſes. Fear, anxiety, and a fretful temper both occaſion and aggravate diſeaſes. The medicine of the mind is too little regarded. In vain do we apply medicines to the body to remove diſeaſes which proceed from the mind. When that is the caſe, the beſt medicine is to ſooth the paſſions, divert the mind from anxious thought, and to cheriſh the hopes of the patient.

Attention ought likewiſe to be paid to the place where the patient lives, the air he breathes, his diet, occupation, &c. Such as live in low marſhy countries are ſubject to many diſeaſes which are unknown to the inhabitants of high countries. Thoſe who breathe the impure air of cities have many maladies, to which the more happy ruſtics are ſtrangers, Such as feed groſs, and indulge in ſtrong liquors are liable to diſeaſes which do not affect the temperate and abſtemious. The ſituation of life, as has been obſerved, likewiſe prediſpoſes men to peculiar diſeaſes. Thus the laborious, the ſedentary, the ſtudious, &c. are liable to particular maladies from the very occupations which they follow.

It is neceſſary to inquire whether or not the patient has been guilty of any exceſs in eating or drinking, if he has overſtrained himſelf, has

drank

drank cold liquor when he was warm, lain on the damp ground, changed his uſual cloathing, or, in a word, done any thing that might obſtruct the perſpiration It will alſo be proper to inquire, if any uſual evacuation, as ſweating of the feet, iſſues, &c. has been ſtopped. The ſtate of the belly ſhould likewiſe be inquired into. Coſtiveneſs alone will occaſion diſeaſes, and the removing of it will cure them.

It is likewiſe neceſſary to inquire what diſeaſes the patient has formerly been moſt liable to, and what medicines were moſt beneficial. If medicines have been adminiſtered, it will be proper to inquire into their effect. It will likewiſe be neceſſary to inquire, what kind of medicines are moſt agreeable to the patient, or if he has an averſion to any particular drug, &c.

It is alſo neceſlary to inquire whether the patient can perform with eaſe all the animal and vital functions, or which of them gives him pain; and alſo to inquire, if all the different ſecretions go duly on, as the perſpiration, diſcharge of urine, &c.

The nature of the diſeaſe is likewiſe to be inquired into, as whether it be primary or ſecondary; whether ſimple or complicated with ſome other diſeaſe; whether it be external or internal; whether epidemic or not; whether it be the effect of age, intemperance, infection, or owing to a vitiated ſtate of the humours, &c. &c. &c.

Of

Of FEVERS in general.

A Fever is the most general disease incident to mankind. It attacks every age, sex, and constitution, and affects every part of the body; nor is the mind itself free from its influence. A fever is known by a quick pulse, an increased heat, and a difficulty in performing some of the vital or animal functions, as breathing, walking, &c.

FEVERS are divided into continual, remitting, and intermitting. By a continual fever is meant that which never leaves the patient during the whole course of the disease, or which shews no remarkable increase or abatement in the symptoms. This kind of fever is likewise divided into acute, slow, and malignant. The fever is called *acute* when its progress is quick, and the symptoms violent; but when these are more gentle, it is generally denominated *slow*. When livid or petechial spots, show a putrid state of the humours, the fever is called *malignant*, *putrid*, or *petechial*.

A remitting fever differs from a continual only in degree. It has frequent increases and decreases, or exacerbations and remissions, but never wholly leaves the patient during the course of the disease. Intermitting fevers, or agues, are those which, during the time that the

the patient may be ſaid to be ill, have evident intervals or remiſſions of the ſymptoms.

As a fever is nothing elſe but an effort of nature to free herſelf from an offending cauſe, it is the buſineſs of thoſe who have the care of the ſick, to obſerve with diligence which way nature points, and to endeavour to aſſiſt her operations. Our bodies are ſo framed as to have a conſtant tendency to expel or throw off whatever is injurious to health. This is generally done by urine, ſweat, ſtool, expectoration, vomit, or ſome other evacuation.

There is reaſon to believe, if the efforts of nature, at the beginning of a fever, were duly attended to and promoted, it would ſeldom continue longer than twenty-four hours; but when her attempts are either neglected, or counteracted, it is no wonder if the diſeaſe be prolonged. There are daily inſtances of perſons who, after catching cold, have all the ſymptoms of a beginning fever; but by keeping warm, drinking diluting liquors, bathing their feet in warm water, &c. the ſymptoms in a few hours diſappear, and the danger is prevented. In a word, almoſt every fever proceeding from an obſtructed perſpiration, might be carried off, or its danger prevented, by timely care.

Our deſign is not to enter into a critical inquiry into the nature, cauſes, &c. of fevers, but to mark their moſt obvious ſymptoms, and to point out the proper treatment of the patient with

with reſpect to his diet, drink, air, warmth, &c. in the different ſtages of the diſeaſe. In theſe articles the inclinations of the patient will, in a great meaſure, direct our conduct.

ALMOST every perſon in a fever complains of great thirſt, and calls out for drink, eſpecially of a cooling nature. This at once points out the uſe of *water*, which we may venture to call the greateſt febrifuge in nature. What is ſo likely to abate the heat, attenuate the humours, remove ſpaſms and obſtructions, promote perſpiration, increaſe the quantity of urine, and, in ſhort, produce every ſalutary effect in an ardent or inflammatory fever, as drinking plentifully of warm water, thin gruel, or any other weak, diluting liquor of which water is the baſis? The neceſſity of diluting liquors is pointed out by the dry tongue, the parched ſkin, and the burning heat, as well as by the unquenchable thirſt of the patient.

MANY cooling liquors, which are extremely grateful to patients in a fever, may be prepared from fruits, roots, and acid vegetables, as decoctions of tamarinds, apple-tea, orange whey, and the like. Mucilaginous liquors might alſo be prepared from marſh mallow roots, linſeed, lime-tree-buds, and many other vegetables. Theſe liquors, eſpecially when acidulated, are highly agreeable to the patient, and ſhould never be denied him.

AT the beginning of a fever the patient generally complains of great laſſitude or weari-

neſs,

neſs, and has no inclination to move. This evidently ſhows the propriety of keeping him eaſy, and, if poſſible, in bed; that relaxes the ſpaſms, abates the violence of the circulation, and gives Nature an opportunity of exerting all her force to overcome the diſeaſe. The bed alone would often remove a fever at the beginning; but when the patient ſtruggles with the diſeaſe, inſtead of driving it off, he only fixes it the deeper, and renders it more dangerous. This obſervation is too often verified in travellers, who happen when on a journey to be ſeized with a fever. Their anxiety to get home induces them to travel with the fever upon them, which conduct ſeldom fails to render it fatal.

In fevers the mind as well as the body ſhould be kept eaſy. Company is ſeldom agreeable to the ſick. Indeed every thing that diſturbs the imagination increaſes the diſeaſe; for which reaſon every perſon in a fever ought to be kept perfectly quiet, and neither allowed to ſee nor hear any thing that may in the leaſt affect or diſcompoſe his mind.

Tho' the patient in a fever has the greateſt inclination for drink, yet he ſeldom has any appetite for ſolid food; from whence we may ſee the impropriety of loading his ſtomach with victuals. Much ſolid food in a fever is every way hurtful to the patient. It oppreſſes nature, and inſtead of nouriſhing the patient, ſerves only to feed the diſeaſe. What food the patient takes

takes ſhould be in ſmall quantity, light, and eaſy of digeſtion. It ought to be chiefly of the vegetable kind, as water pap, roaſted apples, groat-gruel, and ſuch like.

Poor people, when any of their family are taken ill, run directly to their rich neighbours for cordials, and pour wines, ſpirits, &c. into the patient, who perhaps never had been accuſtomed to taſte ſuch liquors when in health. If there be any degree of fever, this conduct muſt increaſe it, and if there be none, this is the ready way to raiſe one. Stuffing the patient with ſweet-meats and other delicacies, is likewiſe very pernicious. Theſe are always harder to digeſt than common food, and cannot fail to hurt the ſtomach.

Nothing is more deſired by a patient in a fever than freſh air. It not only removes his anxiety, but cools the blood, revives the ſpirits, and proves every way beneficial. Many patients are in a manner ſtiffled to death in fevers, for want of freſh air; yet ſuch is the unaccountable infatuation of many people, that the moment they think a perſon in a fever, they imagine he ſhould be kept in a cloſe chamber, into which not one particle of freſh air muſt be admitted. There ought to be a conſtant ſtream of freſh air into a ſick perſon's chamber, ſo as to keep it always in a temperate degree of warmth, which ought never to be greater than is agreeable to one in perfect health.

Nothing ſpoils the air of a ſick perſon's chamber

chamber, or hurts the patient more than a number of people breathing in it. When the blood is inflamed, or the humours in a putrid ſtate, air that has been breathed over and over will greatly increaſe the diſeaſe. Such air not only loſes its ſpring, and becomes unfit for the purpoſes of reſpiration, but acquires a noxious quality, which renders it in a manner poiſonous to the ſick.

In fevers, when the patient's ſpirits are low and depreſſed, he is not only to be ſupported with cordials, but every method ſhould be taken to cheer and comfort his mind. Many, from a miſtaken zeal, when they think a perſon in danger, inſtead of ſolacing his mind with the hopes and conſolations of religion, fright him with the views of hell and damnation, &c. It would be unſuitable here to dwell upon the impropriety and dangerous conſequences of this conduct; it often hurts the body, and there is reaſon to believe ſeldom benefits the ſoul.

Amongst common people, the very name of a fever generally ſuggeſts the neceſſity of bleeding. This notion ſeems to have taken its riſe from moſt fevers having been formerly of an inflammatory nature; but true inflammatory fevers are now ſeldom to be met with. Sedentary occupations, and a different manner of living, has ſo changed the ſtate of diſeaſes in Britain, that there is now hardly one fever in ten where the lancet is neceſſary. In moſt low, nervous, and putrid fevers, which are now ſo common, bleeding is really hurtful, as it weakens the patient, and ſinks his ſpirits, &c. We would recommend this general rule, never to bleed at the beginning of a fever, unleſs there be evident ſigns of an inflammation. Bleeding is an excellent medicine when neceſſary, but ſhould never be wantonly performed.

It is likewiſe a common notion, that it is always neceſſary to raiſe a ſweat in the beginning of a fever. As fevers often proceed from an obſtructed perſpiration, this notion is not ill founded. If the patient only lies in bed, bathes his feet and legs in warm water, and drinks freely of water-gruel, or any other weak, diluting liquor, he will ſeldom fail to perſpire freely. The warmth of the bed, and the diluting drink will relax the univerſal ſpaſm, which generally affects the ſolids at the beginning of a fever; it will open the pores, and promote the perſpiration, by means of which the fever may often be carried off. But inſtead of this, the common practice is to heap cloaths upon the patient, and to give him things of a hot nature, as ſpirits, ſpiceries, &c. which fire his blood, increaſe the ſpaſms, and render the diſeaſe more dangerous.

In all fevers a proper attention ſhould be paid to the patient's longings. Theſe are the calls of nature, and often point out what may be of real uſe. Patients are not to be wantonly indulged in every thing that the ſickly appetite may crave; but it is generally right to let them

have

have a little of what they eagerly defire, tho' it may not feem altogether proper. What the patient longs for, his ftomach will generally digeft; and fuch things have fometimes a very happy effect.

When a patient is recovering from a fever, great care is neceffary to prevent a relapfe. Many perfons, by too foon imagining themfelves well, have relapfed, or contracted fome other difeafe of an obftinate nature. As the body after a fever is weak and delicate, it is neceffary to guard againft catching cold. Moderate exercife in the open air will be of ufe; agreeable company will alfo have a good effect. The diet muft be light, but nourifhing. It fhould be taken frequently, but in fmall quantities. It is very dangerous at fuch a time to eat as much as the ftomach craves.

Of Intermitting FEVERS or AGUES.

Intermitting fevers afford the beft opportunity both of obferving the nature of a fever, and alfo the effects of medicine. No perfon can be at a lofs to diftinguifh an intermitting fever from any other difeafe, and the proper medicine for it is now almoft univerfally known.

The feveral kinds of intermitting fevers, as has been obferved, take their names from the period

period in which the fit returns, as quotidians, tertians, quartans, &c.

CAUSES.——Agues are occaſioned by moiſt air. This is evident from their abounding in rainy ſeaſons, and being moſt frequent in countries where the ſoil is marſhy, as in Holland, the fens of Cambridgeſhire, the Hundreds of Eſſex, &c. This diſeaſe is alſo occaſioned by eating too much ſtone fruit, a poor watery diet, damp houſes, evening dews, lying upon the wet ground, &c. When the inhabitants of a high country remove to a low one, they ſeldom fail to catch an intermitting fever, and to ſuch the diſeaſe is moſt apt to prove fatal. In a word, whatever relaxes the ſolids, diminiſhes the perſpiration, or obſtructs the circulation in the capillary or ſmall veſſels, prediſpoſes the body to agues.

SYMPTOMS.—— An intermitting fever generally begins with a pain of the head and loins, wearineſs of the limbs, coldneſs of the extremities, ſtretching, yawning, with ſometimes great ſickneſs and vomiting; to which ſucceed ſhivering and violent ſhaking. Afterwards the ſkin becomes moiſt, and a profuſe ſweat breaks out, which generally terminates the fit or paroxyſm. Sometimes indeed the diſeaſe comes on ſuddenly, when the perſon thinks himſelf in perfect health; but it is more commonly preceeded by liſtleſsneſs, loſs of appetite, and the ſymptoms mentioned above.

REGIMEN.—— While the fit continues, the

the patient may drink freely of water-gruel, orange whey, weak camomile tea; or, if his spirits be low, small wine-whey, sharpened with the juice of lemon. His drink ought to be a little warm, as that will assist in bringing on the sweat, and consequently shorten the paroxysm.

Between the paroxysms the patient must be supported with food that is nourishing, but light and easy of digestion, as veal or chicken-broths, sago-gruel with a little wine, light puddings, &c. His drink may be small negas, acidulated with the juice of lemons or oranges, and sometimes a little weak punch. He ought also to drink infusions of bitters, as camomile, wormwood, or water trefoil tea, and may now and then take a glass of small wine, in which gentian root, centaury, or some other bitter, has been infused.

As the chief intentions of cure in an ague are to brace the solids, and promote perspiration, the patient ought to take as much exercise between the fits as he can bear. If he be able to go abroad, riding on horseback, or in a machine, will be of great service. But if he cannot bear that kind of exercise, he ought to take such as his strength will permit. Nothing tends more to prolong an intermiting fever, than indulging a lazy indolent disposition.

Intermitting fevers, under a proper regimen, will generally cure of themselves; and when the disease is mild, in an open dry country, there is seldom any danger from allowing it to take

take its courſe; but when the patient's ſtrength is exhauſted, and the paroxyſms are ſo violent, that his life is in danger, medicine ought immediately to be adminiſtered. This however ſhould never be done till the diſeaſe be properly formed, that is to ſay, till the patient has had ſeveral fits of ſhaking and ſweating.

MEDICINE.—— The firſt thing to be done in the cure of an intermitting fever, is to cleanſe the firſt paſſages. This not only renders the application of other medicines more ſafe, but likewiſe more efficacious. In this diſeaſe the ſtomach is generally overcharged with cold viſcid phlegm, and frequently great quantities of bile are diſcharged by vomit; which plainly points out the neceſſity of ſuch evacuations. Vomits are therefore to be adminiſtered before the patient takes any other medicine. A doſe of ipecacoanha will generally anſwer this purpoſe very well. Half a dram of the powder will be ſufficient for an adult, and for a younger perſon the doſe muſt be leſs in proportion. After the vomit begins to operate, it may be wrought off by drinking plentifully of weak camomile tea. The vomit ſhould be taken two or three hours before the coming on of the fit, and may be repeated two or three times at the diſtance of three or four days from each other. Vomits not only cleanſe the ſtomach, but increaſe the perſpiration, and all the other ſecretions, which render them of ſuch importance, that they often cure intermitting fevers without

out the aſſiſtance of any other medicine. Of this I have ſeen many inſtances, and remember myſelf to have been compleatly cured of a regular tertian, by taking two vomits of ipecacoanha, and obſerving proper regimen.

Purging medicines are likewiſe uſeful, and often neceſſary, in intermitting fevers. A ſmart purge has been known to cure an obſtinate ague, after the jeſuites bark and other medicines had been uſed in vain. Vomits however are more ſuitable in this diſeaſe, and render purging leſs neceſſary; but if the patient be afraid to take a vomit, he ought in this caſe to cleanſe the bowels by a doſe or two of glaubers ſalts, jalap, or rhubarb, &c.

Bleeding may ſometimes be proper at the beginning of an intermitting fever, when exceſſive heat, a delirium, &c. give reaſon to ſuſpect an inflammation; but as the blood is very ſeldom in an inflammatory ſtate in intermitting fevers, this operation is rarely neceſſary.

After proper evacuations, the patient may ſafely uſe the jeſuites bark, which may be taken in any way that is moſt agreeable to him. As it would anſwer no purpoſe to multiply forms, we ſhall only mention the following.

Two ounces of the beſt jeſuites bark, half an ounce of virginian ſnake-root, and a quarter an ounce of ginger, all finely powdered, may be divided into twenty-four doſes. Theſe may be be either made into bolusses, as they are used, with a little syrup of lemon, or mixed in a glass of red wine, a cup of camomile-tea, water-gruel, or the like.

In an ague which returns every day, a dose of the above may be taken every two hours during the interval of the fit. By this method the patient will be able to take five or six doses between each paroxysm. In a tertian, or third-day ague, it will be sufficient to take a dose every third hour, during the interval, and in a quartan every fourth. If the patient cannot take so large a dose of the bark, he may divide each of the powders into two parts, and take one every hour. For a young person, a smaller quantity of this medicine will be sufficient, and the dose must be adapted to the age, constitution, &c.

The above will seldom fail to remove an ague; but the patient ought not to leave off taking the medicine so soon as the paroxysms are stopped, but should continue to use it till such time as there is reason to believe the disease is intirely overcome. Most of the failures in the cure of this disease are owing to the patients not continuing to use the medicine long enough. They are generally directed to take it till the fits are stopped, then to leave it off, and begin again at some distance of time; by which means the disease gathers strength, and often returns with as much violence as before. A

relapse

relapſe may always be prevented by the patient's continuing to take ſmall doſes of the medicine for ſome time after the ſymptoms diſappear. This is both the moſt ſafe and effectual method of cure.

Though the bark alone will generally cure intermitting fevers; yet it may be aſſiſted by alkaline ſalts, acid and aſtringent vegetables, &c. Many have been cured of an intermitting fever, after the bark had failed, by taking twice or thrice a-day a dram of the ſalt of wormwood in water-gruel. Some have ſtopped an ague by eating a boiled lemon with the rind immediately before the coming on of the fit. We would rather recommend a medicine which is the reſult of theſe two when joined together, than either of them ſeparately. Thus, a dram of ſalt of wormwood may be diſſolved in an ounce and half of freſh lemon-juice, to which may be added three or four ounces of boiling water, and half a glaſs of brandy. Theſe will make an agreeable medicine; a tea cupful of which may be taken three or four times a-day.

An ounce of gentian root, calamus aromaticus, and orange-peal, of each half an ounce, with three or four handfuls of chamomile flowers, and an handful of coriander-ſeed, all bruiſed together in a mortar, may be uſed in form of infuſion or tea. About half an handful of theſe ingredients may be put into a tea pot, and an Engliſh pint of boiling water poured on them.

them. A cup of this infuſion may be drank three or four times a day. This ſtrengthens the ſtomach, rectifies the blood, and greatly promotes the cure. Such patients as cannot drink the watry infuſion, may put two handfuls of the ſame ingredients into a bottle of white wine, and take a glaſs of it twice or thrice a-day. If patients drink freely of the above, or any other proper infuſion of bitters, a much ſmaller quantity of bark than is generally uſed, will be ſufficient to cure an ague.

THERE is reaſon to believe, that ſundry of our own plants or barks, which are very bitter and aſtringent, would ſucceed well enough in the cure of intermitting fevers, eſpecially when aſſiſted by aromatics. But as the jeſuits bark has been long approved in the cure of this diſeaſe, and is now to be obtained at a very reaſonable rate, it is of leſs importance to ſearch after new medicines. We cannot however omit taking notice, that the jeſuits bark is very often adulterated, and that it requires conſiderable ſkill to diſtinguiſh between the genuine and the falſe. This ought to make people very cautious of whom they purchaſe it.

THOSE who cannot ſwallow the bark in ſubſtance, may take it in decoction or infuſion. An ounce of bark in powder may be infuſed in a bottle of white wine for four or five days, frequently ſhaking the bottle, afterwards let the powder ſubſide, and pour off the clear liquor. A wine glaſs may be drank three or four

four times a day, or oftener, as there is occasion. If a decoction be more agreeable, an ounce of the bark, and two drams of snake-root bruised, with a dram of salt of wormwood, may be boiled in a proper quantity of water, into half an English pint. To the strained liquor may be added an equal quantity of red wine, and a glass of it taken thrice a-day, or oftener if necessary

In obstinate agues the bark will be found much more efficacious when assisted by warm cordials, than if taken alone. This I have had frequently occasion to observe in a country where intermitting fevers were endemical. The bark seldom succeeded unless assisted by snake-root, ginger, canella alba, or some other warm aromatic. When the fits are very frequent and violent, in which case the fever often approaches towards an inflammatory nature, it will be safer to leave out the ginger, and to add in its place half an ounce of salt of wormwood. But in obstinate tertians or quartans, in the end of autumn or beginning of winter, warm and cordial medicines are absolutely necessary.

As autumnal and winter agues generally prove much more obstinate than those which attack the patient in spring or summer; it will be necessary to continue the use of medicines longer in the former than in the latter A person who is seized with an intermitting fever in the beginning of winter, ought frequently, if the season proves rainy, to take a little medicine,

cine, altho' the diſeaſe be cured, to prevent a relapſe, till the return of the warm ſeaſon. He ought likewiſe to take care not to be much abroad in wet weather, eſpecially in cold moiſt eaſterly winds.

WHEN agues are not properly cured, they often degenerate into obſtinate chronical diſeaſes, as the dropſy, jaundice, &c. For this reaſon all poſſible care ſhould be taken to have them radically cured, before the humours be vitiated, and the conſtitution ſpoiled.

THO' nothing is more rational than the method of treating intermitting fevers, yet, by ſome ſtrange infatuation, more charms and whimſical remedies are daily uſed for removing this than any other diſeaſe. There is hardly an old woman who is not poſſeſſed of a noſtrum for ſtopping an ague; and there is reaſon to fear, that many by truſting to them loſe their lives. Thoſe in diſtreſs eagerly graſp at any thing that promiſes ſudden relief; but the ſhorteſt way is not always the ſafeſt in the treatment of diſeaſes. The only method to obtain a ſafe and laſting cure, is gradually to aſſiſt nature in removing the cauſe of the diſeaſe.

SOME people try bold, or rather fool-hardy experiments to cure agues, as drinking ſtrong liquors, jumping into a river, &c. Theſe may ſometimes have the deſired effect, but muſt always be attended with danger. When there is any degree of inflammation, or the leaſt tendency to it, ſuch experiments may prove fatal

The

The only person whom I remember to have seen die in an intermitting fever, evidently killed himself by drinking strong liquor, which some person had persuaded him would prove an infallible remedy.

MANY out-of-the-way things are extolled for the cure of intermitting fevers, as cobwebs, snuffings of candles, &c. Though these may sometimes succeed, yet their very nastiness is sufficient to set them aside, especially when cleanly medicines will answer the purpose better. The only medicine that can be depended upon, for thoroughly curing an intermitting fever, is the jesuites bark. It may always be used with safety: And I can honestly declare, that in all my practice I never knew it fail, when properly applied, and duly persisted in.

WHERE agues are endemical, even children are often afflicted with that disease. Such patients are very difficult to cure, as they can seldom be brought to take the bark, or any other disagreeable medicine. One method of rendering this medicine more palatable is, to make it into a mixture with distilled waters and syrup, and afterward to give it an agreeable sharpness with the elixir or spirit of vitriol. This both improves the medicine, and takes off the nauseous taste. The bark may be administered to children in form of clyster when they will not take it by the mouth. Wine-whey is a very proper drink for a child in an ague;

to

to half an Engliſh pint of which may be put a tea-ſpoonful of the ſpirit of hartſhorn. Exerciſe is likewiſe of conſiderable ſervice; and when the diſeaſe proves obſtinate, the child ought, if poſſible, to be removed to a warm dry air. Their food ought to be nouriſhing, and they ſhould ſometimes have a little generous wine.

We have been the more full upon this diſeaſe becauſe it is very common, and becauſe few patients in an ague apply to phyſicians unleſs in extremities. There are however many caſes in which the diſeaſe is very irregular, being complicated with other diſeaſes, or attended with ſymptoms which are both very dangerous, and difficult to underſtand. All theſe we have purpoſely paſſed over, as they would only bewilder the generality of readers. When the diſeaſe is very irregular, or the ſymptoms dangerous, the patient ought immediately to apply to a phyſician, and ſtrictly to follow his advice.

To prevent agues, people muſt avoid their cauſes. Theſe have been already pointed out in the beginning of this ſection; we ſhall therefore only add one preventive medicine, which may be of uſe to ſuch as are obliged to live in low marſhy countries, or who are liable to frequent attacks of this diſeaſe.

Take an ounce of the beſt jeſuites bark, half an ounce of virginian ſnake-root, and half an ounce of orange-peel, bruiſe them all together, and infuſe for five or ſix days in a bottle of brandy,

brandy, Holland gin, or any good ſpirit; afterwards pour off the clear liquor, and take a wine glaſs of it twice or thrice a-day. This indeed is recommending a dram; but the bitter in a great meaſure takes off the ill effects of the ſpirit. Thoſe who do not chuſe it in brandy may infuſe it in wine; and ſuch as can bring themſelves to chew the bark, will find that method ſucceed very well. Gentian-root, or calamus-aromaticus, may alſo be chewed by turns for the ſame purpoſe. All bitters ſeem to be antidotes to agues, eſpecially thoſe that are warm and aſtringent.

Of an ACUTE CONTINUAL FEVER.

THIS fever is denominated acute, ardent, or inflammatory. It moſt commonly attacks the young, or thoſe about the prime or vigour of life, eſpecially ſuch as live full, abound with blood, and whoſe fibres are ſtrong and elaſtic. It ſeizes people at all ſeaſons of the year; but is moſt frequent in the ſpring and beginning of ſummer.

CAUSES.—— An ardent fever may be occaſioned by any thing that overheats the body, as violent exerciſe, ſleeping in the ſun, drinking ſtrong liquors, eating ſpiceries, &c. It may likewiſe be occaſioned by any thing that obſtructs the perſpiration, as lying on the damp

damp ground, drinking cold liquor when the body is hot, night-watching, or ſuch like.

SYMPTOMS.—— A rigor or chillneſs generally uſhers in this fever, which is ſoon ſucceeded by great heat, a frequent and full pulſe, a pain of the head, dry ſkin, redneſs of the eyes, a florid countenance, pains in the back, loins, &c. To theſe ſucceed difficulty of breathing, ſickneſs, with an inclination to vomit. The patient complains of great thirſt, has no appetite for ſolid food, is reſtleſs, and his tongue generally appears black and rough.

A delirium, exceſſive reſtleſsneſs, great oppreſſion of the breaſt, with laborious reſpiration, ſtarting of the tendons, hiccup, cold, clammy ſweats, and an involuntary diſcharge of urine, are generally the forerunners of death.

As this diſeaſe is always attended with danger, the beſt medical aſſiſtance ought to be procured as ſoon as poſſible. A phyſician may be of uſe at the beginning, but his ſkill is often of no avail afterwards.

WE cannot here omit, once for all, taking notice of the unaccountable conduct of thoſe who have it in their power, at the beginning of a fever, to procure the beſt medical aſſiſtance, yet put it off till things come to an extremity. When the diſeaſe, by delay or wrong treatment, has become incurable, and has exhauſted the ſtrength of the patient, it is in vain to hope for relief from medicine. Phyſicians may indeed aſſiſt nature; but their attempts muſt ever prove fruitleſs, when ſhe is no longer able to co-operate with their endeavours.

REGIMEN.—From the ſymptoms of this diſeaſe it is evident, that the blood muſt be thick and viſcous, by which its circulation thorough the ſmall veſſels is impeded; that the perſpiration, urine, and all the other ſecretions, are in too ſmall quantity; that the veſſels are too rigid, and the heat of the whole body too great: All theſe clearly point out the neceſſity of a regimen, calculated to dilute the blood, allay the exceſſive heat, remove the ſpaſmodic ſtricture of the veſſels, and promote the ſecretions.

THESE important purpoſes may be greatly promoted by drinking plentifully of diluting liquors, as thin water-gruel, oatmeal-tea, clear whey, barley-water, balm-tea, apple-tea, &c. Theſe ſhould be ſharpened with juice of orange, jelly of currants, raſpberries, and ſuch like: Orange whey is likewiſe an excellent cooling drink. It is made by boiling a bitter orange ſliced among milk and water, till the curd ſeparates. If no orange can be had, a lemon, a little cream of tartar, or a few ſpoonfuls of vinegar, will have the ſame effect. Two or three ſpoonfuls of white wine may be occaſionally added to the liquor when boiling.

IF the patient be coſtive, an ounce of tamarinds, with two ounces of ſtoned raiſins of the ſun, and a couple of figs, may be boiled in three

Engliſh pints of water to a quart. This makes a very pleaſant drink, and may be uſed at diſcretion. The common pectoral decoction is likewiſe a very proper drink in this diſeaſe. It is made by boiling barley, ſtoned raiſins and figs, of each two ounces, with half an ounce of liquorice-root ſliced, in two Engliſh quarts of water, till one half be conſumed. The barley ſhould be boiled ſome time before the other ingredients are put in. This, with the addition of two or three drams of purified nitre, or ſal-prunel, will not only be a proper drink, but prove an exceeding good medicine. A tea-cupful of it may be taken every two hours, or oftner, if the patient's heat and thirſt be very great.

The above liquors muſt all be drank a little warm. They may be uſed in ſmaller quantities at the beginning of a fever, but more freely afterwards, in order to aſſiſt in carrying off the morbid matter by the different excretions. We have mentioned a variety of liquors, that the patient may have it in his power to chuſe that which is moſt agreeable; and that, when tired of one, he may have recourſe to another.

The patient's diet muſt be very ſpare and light. All ſorts of meats, and even chicken-broths, are to be avoided. He may be allowed groat-gruel, panada, or light bread boiled in water, and afterwards ſtrained; to which may be added a few grains of common ſalt, and a little a little ſugar, which will render it more palatable. He may eat roaſted apples with ſugar, toaſted bread with jelly of currants ſpread upon it, boiled prunes, &c.

It will greatly relieve the patient, eſpecially in an hot ſeaſon, to have freſh air frequently let into his chamber. This however muſt always be done in ſuch a manner as not to endanger his catching cold.

It is a common practice to load the patient with bed-cloaths, under the pretence of making him ſweat, or defending him from the cold. This cuſtom has many ill effects. It increaſes the heat of the body, fatigues the patient, and retards, inſtead of promoting, the perſpiration.

Sitting upright in bed, if the patient be able to bear it, will often have a good effect. It relieves the head, by retarding the motion of the blood to the brain. But this poſture ought never to be continued too long: And if the patient be inclined to ſweat, it will be more ſafe to let him lie ſtill, only raiſing his head with pillows, &c.

Sprinkling the chamber with vinegar, juice of lemon, or vinegar and roſe-water, with a little nitre diſſolved in it, will greatly refreſh the patient. This ought to be done frequently, eſpecially if the weather be hot.

The patient's mouth ſhould be often waſhed with warm water, mixed with honey, and a little vinegar; or a decoction of figs in barley-water, &c.

His

His feet and hands ought likewiſe frequently to be bathed in lukewarm water; eſpecially if the head be affected.

THE patient ſhould be kept as quiet and eaſy as poſſible. Company, noiſe, and every thing that diſturbs the mind is hurtful. Even too much light, or any thing that affects the ſenſes, is to be avoided His attendants ſhould be as few as poſſible, and they ought not to be too often changed. His inclinations ought rather to be ſoothed than contradicted; even the promiſe of what he craves will often ſatisfy him as much as its reality.

MEDICINE.—— In this and all other fevers ariſing from too great a quantity, and too rapid a motion of the blood, bleeding is of the greateſt importance. This operation ought always to be performed as ſoon as the ſymptoms of an inflammatory fever appear. The quantity of blood to be let muſt be in proportion to the ſtrength of the patient, and the violence of the diſeaſe. If after the firſt bleeding the fever ſeems to riſe, and the pulſe feels hard, there will be a neceſſity for repeating it a ſecond, and perhaps a third time, which may be done at the diſtance of twelve, eighteen, or twenty-four hours, as the ſymptoms require. If the pulſe continues ſoft, and the patient is tolerably eaſy after the firſt bleeding, it ought not to be repeated till neceſſary.

THE cooling febrifuge draught, recommended in the intermitting fever, page 177. will likewiſe

wiſe be very proper here; only the brandy muſt be left out, and half a dram of purified nitre added in its ſtead.

If the above cannot be conveniently obtained, forty or fifty drops of the dulcified or ſweet ſpirit of vitriol may be made into a draught, with an ounce of roſe-water, two ounces of common water, and half an ounce of ſimple ſyrup, or a bit of loaf-ſugar. This draught may be given to the patient every three hours while the fever is violent; afterwards, once in five or ſix hours will be ſufficient.

If the patient be afflicted with reaching, or an inclination to vomit, it will be right to aſſiſt Nature's attempts, by giving him weak camomile tea or lukewarm water to drink.

If the belly be bound, the patient ought daily to receive a clyſter of milk and water with a little ſalt, and a ſpoonful of ſweet oil or freſh butter. If this has not the deſired effect, a tea-ſpoonful of magneſia alba, or cream of tartar, may be frequently put into his drink. He may likewiſe eat tamarinds, boiled prunes, roaſted apples, and the like.

If about the 10th, 11th, or 12th day, the pulſe becomes more ſoft, the tongue moiſter, and the urine begins to let fall a reddiſh ſediment, there is reaſon to expect a favourable iſſue to the diſeaſe. But if, inſtead of thoſe ſymptoms, the patient's ſpirits grow languid, his pulſe ſinks, and his breathing becomes difficult; with a ſtupor, tremors

mors of the nerves, ſtarting of the tendons, &c. there is reaſon to fear that the conſequences will be fatal. In this caſe bliſtering plaiſters muſt be applied to the head, ancles, inſide of the thighs, &c. and the patient muſt be ſupported with cordials, as ſtrong wine-whey, negas, ſago-gruel, and ſuch like.

A proper regimen is not only neceſſary during the fever, but likewiſe after the patient begins to recover. By neglecting that, many relapſe, or fall into other diſeaſes, and continue valetudinary for life. Tho' the body be weak after a fever, yet the food for ſome time ought to be rather cleanſing than of too nouriſhing a nature. The perſon ſhould take great care not to exceed in any thing. Too much food, drink, ſleep, exerciſe, company, &c. are carefully to be avoided. The mind ought likewiſe to be kept eaſy, and the perſon ſhould not attempt to purſue ſtudy, or any thing that requires intenſe thinking.

If the digeſtion be bad, or the perſon be troubled at times with feveriſh heats, an infuſion of the jeſuites bark in cold water will be of uſe. It will ſtrengthen the ſtomach, and help to ſubdue the remains of the fever.

When the patient's ſtrength is pretty well recovered, he ought to take ſome gentle laxative. An ounce of tamarinds and a dram of ſenna, may be boiled for a few minutes in an Engliſh pint of water, and an ounce of manna diſſolved in the decoction; afterwards it may be ſtrained, and a tea-cupful drank every hour till it operates. This doſe may be repeated twice or thrice, five or ſix days interveening betwixt each doſe.

THOSE who follow laborious employments ought not to return too ſoon to their labour after a fever, but ſhould keep eaſy till their ſtrength and ſpirits be recruited.

Of the PLEURISY.

THE true pleuriſy is an inflammation of that membrane, called *the pleura*, which lines the inſide of the breaſt. It is diſtinguiſhed into the moiſt and the dry. In the former, the patient ſpits freely; but in the latter, little or none at all. There is likewiſe a ſpecies of this diſeaſe, which is called the *ſpurious* or *baſtard pleuriſy*, in which the pain is more external, and chiefly affects the muſcles between the ribs. This diſeaſe abounds among labouring people, eſpecially ſuch as work without doors, and are of a ſanguine conſtitution. It is moſt frequent in the ſpring-ſeaſon.

CAUSES.—— The pleuriſy is occaſioned by whatever obſtructs the perſpiration; as cold northerly winds, drinking cold liquors when the body is hot, ſleeping without doors on the damp ground; wet cloaths; plunging the body into cold water, or expoſing it to the cold air when

when covered with ſweat, &c. It may likewiſe be occaſioned by drinking ſtrong liquors; by the ſtoppage of uſual evacuations; as old ulcers, iſſues, ſweating of the feet or hands, &c.; the ſudden ſtriking in of any eruption, as the itch, the meaſles, or the ſmall pox. Thoſe who have been accuſtomed to bleed at a certain ſeaſon of the year, are apt, if they neglect it, to be ſeized with a pleuriſy. Keeping the body too warm by means of fire, cloaths, &c. renders it more liable to this diſeaſe. A pleuriſy may likewiſe be occaſioned by voilent exerciſe, as running, wreſtling, leaping, or by ſupporting great weights, eſpecially on the breaſt. The very make of the body ſometimes prediſpoſes perſons to this diſeaſe, as a narrow cheſt, a ſtraitneſs of the arteries of the pleura, &c.

SYMPTOMS.—— This, like moſt other fevers, begins with chillneſs and ſhivering, which are followed by heat, thirſt, and reſtleſsneſs. To theſe ſucceed a violent pricking pain in one of the ſides amongſt the ribs. Sometimes the pain extends towards the backbone, ſometimes towards the forepart of the breaſt, and at other times towards the ſhoulder-blades. The pain is generally moſt violent when the patient draws in his breath.

The pulſe in this diſeaſe is generally hard, the urine high coloured; and if blood be let, it is covered with a tough cruſt, or buffy coat. The patient's ſpittle is at firſt thin, but afterwards it it becomes groſſer, and is often ſtreaked with blood.

REGIMEN.—— Nature endeavours to carry off this diſeaſe either by a critical diſcharge of blood from the noſe, &c. or by expectoration, ſweat, looſe ſtools, thick urine, &c. When the violence of the fever is not broken by theſe, or other evacuations, it often ends in an abſceſs or ſuppuration ; to which enſues an ulcer, mortification, and death.

THE violence of this diſeaſe may generally be checked by leſſening the force of the circulation, relaxing the veſſels, diluting the humours, and promoting expectoration, &c.

FOR theſe purpoſes the diet, as in the former diſeaſe, muſt be cool, ſlender, and diluting. The patient muſt avoid food that is viſcid, hard of digeſtion, or that affords much nouriſhment, as fleſh, butter, cheeſe, eggs, milk, and alſo every thing that is of a heating nature. His drink muſt be ſweat whey, or decoctions and infuſions of the pectoral and balſamic vegetables.

TAKE a table-ſpoonful of linſeed, a quarter of an ounce of liquorice-root ſliced, and half an ounce of the leaves of coltsfoot. Put theſe ingredients in a cloſe veſſel, pour on them a quart of boiling water, and let them ſtand near a fire for eight or ten hours; afterwards ſtrain off the liquor; of which the patient may take a cupful frequently for his ordinary drink.

BARLEY WATER ſweetened with honey, or ſharpened with the jelly of currants, is like-

 wiſe

wiſe a very proper drink in this diſeaſe. It is made by boiling an ounce of pearl barley in three Engliſh pints of water to two, which muſt afterwards be ſtrained. The decoction of figs, raiſins, and barley, &c. recommended in the continual fever, page 186. is here likewiſe very proper. Theſe and other diluting liquors are not to be drank in large quantities at a time, but the patient ought, in a manner, to keep continually ſipping them, ſo as to render his mouth and throat always moiſt. All his food and drink muſt be taken a little warm.

THE patient ſhould be kept quiet, cool, and every way eaſy, as directed under the foregoing diſeaſe. His feet and hands ought daily to be bathed in warm water; and he may ſometimes ſit up in bed for a ſhort ſpace, in order to relieve his head.

MEDICINE.—— Almoſt every perſon knows when a fever is attended with a violent pain of the ſide, and a quick, hard pulſe, that bleeding is neceſſary. When theſe ſymptoms appear, the ſooner this operation is performed the better; and the quantity at firſt muſt be pretty large, provided the patient be able to bear it. A large quantity of blood let at once, in the beginning of a pleuriſy, has a much greater effect than ſeveral repeated ſmall bleedings. An adult perſon may loſe ten or twelve ounces of blood as ſoon as it is certainly known that he is ſeized with a pleuriſy. For a younger a younger perſon, or one of a delicate conſtitution, the quantity muſt be leſs.

If after the firſt bleeding, the ſtitch, with the other violent ſymptoms, ſhould continue, it will be neceſſary, at the diſtance of twelve or eighteen hours, to let eight or nine ounces more. If the ſymptoms do not then abate, and the blood ſhows a ſtrong buffy coat, a third or even a fourth bleeding may be requiſite. If the pain of the ſide abates, the pulſe becomes ſofter, or the patient begins to ſpit freely of a brown or reddiſh colour, bleeding ought not to be repeated. This operation is ſeldom neceſſary after the third or fourth day of the fever, and ought not then to be performed without the advice of a phyſician, unleſs in the moſt urgent circumſtances.

The blood may be many ways attenuated without letting it off. There are likewiſe many things that may be done to eaſe the pain of the ſide beſides bleeding. Thus, after the firſt or ſecond bleeding, emollient fomentations may be applied to the part affected. Theſe may be made by boiling a handful of the flowers of elder, camomile, and common mallows, or any other ſoft vegetables, in a proper quantity of water. The herbs may be either put into a bag, and applied warm to the ſide, or flannels may be dipped in the decoction, afterwards wrung out, and applied to to the part affected, with as much warmth as the patient can eaſily bear. As the cloths grow cool,

cool, they muſt be changed, and great care taken that the patient do not catch cold. An ox's bladder may be half filled with warm milk and water, and applied to the ſide, if the above method of fomenting be found inconvenient. Fomentations not only eaſe the pain, but by relaxing the veſſels, prevent the ſtagnation of the blood and other humours.

THE ſide may likewiſe be frequently rubbed with a little of the following liniment. Take two table-ſpoonfuls of the oil of ſweet almonds, olives, or any other ſweet oil, and two tea ſpoonfuls of ſpirit of hartſhorn: Shake them well together, and rub about a tea ſpoonful upon the ſide, with a warm hand, three or four times a-day.

SOME recommend dry applications to the affected ſide, as burnt oats, toaſted bread, &c. But theſe, tho' they may be uſeful, are not ſo proper as moiſt ones. Could it be properly conducted, we would recommend putting the patient into a bath of warm milk and water, in which emollient vegetables had been boiled; but as this cannot always be obtained, we ſhall recommend what is in every perſon's power, viz. to apply ſoft poultices, or cataplaſms to the part affected. Theſe may be made of wheat-bread and milk, ſoftened with oil or freſh butter.

LEAVES of various plants might likewiſe be applied to the patient's ſide with advantage. We have often ſeen, and even felt, the benefit of young cabbage-leaves applied warm to the

ſide

ſide in a pleuriſy. Theſe not only relax, but likewiſe draw off a little moiſture, and may prevent the neceſſity of bliſtering plaiſters; which, however, when other things fail, muſt be applied.

If the ſtitch continues after repeated bleedings, fomentations, &c. a bliſtering plaiſter muſt be laid upon the part affected, and ſuffered to remain for two days. This not only procures a diſcharge from the ſide, but actually thins the blood, and by that means aſſiſts in removing the cauſe of the diſeaſe.

To prevent a ſtrangury when the bliſtering plaiſter is on, the patient may drink freely of the following emulſion. Take an ounce of ſweet almonds blanched, and beat them well in a mortar, with an equal quantity of fine ſugar. Then diſſolve half an ounce of gum-arabic in an Engliſh quart of barley-water warm. Let it ſtand till cool, and afterwards pour it by little and little upon the almonds and ſugar, continually rubbing them till the liquor becomes uniformly white or milky. Afterwards ſtrain it, and let the patient uſe it for ordinary drink. A quart bottle, at leaſt, may be drank daily.

If the patient be coſtive, a clyſter of warm water, or of barley-water in which a handful of mallows, or any other emollient vegetable, has been boiled, may be daily adminiſtered. This will not only empty the bowels, but have the effect of a warm fomentation applied to the inferior

ferior viſcera, which will help to make a derivation from the breaſt.

The expectoration, or ſpitting, may be promoted by ſharp, oily, and mucilaginous medicines. For this purpoſe, an ounce of the oxymel or vinegar of ſquills may be added to ſix ounces of the pectoral decoction, and two table-ſpoonfuls of it taken every two hours.

Should the ſquill diſagree with the ſtomach, two ounces of the oil of ſweet almonds, or oil of olives, and two ounces of the ſyrup of violets, may be mixed with as much ſugar-candy powdered as will make an electuary of the conſiſtence of honey. The patient may take a little of this frequently, when the cough is troubleſome,

Should oily medicines happen to prove nauſeous, which is ſometimes the caſe, two drams of gum ammoniac may be diſſolved in half an Engliſh pint of barley-water, in the following manner: The gum muſt be well rubbed in a mortar, and the water gradually poured upon it till it be quite diſſolved. Three or four ounces of ſimple pennyroyal water may be added to the above quantity, and two table-ſpoonfuls of it taken three or four times a-day.

If the patient does not perſpire, but has a burning heat upon his ſkin, and paſſes very little water, ſome ſmall doſes of purified nitre and camphire will be of uſe. Two drams of the former may be rubbed with five or ſix grains of the latter in a mortar, and the whole divided

divided into ſix doſes, one of which may be taken every five or ſix hours, in a little of the patient's ordinary drink.

But the beſt medicine, which ſome indeed reckon almoſt a ſpecific in the pleuriſy, is the decoction of the ſeneka rattle ſnake root. Two ounces of the root groſsly powdered muſt be boiled in two Engliſh pints and a half water, till one half the water be conſumed. It muſt not be boiled quickly, but gradually ſimmered over a flow fire. After bleeding, and other evacuations have been premiſed, the patient may take two, three, or four table-ſpoonfuls of this decoction, according as his ſtomach will bear it, three or four times a-day. If it ſhould occaſion vomiting, two or three ounces of ſimple cinnamon-water may be mixed with the quantity of decoction above mentioned, or it may be taken in ſmaller doſes. As this medicine at once promotes perſpiration, urine, and keeps the belly eaſy, it bids the faireſt of any thing yet known to anſwer all the intentions of cure in a pleuriſy, or any other inflammation of the breaſt.

No one will imagine, that theſe medicines are all to be uſed at the ſame time. We have mentioned different things, on purpoſe that people may have it in their power to chuſe; and likewiſe, that when one thing cannot be obtained, they may make uſe of another. Different medicines are no doubt neceſſary in the different periods of a diſorder; and where one fails of ſucceſs,

ſucceſs, or diſagrees with the patient, it will be proper to try another.

WHAT is called the criſis, or height of the fever, is ſometimes attended with very alarming ſymptoms, as difficulty of breathing, an irregular pulſe, convulſive motions, &c. Theſe are apt to fright the attendants, and induce them to do improper things, as bleeding the patient, giving him ſtrong ſtimulating medicines, or the like. But they are only the ſtruggles of nature to overcome the diſeaſe, in which ſhe ought to be aſſiſted by plenty of diluting drink, which is then peculiarly neceſſary, as the febrile matter is now ready to be diſcharged. If the patient's ſtrength however be much exhauſted by the diſeaſe, it may be neceſſary at this time to ſupport him with frequent ſmall draughts of wine-whey, or the like.

WHEN the pain and fever are gone, it will be proper, after the patient has gathered ſufficient ſtrength, to give him ſome gentle purges, as thoſe directed under the acute continual fever, page 190. He ought likewiſe to uſe a light diet of eaſy digeſtion, and his drink ſhould be butter-milk, whey, and other things of a cleanſing nature.

THAT ſpecies of pleuriſy which is called the *baſtard* or *ſpurious*, generally goes off by keeping warm for a few days, drinking plenty of diluting liquors, and obſerving a proper regimen.

IT is known by a dry cough, a quick pulſe, and a difficulty of lying on the affected ſide,

ſide, which laſt does not always happen in the true pleuriſy. Sometimes indeed this diſeaſe proves obſtinate, and requires bleeding, with cupping, and ſcarifications of the affected ſide. Theſe, together with the uſe of nitrous, and other cooling medicines, ſeldom fail to effect a cure.

THE *paraphrenitis*, or inflammation of the diaphragm, is ſo nearly connected with the pleuriſy, and reſembles it ſo much in the manner of treatment, that it is ſcarce neceſſary to conſider it as a ſeparate diſeaſe.

IT is attended with a very acute fever, and an extreme pain of the part affected, which is generally augmented by coughing, ſneezing, drawing in the breath, taking food, going to ſtool, making water, &c. Hence the patient breathes quick, and draws in his bowels to prevent the motion of the diaphragm, is reſtleſs, anxious, has a dry cough, a hiccup, and often a delirium. A convulſive laugh, or rather a kind of involuntary grin, is no uncommon ſymptom of this diſeaſe.

EVERY method muſt be taken to prevent a ſuppuration, as it is impoſſible to ſave the patient's life when that happens. The regimen and medicine are in all reſpects the ſame as in the pleuriſy. We ſhall only add, that in this diſeaſe emollient clyſters are peculiarly uſeful, as they relax the bowels, and by that means draw the humours from the part affected.

Of a PERIPNEUMONY, or INFLAMMATION of the LUNGS.

As this diſeaſe affects an organ which is abſolutely neceſſary to life, it muſt always be attended with danger. Thoſe who abound with thick blood, whoſe fibres are tenſe and rigid, who feed upon groſs aliment, and drink ſtrong viſcid liquors, are moſt liable to this diſeaſe. It is generally fatal to perſons of a flat breaſt, or narrow cheſt, and to ſuch as are afflicted with an aſthma, eſpecially in the decline of life. Sometimes the inflammation reaches to one lobe of the lungs only, at other times the whole of that organ is affected; in which caſe the diſeaſe can hardly fail to prove fatal.

When the diſeaſe proceeds from a viſcid pituitous matter, obſtructing the veſſels of the lungs, it is called a *ſpurious*, or *baſtard peripneumony*. When it ariſes from a thin acrid defluction on the lungs, it is denominated a *catarrhal peripneumony*, &c.

CAUSES.—— An inflammation of the lungs is ſometimes a primary diſeaſe, and ſometimes it ſucceeds to other diſeaſes, as a quinſy, a pleuriſy, &c. It ariſes from the ſame cauſes as a pleuriſy, viz. an obſtructed perſpiration from cold, wet cloaths, &c.; or from an increaſed circulation of the blood by violent exerciſe, the uſe of ſpiceries, ardent ſpirits, and ſuch like. The

The pleurify and peripneumony are often complicated; in which cafe the difeafe is called a *pleuro-peripneumony*.

SYMPTOMS.—— Moft of the fymptoms of a pleurify likewife attend an inflammation of the lungs; only in the latter the pulfe is more foft, and the pain lefs acute; but the difficulty of breathing, and oppreffion of the breaft, are generally greater.

REGIMEN.—— As the regimen and medicine are in all refpects the fame in the true peripneumony as in the pleurify, we fhall not here repeat them, but refer the reader to the treatment of that difeafe. It may not however be improper to add, that the aliment ought to be more flender and thin in this than in any other inflammatory difeafe. The learned Dr Arbuthnot afferts, that even common whey is fufficient to fupport the patient, and that decoctions of barley, and infufions of fennel-roots in warm water with milk, are the moft proper both for drink and nourifhment. He likewife recommends the fteam of warm water taken in by the breath, which ferves as a kind of internal fomentation, and helps to attenuate the impacted humours. If the patient has loofe ftools, but is not weakened by them, they are not to be ftopped, but rather promoted by the ufe of emollient clyfters.

It has already been obferved, that the *fpurious* or *baftard* peripneumony is occafioned by a vifcid pituitous matter obftructing the vef-

fels

ſels of the lungs. It commonly attacks the old, infirm, and phlegmatic, in winter or wet ſeaſons.

THE patiert at the beginning is cold and hot by turns, has a ſmall quick pulſe, feels a ſenſe of weight upon his breaſt, breathes with difficulty, and ſometimes complains of a pain and giddineſs of his head. His urine is commonly pale, and his colour very little changed.

THE diet in this, as well as in the true peripneumony, muſt be very ſlender, as weak broths ſharpened with the juice of orange or lemon, &c. His drink may be thin water-gruel ſweetened with honey, or a decoction of fennel root, liquorice, and roots of quick graſs. An ounce of each of theſe may be boiled in three Engliſh pints of water to a quart, and ſharpened with a little currant jelly, or the like.

BLEEDING and purging are generally proper at the beginning of this diſeaſe; but if the patient's ſpittle be pretty thick, or well concocted, neither of them are neceſſary. It will be ſufficient to aſſiſt the expectoration by ſome of the ſoft balſamic medicines, recommended for that purpoſe in the pleuriſy. Bliſtering plaiſters have generally a good effect, and ought to be applied pretty early. They may either be applied to the neck or ancles, or both, if neceſſary.

IF the patient does not ſpit, he muſt be bled, if his ſtrength will permit, and have a gentle purge adminiſtered. Afterwards his belly may be be kept open by clysters, and the expectoration promoted, by taking every four hours two table-spoonfuls of the solution of gum-ammoniac, recommended in the pleurisy, page 198.

When an inflammation of the breast does not yield to bleeding, blistering, and the other means mentioned above, it commonly ends in a suppuration, which is more or less dangerous, according to the part where it is situate. When this happens in the pleura, it sometimes breaks outwardly, and the matter is discharged by the wound.

Sometimes the suppuration happens within the substance or body of the lungs; in which case the matter may be discharged by expectoration; but if the matter floats in the cavity of the breast, between the pleura and the lungs, it can only be discharged by an incision made betwixt the ribs.

If the patient's strength does not return after the inflammation is to all appearance removed; if his pulse continues quick tho' soft, his breathing difficult and oppressed; if he has cold shiverings at times, his cheeks flushed, his lips dry; and if he complains of thirst, and want of appetite; there is reason to fear that a suppuration is going on, and that a phthisis or consumption of the lungs will ensue. We shall therefore proceed to consider the proper treatment of that disease.

Of CONSUMPTIONS.

A consumption is a wasting or decay of the whole body from an ulcer, tubercles, or concretion of the lungs; from an empyema, a nervous atrophy, &c.

Dr Arbuthnot observes, that in his time consumptions made up above one tenth part of the bills of mortality about London. There is reason to believe they have rather increased since that time; and we know for certain, that they are not less fatal in several other towns in England than in London.

Young persons betwixt the age of fifteen and thirty, of a slender make, long neck, high shoulders, and flat breasts, are most liable to this disease.

Consumptions prevail more in England than in any other part of the world, owing perhaps to the great use of animal food, and strong liquors, the general application to sedentary employments, and the great quantity of pit-coal which is there burnt; to which we may add the perpetual changes in the atmosphere, or variableness of the weather.

CAUSES.—— It has already been observed, that inflammations of the breast often end in an imposthume: Consequently whatever predisposes

diſpoſes to thoſe diſeaſes muſt likewiſe be conſidered as a cauſe of conſumptions.

MANY other diſeaſes, by vitiating the humours, may likewiſe occaſion conſumptions; as the ſcurvy, the ſcrophula or king's evil, the venereal diſeaſe, the aſthma, ſmall pox, meaſles, &c.

As this diſeaſe is ſeldom cured, it will be neceſſary to point out its cauſes more particularly, in order that people may be the better enabled to avoid it. Theſe are:

——WANT of exerciſe. Hence it comes to paſs, that this diſeaſe is ſo common amongſt the inhabitants of great towns, who follow ſedentary employments, and likewiſe amongſt the rich, who are not under the neceſſity of labouring for their bread.

——CONFINED or unwholeſome air. Air which ſtagnates, or is impregnated with the fumes of metals or minerals, is extremely hurtful to the lungs, and often corrodes the tender veſſels of that neceſſary organ.

——VIOLENT paſſions, or affections of the mind as grief, diſappointment, anxiety, or cloſe application to the ſtudy of abſtruſe arts or ſciences, &c.

——EXCESSIVE evacuations; as ſweating, diarrhœas, diabetes, exceſſive venery, the fluor albus, an over-diſcharge of the menſtrual flux, giving ſuck too long, &c.

——THE

—— The ſudden ſtoppage of cuſtomary evacuations; as the bleeding piles, ſweating of the feet, bleeding of the noſe, the menſes, iſſues, ulcers, or eruptions of any kind.

—— Changing ſuddenly from a hot to a very cold climate, or whatever greatly leſſens the perſpiration.

—— Frequent and exceſſive debaucheries. Late watching, and drinking of ſtrong liquors, which generally go together, can hardly fail to deſtroy the lungs. Hence the *bon companion* generally falls a ſacrifice to this diſeaſe.

—— Infection. Conſumptions are often caught by ſleeping with the diſeaſed; for which reaſon this ſhould be carefully avoided. It cannot be of great benefit to the ſick, and muſt hurt thoſe in health.

—— Occupations in life. Thoſe artificers who ſit much, and are conſtantly leaning forward, or preſſing upon their ſtomachs and breaſts, as cutlers, taylors, ſhoemakers, &c. often die of conſumptions.

——Cold. More conſumptive patients date their diſorders from wet feet, damp beds, night-air, wet cloaths, and ſuch like, than from all other cauſes.

Sharp, ſaline, and aromatic aliments, which heat and inflame the blood, are likewiſe frequently the cauſe of conſumptions.

We ſhall only add, that this diſeaſe is of-often owing to an hereditary taint; in which caſe it is generally incurable.

SYMP-

SYMPTOMS.—— This diſeaſe generally begins with a dry cough, which often continues for ſome months. If a diſpoſition to vomit after eating be excited by it, there is great reaſon to fear an approaching conſumption. The patient complains of a more than uſual degree of heat, a pain and oppreſſion of the breaſt, eſpecially after motion; his ſpittle is of a ſaltiſh taſte, and ſometimes mixed with blood. He is apt to be ſad; his appetite is bad, and his thirſt great. There is generally a ſenſe of weight on the breaſt, with a quick, ſoft, ſmall pulſe; tho' ſometimes the pulſe is pretty full, and rather hard. Theſe are the common ſymptoms of a beginning conſumption.

AFTERWARDS the patient begins to ſpit a greeniſh, white, or bloody matter. His body is extenuated by the hectic fever and colliquative ſweats, which mutually ſucceed one another, viz. the one towards the night, and the other in the morning. A looſeneſs, and exceſſive diſcharge of urine, are often troubleſome ſymptoms at this time, and greatly weaken the patient. There is a burning heat in the palms of the hands, and the face generally fluſhes after eating; the fingers become remarkably ſmall, the nails are bent inwards, and the hairs fall off.

AT laſt the ſwelling of the feet and legs, the total loſs of ſtrength, the ſinking of the eyes, the difficulty of ſwallowing, and the coldneſs of the extremities, ſhow the immediate approach of death, which however the patient ſeldom believes to be ſo near. Such is the uſual progreſs of this fatal diſeaſe, which, if not early checked, commonly ſets all medicine at defiance.

REGIMEN.—— On the firſt appearance of this diſeaſe, if the patient lives in a large town, or any place where the air is confined, he ought immediately to quit it, and to make choice of a ſituation in the country, where the air is pure, dry and free. Here he muſt not remain inactive, but take every day as much exerciſe as he can bear.

THE beſt method of taking exerciſe is to ride on horſeback, as this gives the body a great deal of motion without much fatigue. Such as cannot bear this kind of exerciſe, muſt make uſe of a machine. A long journey, as it amuſes the mind by a continual change of objects, is greatly preferable to riding the ſame ground over and over. Care however muſt be taken to avoid catching cold from wet cloaths, damp beds, or ſuch like. At any rate, the patient muſt ride; his life depends upon it; and it is almoſt an infallible remedy, if begun in time, and duly perſiſted in.

IT is pity thoſe who attend the ſick ſeldom recommend riding in this diſeaſe, till the patient is either unable to bear it, or the malady is become incurable. Patients are always apt

to

to trifle with every thing that is in their own power. They cannot ſee how one of the common actions of life ſhould prove a remedy in an obſtinate diſeaſe, and therefore they reject it, while they greedily hunt after relief from medicine, merely becauſe it is unknown.

THOSE who have ſtrength and courage to undertake a pretty long voyage, may expect great advantage from it. This has frequently cured a conſumption after the patient was thought to be in the laſt ſtage of that diſeaſe, and where medicine had proved ineffectual. It is reaſonable from hence to conclude, that if a voyage were undertaken in due time, it would ſeldom fail to perform a cure.

SUCH as try this method of cure ought to carry as much freſh proviſions along with them as will ſerve for the whole time they are at ſea. As milk is not to be obtained in this ſituation, they ought to live upon fruits and the broth of chickens, or other young animals which can be kept alive on board. It is ſcarce neceſſary to add, that ſuch voyages ſhould be undertaken, if poſſible, in the mildeſt ſeaſon, and that they ought to be towards a warmer climate.

THOSE who have not courage for a long voyage may travel into a more ſouthern climate, as the ſouth of France, Spain, or Portugal; and if they find the air of theſe countries agree with them, they ſhould continue there, at leaſt till their health be confirmed.

NEXT

Next to proper air and exercise, we would recommend a due attention to the diet. The patient must eat nothing that is either heating or hard of digestion, and his drink must be of a soft and cooling nature. All the diet must be calculated to lessen the acrimony of the humours, and abate the rapid motion of the blood. For this purpose the patient must keep strictly to the use of vegetables and milk. Milk alone is of more value in this disease than the whole *materia medica.*

Asses milk is generally reckoned preferable to any other; but it cannot always be obtained; besides, it is generally taken as a medicine, whereas, to produce any considerable effects, it ought in a manner to make the principal part of the patient's food. It is hardly to be expected, that a gill or two of asses milk, drank in the space of twenty-four hours, should be able to produce any considerable change in the humours in a short time; but when people do not perceive its effects soon, they lose hope, and so leave it off. Hence it comes to pass that this medicine, however valuable, very seldom performs a cure. The reason is obvious; it is commonly used too late, is taken in too small quantities, and is not duly persisted in

I have known very extraordinary effects from asses milk in obstinate coughs, which threatened a consumption of the lungs; and do verily believe, if used at this period, that it would seldom fail; but if it be delayed till

till an ulcer is formed, which is generally the cafe, how can it be expected to fucceed?

Asses milk ought to be drank, if poffible, in its natural warmth, and in the quantity of half an Englifh pint at a time. Inftead of taking this quantity night and morning only, the patient ought to take it four times, or at leaft thrice a-day, and to eat a little light bread along with it, fo as to make it a kind of meal.

If affes milk fhould happen to purge the patient, it may be mixed with old conferve of rofes, which is itfelf a valuable medicine in this difeafe. If that cannot be obtained, the powder of crabs claws may be ufed in its ftead. Affes milk is ufually ordered to be drank warm in bed; but as it generally throws the patient into a fweat when taken in this way, it would be proper to give it after he rifes.

Some extraordinary cures in confumptive cafes have been performed by breaft-milk. Could this be obtained in fufficient quantity, we would recommend it preferably to any other. It is better if the patient can fuck it from the breaft than to drink it afterwards. I knew a man who was reduced to fuch a degree of weaknefs in a confumption, as not to be able to turn himfelf in bed. His wife was at that time giving fuck, and the child happening to die, he fucked her breafts, not with a view to reap any advantage from the milk, but to make her eafy. Finding himfelf however greatly benefited by it,

he

he continued to ſuck her till perfectly recovered, and is at preſent a ſtrong and healthy man.

Some prefer butter milk to any other, and it certainly is a very valuable medicine, if the ſtomach be able to bear it. It does not agree with every perſon at firſt; and is therefore often laid aſide without a ſufficient trial. It ſhould at firſt be taken ſparingly, and the quantity gradually increaſed, until it comes to be almoſt the ſole food. I never knew it ſucceed unleſs where the patient almoſt entirely lived upon it.

Cows milk is moſt readily obtained of any, and tho' it be not ſo eaſily digeſted as that of aſſes or mares, it may be rendered lighter by adding to it an equal quantity of barley-water, or allowing it to ſtand for ſome hours, and afterwards taking off the cream. If it ſhould notwithſtanding lie heavy on the ſtomach, a table-ſpoonful of rum or brandy, and a bit of loaf-ſugar, may be put into half an Engliſh pint.

It is not to be wondered, that milk ſhould, for ſome time, diſagree with a ſtomach that has not been accuſtomed to digeſt any thing but fleſh and ſtrong liquors, which is the caſe of moſt of thoſe who fall into conſumptions. We do not however adviſe thoſe who have been accuſtomed to animal food and ſtrong liquors, to leave them off all at once. This might be dangerous. It will be neceſſary for ſuch to eat a little once a-day

day of the flesh of some young animal, or rather to use the broth made of chickens, veal, lamb, or such like. They ought likewise to drink a little wine made into negas, or diluted with twice or thrice its quantity of water, and to make it gradually weaker till they can leave it off altogether.

THESE must be used only as preparatives to a diet consisting solely of milk and vegetables, which the sooner the patient can be brought to bear, the better. Rice and milk, or barley and milk boiled, with a little sugar, is very proper food. Ripe fruits roasted, baked, or boiled, are likewise proper, as goose or currant-berry tarts, apples roasted, or boiled in milk, &c. The jellies, conserves, and preserves, &c. of ripe subacid fruits, ought to be eat plentifully, as the jelly of currants, conserve of roses, preserved plumbs, cherries, &c.

WHOLESOME air, proper exercise, and a diet consisting solely of these and other vegetables, with milk, is the only course that can be depended on in a beginning consumption. If the patient has strength and sufficient resolution to persist in this course, he will seldom be disappointed of a cure.

IN a populous town in England, where consumptions are very common, I have frequently seen consumptive patients, who had been sent to the country with orders to ride, and live upon milk and vegetables, return in a few months quite plump, and free of any complaint.

This

This indeed was not always the caſe, eſpecially when the diſeaſe was hereditary, or far advanced; but it was the only method in which ſucceſs was to be expected; where it failed, I never knew medicine ſucceed.

If the patient's ſtrength and ſpirits flag, he muſt be ſupported by rich broths and jellies, &c. Some recommend ſhell fiſh in this diſorder, and we are inclined to think with reaſon; they are very nouriſhing, at the ſame time that they cool the blood, and blunt the acrimony of the humours. All the food and drink ought to be taken in ſmall quantities, leſt an overcharge of freſh chyle ſhould oppreſs the lungs, and too much accelerate the circulation of the blood.

The patient's mind ought to be kept as eaſy and chearful as poſſible. Conſumptions are often occaſioned by a melancholly caſt of mind; for which reaſon, muſic, chearful company, and every thing that inſpires mirth, are highly beneficial. The patient ought ſeldom to be left alone, as brooding over his calamities is ſure to render them worſe.

MEDICINE.—— Tho' we know no medicine that will cure a confirmed conſumption; yet the following things may be of ſervice, in abating ſome of the more violent ſymptoms.

In the firſt ſtage of a conſumption, the cough may ſometimes be appeaſed by bleeding; and expectoration promoted by the following medicines. Take freſh ſquills, gum-ammoniac, and pow-

powdered cardamum ſeeds, of each a quarter of an ounce; beat them together in a mortar, and if the maſs proves too hard for pills, a little of any kind of ſyrup may be added to it. This may be formed into pills of a moderate ſize, and four, or five of them taken twice or thrice a-day, according as the patient's ſtomach will bear them.

THE lac-ammoniacum, or milk of gum-ammoniac, as it is called, is likewiſe a proper medicine in this ſtage of the diſeaſe. It may be prepared and uſed as directed page 198.

A ſyrup made of equal parts of lemon-juice, fine honey, and ſugar candy may likewiſe be uſed. Four ounces of each of theſe may be ſimmered together in a ſauce-pan, over a ſlow fire, and a table-ſpoonful of it taken at any time when the cough is troubleſome.

IT is common in this ſtage of the diſeaſe to load the patient's ſtomach with balſamic medicines, and at the ſame time to drench him with decoctions, infuſions, &c. of the pectoral vegetables. The former of theſe, inſtead of removing the cauſe of the diſeaſe, tend rather to increaſe it, by heating the blood, while the latter pall the appetite, relax the ſolids, and prove every way hurtful to the patient. Whatever is uſed for removing the cough, beſides riding and other proper regimen, ought to be medicines of a ſharp and cleanſing nature.

FOR the patient's drink, we would recommend infusions of the bitter plants, as ground-ivy, the lesser centaury, camomile flowers, or water trefoil. These infusions may be drank at pleasure. They strengthen the stomach, promote digestion, rectify the blood, and at the same time answer all the purposes of dilution, and quench thirst much better than things that are luscious or sweet.

But if the patient spits blood, he ought to use the following decoction for his ordinary drink. Take an ounce of comfrey-root, of liquorice and marsh mallow roots, each half an ounce. Boil them in two English quarts of water to one. If a tea spoonful of the acid elixir of vitriol be added to this decoction when cold, it will be a very proper medicine. A tea-cupful of it may be taken at pleasure.

There are many other mucilaginous plants and seeds, of a healing and agglutinating nature, from which decoctions or infusions may be prepared with the same intention, as the orches, the quince seed, coltsfoot, linseed, sarsaparilla, &c. It is not necessary to mention the different forms in which these may be used. Simple infusion or boiling is all that is necessary, and the dose may be at discretion.

The conserve of roses is here peculiarly proper. It may either be put into the decoction above prescribed, or eat by itself. No benefit is to be expected from trifling doses of this medicine. I never knew it of any service unless where

where three or four ounces at leaſt were uſed daily. In this way I have ſeen it produce very extraordinary effects, and would recommend it wherever there is a diſcharge of blood from the lungs.

WHEN the ſpitting up of groſs matter, oppreſſion of the breaſt, and the hectic ſymptoms ſhow that an impoſthume is formed in the lungs, we would recommend the jeſuites bark, that being the only drug which has any chance to counteract the tendency which the humours then have to putrefaction.

AN ounce of the bark in powder may be divided into eighteen or twenty doſes, of which one may be taken every three hours through the day, in a little ſyrup, or a cup of the patient's ordinary drink.

IF the bark ſhould happen to purge, it may be made into an electuary, with the conſerve of roſes, thus. Take old conſerve of roſes a quarter of a pound, jeſuites bark in powder an ounce, ſyrup of orange or lemon, as much as will make it of the conſiſtence of honey. This quantity will ſerve the patient four or five days, and may be repeated as there is occaſion.

SUCH as cannot take the bark in ſubſtance, may infuſe it in cold water. This ſeems to be the beſt medium for extracting the virtues of that drug. Half an ounce of bark in powder may be infuſed for twenty-four hours in half an Engliſh pint of water. Afterwards let it be paſſed through a fine ſtrainer, and an ordinary

tea-

tea cupful of it taken three or four times a-day.

We would not recommend the bark while there are any symptoms of an inflammation of the breast; but when it is certainly known, that matter is collecting there, it is the only medicine upon which any stress can be laid. Few patients have resolution enough to give the bark a fair trial at this period of the disease, otherwise we have reason to believe, that great benefit might be reapt from it.

When it is evident, that there is an imposthume in the breast, and the matter can neither be spit up nor carried off by absorption, the patient must endeavour to make it break inwardly, by drawing in the steams of warm water or vinegar with his breath, coughing, laughing, or bawling aloud, &c. When it happens to burst within the lungs, the matter may be discharged by the mouth. Sometimes indeed the bursting of the vomica occasions immediate death, by suffocating the patient. When the quantity of matter is great, and the patient's strength exhausted, this is apt to happen. At any rate, the patient is ready to fall into a swoon, and should have volatile spirits or salts held to his nose.

If the matter discharged be thick, and the cough and breathing become easier, there may be some hopes of a cure. The diet at this time ought to be light, but restorative, as small chicken broths, sago gruel, rice-milk, &c. the drink, butter-milk, or whey sweetened with honey. This

This is likewiſe a proper time for uſing the jeſuites bark, which may be taken as before directed.

IF the vomica or impoſthume ſhould diſcharge itſelf into the cavity of the breaſt, betwixt the pleura and the lungs, there is no way of getting the matter out but by an inciſion, as has already been obſerved. As this operation muſt always be performed by a ſurgeon, it is not neceſſary for us to deſcribe it. We ſhall only obſerve, that it is not ſo dreadful as people are apt to imagine, and that it is the only chance the patient has for his life. It is indeed a pity that this operation, like moſt others, is generally delayed till too late. When the whole maſs of humours is tainted, the body waſted, and the ſtrength decayed, it is in vain to attempt to ſave the patient's life by an operation.

A NERVOUS CONSUMPTION, is a waſting or decay of the whole body, without any conſiderable degree of fever, cough, or difficulty of breathing. It is attended with indigeſtion, weakneſs, and want of appetite, &c.

THOSE who are of a fretful temper, who indulge in ſpirituous liquors, or who breathe an unwholeſome air, are moſt liable to this diſeaſe.

WE would chiefly recommend, for the cure of a nervous conſumption, a light and nouriſhing diet, enough of exerciſe in a free open air, and the uſe of ſuch bitters as brace and ſtrengthen the ſtomach; as the jeſuites bark, gentian-

root,

root, camomile, &c. Theſe may be infuſed in wine, and a glaſs of it drank frequently.

It will greatly aſſiſt the digeſtion, and promote the cure of this diſeaſe, to take twice a-day twenty or thirty drops of the elixir of vitriol in a glaſs of wine or water.

The chalybeate wine is likewiſe an excellent medicine in this caſe. It ſtrengthens the ſolids, and powerfully aſſiſts nature in the preparation of good blood. It is made by putting three ounces of the filings of ſteel or iron into a bottle of Rheniſh wine, and allowing it to digeſt for three weeks, frequently ſhaking the bottle. Afterwards the wine muſt be filtered for uſe. A table-ſpoonful of it may be taken twice or thrice a-day.

Agreeable amuſements, chearful company, and riding about, are however preferable to all medicines in this diſeaſe. For this reaſon, when the patient can afford it, we would recommend a long journey of pleaſure, as the moſt likely means to reſtore his health.

What is called a *ſymptomatic conſumption* cannot be cured without firſt removing the diſeaſe by which it is occaſioned. Thus, when a conſumption proceeds from the ſcrophula or king's evil, from the ſcurvy, the aſthma, the veneral diſeaſe, &c. a due attention muſt be paid to the malady from whence it ariſes, and the regimen and medicine directed accordingly.

When exceſſive evacuations of any kind occaſion a conſumption, they muſt not only be reſtrained,

reſtrained, but the patient's ſtrength muſt be reſtored by gentle exerciſe, nouriſhing diet, and generous cordials, &c. Young and delicate mothers often fall into conſumptions, by giving ſuck too long. As ſoon as they perceive their ſtrength and appetite begin to fail, they ought immediately to wean the child, or give it another nurſe, otherwiſe they cannot expect a cure.

BEFORE quitting this ſubject, we would earneſtly recommend it to all who wiſh to avoid conſumptions, to take as much exerciſe without doors as they can, to avoid unwholeſome air, and to ſtudy ſobriety. Conſumptions owe their preſent increaſe not a little to the faſhionable mode of ſpending every evening over a punch-bowl, or a bottle of wine. These liquors not only ſpoil the appetite, and hurt the digeſtion, but heat and inflame the blood, and ſet the whole conſtitution on fire.

The SLOW or NERVOUS FEVER.

NERVOUS fevers have increaſed greatly of late years in this iſland, owing doubtleſs to the increaſe of luxury and ſedentary employments; as this diſeaſe commonly attacks perſons of a weak relaxed habit, who neglect exerciſe, eat little ſolid food, ſtudy hard, or indulge in ſpiritous liquors.

CAUSES.—— Nervous fevers are occaſioned

oned by whatever depreſſes the ſpirits, or impoveriſhes the blood; as grief, fear and anxiety, want of ſleep, intenſe thought; living on poor watery diet, as unripe fruits, cucumbers, melons, muſhrooms, &c. They are likewiſe occaſioned by damp, confined, or unwholeſome air. Hence they are very common in rainy ſeaſons, and prove moſt fatal to thoſe who live in dirty, low houſes, crouded ſtreets, hoſpitals, jails, or ſuch like places.

PERSONS whoſe conſtitutions have been broken by exceſſive venery, frequent ſalivations, too free an uſe of purgative medicines, or the like, are very liable to this diſeaſe.

KEEPING on wet cloaths, ſleeping in the ſun, lying on the damp ground, exceſſive fatigue, and whatever obſtructs the perſpiration, or cauſes a ſpaſmodic ſtricture of the ſolids, may likewiſe occaſion nervous fevers. We ſhall only add frequent and great irregularities in eating and drinking. Too great abſtinence as well as exceſs is hurtful. Nothing tends ſo much to preſerve the humours in a ſound ſtate as a regular diet; nor can any thing contribute more to occaſion fevers of the worſt kind than its contrary.

SYMPTOMS—— Low ſpirits, want of appetite, weakneſs, wearineſs after motion, watchfulneſs, deep ſighing, and dejection of mind, are generally the forerunners of this diſeaſe. Theſe are ſucceeded by a quick low pulſe, a dry tongue without any conſiderable thirſt, chillneſs and fluſhing in turns, &c.

After ſome time the patient complains of a giddineſs and pain of his head, has a nauſea, with reachings and vomiting; his pulſe is quick, and ſometimes intermitting; his urine pale, reſembling dead ſmall bear, and his breathing is difficult, with oppreſſion of the breaſt, and ſlight alienations of mind.

If towards the ninth, tenth, or twelfth day, the tongue becomes more moiſt, with a plentiful ſpitting, a gentle diarrhœa, or a moiſture upon the ſkin; or if a ſuppuration happens in one or both ears, or large puſtules break out about the lips and noſe, there is reaſon to hope for a favourable criſis.

But, if there be an exceſſive looſeneſs, or waſting ſweats, with frequent fainting fits; if the tongue, when put out, trembles exceſſively, and the extremities feel cold, with a fluttering or ſlow creeping pulſe; if there be a ſtarting of the tendons, an almoſt total loſs of ſight and hearing, and an involuntary diſcharge by ſtool and urine, there is great reaſon to fear that death is approaching.

REGIMEN.——It is highly neceſſary in this diſeaſe to keep the patient eaſy and quiet. The leaſt motion will fatigue him, and will be apt to occaſion weerineſs, and even faintings. His mind likewiſe ought not only to be kept eaſy, but ſoothed and comforted with the hopes of a ſpeedy recovery. Nothing is more hurtful in low fevers of this kind, than preſenting to the patient's mind gloomy or frightful ideas. These often occasion nervous fevers, and it is not to be doubted but they will likewise increase the danger.

THE patient must not be kept too low. His strength and spirits ought to be supported by nourishing diet and generous cordials. For this purpose his gruels, panadas, or whatever food he takes, must be strengthened with wine according as the symptoms may require. Pretty strong wine whey, or small negas sharpened with the juice of orange or lemon, will be proper for his drink.

WINE in this disease, if it could be obtained genuine, would be almost the only medicine that we should need. Good wine possesses all the virtues of the cordial medicines, while it is free from many of their bad qualities. I say good wine; for however common that article of luxury is now become, it is rarely to be obtained genuine, especially by the poor, or such as purchase it in small quantities.

I have seen a patient in a low nervous fever, whose pulse could hardly be felt, with a constant delirium, coldness of the extremities, and almost every other mortal symptom, recover by using, in whey, gruel, and negas, a bottle of strong wine every day. Good wine is not only the most proper cordial, but seems also to be an excellent antispasmodic medicine; and consequently it must be highly proper in all diseases arising from a poor vapid state of the blood, and too great a stricture of the solids.

MUSTARD

MUSTARD whey is a very proper drink in this fever. It is made by tying in a linen rag a table-ſpoonful of common muſtard bruiſed, and boiling it a little in half an Engliſh pint of water, with an equal quantity of milk. Two or three ſpoonfuls of wine may be added to it when boiling, to make the curd ſeparate more perfectly, and to render the whey more cordial. A tea-cupful of this may be given frequently for the patient's ordinary drink.

IN a word, the great aim in this diſeaſe is to ſupport the patient's ſpirits, by giving him frequently ſmall quantities of the above, or other drinks of a warm and cordial nature. He is not however to be over-heated either with liquor or cloaths; and his food ought to be light, and given in ſmall quantities.

MEDICINE. — Where a nauſea, load, and ſickneſs at ſtomach prevail at the beginning of the fever, it will be neceſſary to give the patient a gentle vomit. Fifteen or twenty grains of ipecacoanha will generally anſwer this purpoſe very well. This may be repeated any time before the third or fourth day, if the above ſymptoms continue. Vomits not only clean the ſtomach, but, by the general ſhock which they give promote the perſpiration, and have many other excellent effects in ſlow fevers. where there are no ſigns of inflammation, and nature wants rouſing.

SUCH as dare not venture upon a vomit, may clean the bowels by a ſmall doſe of Turkey

key rhubarb, or an infusion of senna and manna.

In all fevers, the great point is to regulate the symptoms, so as to prevent their going to either extreme. Thus, in fevers of the inflammatory kind, where the force of the circulation is too great, or the blood dense, and the fibres too rigid, bleeding and other evacuations are necessary. But where nature flags, where the blood is vapid and poor, and the solids weak and relaxed, there the lancet is to be avoided. Hence bleeding is never to be permitted in nervous fevers unless there be evident signs of an inflammation, which very seldom happens.

It is the more necessary to caution people against bleeding in this disease, as there is generally at the beginning an universal stricture upon the vessels, which even to the patient himself often gives the idea of a plethora, or too great a quantity of blood. I have known some of the profession deceived by their own feelings in this respect, so far as to insist upon being bled, when it was evident that the operation was improper.

I remember to have attended an apothecary in a nervous fever, who at the beginning was so fully persuaded of the existence of a plethora, and the necessity of bleeding, that when I objected to it, he told me he was so certain of the necessity of that operation from his own feelings, that if it was not performed he could not live; and that if no body else would bleed

bleed him, he was determined to do it himſelf. He was accordingly bled, but was ſoon convinced of his error. The blood ſhewed no ſigns of inflammation, and he was ſo remarkably worſe after the operation, that he narrowly eſcaped with his life. His pulſe and ſpirits ſunk exceedingly, ſo that he could hardly be ſupported by a bottle of ſtrong wine in the day, beſides other cordial medicines.

Tho' bleeding be improper in this diſeaſe, yet bliſtering is highly neceſſary. Bliſtering plaiſters may be applied at all times of the fever with great advantage; we would however adviſe people not to make too free with them at the beginning, leſt there ſhould be more occaſion for them afterwards. If the patient be delirious, he ought to be bliſtered on the neck, and it will be the ſafeſt courſe, while the fever continues, as ſoon as the diſcharge occaſioned by one plaſter abates, to apply another ſome where elſe, and by that means keep up a continual ſucceſſion of them till the patient be out of danger.

I have been more ſenſible of the advantage of bliſtering in this diſeaſe than of any other medicine. It not only promotes the circulation by ſtimulating the ſolids, but likewiſe occaſions a continual diſcharge, which may in ſome meaſure ſupply the want of critical evacuations, which ſeldom happen in this kind of fever.

If the patient be coſtive through the courſe of the diſeaſe, it will be neceſſary to procure a ſtool,

ſtool, by giving him every other day a clyſter of milk and water, with a little ſugar, to which may be added a ſpoonful of common ſalt, if it be neceſſary.

SHOULD a violent looſeneſs come on, it may be checked, by giving the patient frequently a ſmall quantity of Venice treacle, or any thing that will promote the perſpiration.

THO' bliſtering and cordial liquors are the only medicines to be depended on in this kind of fever, yet, for thoſe who may chuſe to uſe them, we ſhall mention one or two of the forms of medicine which are commonly preſcribed in it.

THUS, when the patient is low, ten grains of Virginian ſnake root, and the ſame quantity of contrayerva root, with five grains of Ruſſian caſtor, all in fine powder, may be made into a bolus with a little of the cordial confection, or ſyrup of ſaffron. One of theſe may be taken every four or five hours.

THE following powder may be uſed for the ſame intention. Take wild Valerian root in powder one ſcruple, ſaffron and caſtor each four grains. Mix theſe by rubbing them together in a mortar, and give one in a cup of wine-whey three or four times a-day.

IN deſperate caſes, where the hiccup and ſtarting of the tendons have already come on, we have ſometimes ſeen extraordinary effects from large doſes of muſk frequently exhibited. This is doubtleſs a great antiſpaſmodic, and may

may be given to the quantity of a ſcruple three or four times a-day. Sometimes it may be proper to add to the muſk a few grains of camphire, and ſalt of hartſhorn, as theſe tend to promote perſpiration and urine. Thus fifteen grains of muſk, with three grains of camphire, and ſix grains of ſalt of hartſhorn, may be made into a doſe and given as above.

If the fever ſhould happen to intermit, which it frequently does towards the decline, or if the patient's ſtrength ſhould be waſted with colliquative ſweats, it will be neceſſary to give him an infuſion of the jeſuites bark with ſnake-root, in wine or brandy.

Half an ounce of the bark, with a dram of Virginian ſnake-root, half a dram of ſaffron, and half an ounce of orange-peal, all groſsly powdered, may be infuſed in half an Engliſh pint of brandy for three or four days. Afterwards ſtrain it, and give the patient two tea-ſpoonfuls in a glaſs of water, or ſmall wine, three or four times a-day.

Such as don't chuſe ſpirits may infuſe the above ingredients in a bottle of Liſbon wine, and take a glaſs of it frequently; this will reſtore the ſtrength, prevent a relapſe, and help to carry off the remains of the fever.

It will likewiſe be proper at this time, to interpoſe now and then a gentle doſe of rhubarb, or ſome other mild opening medicine, taking care at the ſame time to ſupport the patient's tient's ſtrength with chicken-broth, jellies, and ſuch like.

Of the MALIGNANT, PUTRID, or SPOTTED FEVER.

THIS may be called the *peſtilential fever* of Europe, as in many of its ſymptoms it bears a great reſemblance to that dreadful diſeaſe.

PERSONS of a lax habit, a melancholy diſpoſition, and thoſe whoſe vigour has been waſted by long faſting, watching, hard labour, exceſſive venery, or frequent ſalivations, &c. are moſt liable to this diſeaſe.

CAUSES.—— This fever is occaſioned by an unwholeſome, putrid, or ſtagnating air. Hence it prevails in jails, hoſpitals and infirmaries, eſpecially where ſuch places are greatly crouded, and cleanlineſs is neglected.

A cloſe conſtitution of the air, with long rainy or foggy weather, likewiſe occaſions putrid fevers. Hence they often ſucceed great inundations in low and marſhy countries, eſpecially when theſe are preceeded or followed by a hot and ſultry ſeaſon.

LIVING too much upon animal food, without a proper mixture of vegetables, or eating fiſh or fleſh that has been kept too long, are likewiſe apt to occaſion this kind of fever. Hence ſailors on long voyages, and the inhabitants of beſieged

ſieged cities, are very often viſited with putrid fevers.

CORN that has been greatly damaged by rainy ſeaſons, or long keeping, and water that has become putrid by ſtagnation, will likewiſe occaſion putrid fevers. The exceſſive uſe of alkaline ſalts will alſo have this effect.

DEAD carcaſes tainting the air, eſpecially in hot ſeaſons, are very apt to occaſion putrid fevers. Hence this kind of fever often prevails in camps, and ſuch countries as are the ſcenes of war and bloodſhed. This ſhews the neceſſity of removing church-yards, ſlaughter houſes, &c. at a proper diſtance from great towns.

WANT of cleanlineſs is a very general cauſe of putrid fevers. Hence they prevail amongſt the poor inhabitants of large towns, who breathe a confined unwholeſome air, neglect cleanlineſs, and are forced to live upon ſpoiled or unwholeſome proviſions, &c. Such mechanics as carry on dirty employments, and are conſtantly confined within doors, are likewiſe very liable to putrid fevers.

WE ſhall only add, that all putrid, malignant, or ſpotted fevers, are very infectious; and are therefore often communicated in this way. For which reaſon all perſons ought to keep at a diſtance from ſuch as are affected with thoſe diſeaſes, unleſs thoſe whoſe attendance is abſolutely neceſſary.

SYMPTOMS.—— The malignant fever is

is generally preceded by a remarkable weakneſs, or loſs of ſtrength, without any apparent cauſe. This is ſometimes ſo great, that the patient can ſcarce walk, or even ſit upright, without being in danger of fainting away. His mind too is greatly dejected; he ſighs, and is full of dreadful apprehenſions.

THERE is a nauſea, and ſometimes vomiting of bile; a violent pain of the head, with a ſtrong pulſation or throbbing of the temporal arteries; the eyes often appear red and inflamed, with a pain at the bottom of the orbit; there is a noiſe in the ears, the breathing is laborious, and often interrupted with a ſigh; the patient complains of pain about the region of the ſtomach, and in his back and loins; his tongue is at firſt white, but afterwards it appears black and chap'd; and his teeth are covered with a black cruſt. He ſometimes paſſes worms both upwards and downwards, is affected with tremors, or ſhaking, and often becomes delirious.

IF blood be let, it appears diſſolved, or with a very ſmall degree of coheſion, and ſoon becomes putrid; the ſtools ſmell extremely fœtid, and are ſometimes of a greeniſh, black, or rediſh caſt. Spots of a pale, purple, dun, or black colour often appear upon the ſkin, and ſometimes violent hæmorrhages, or diſcharges of blood from the mouth, eyes, noſe, &c. happen.

PUTRID fevers may be diſtinguiſhed from the inflammatory, by the ſmallneſs of the pulſe, the dejection

dejection of mind, the diſſolved ſtate of the blood, the petechiæ, or purple ſpots, and the putrid ſmell of the excrements. They may likewiſe be diſtinguiſhed from the low or nervous fever by the heat and thirſt being greater, the urine of a higher colour, and the other ſymptoms more violent.

IT ſometimes however happens, that the inflammatory, nervous, and putrid ſymptoms are ſo blended together, as to render it very difficult to determine to which claſs the fever belongs. In this caſe the greateſt caution and ſkill are requiſite. All endeavours muſt be uſed to relieve the moſt urgent ſymptoms; and the efforts of nature are carefully to be watched, in order that we may give her what aſſiſtance we can in expelling the cauſe of the diſeaſe in her own way.

INFLAMMATORY and nervous fevers are often converted into malignant and putrid, by too hot a regimen, or improper medicines.

THE period of putrid fevers is extremely uncertain; ſometimes they terminate betwixt the ſeventh and fourteenth day, and at other times they are prolonged for five or ſix weeks. Their duration depends greatly upon the conſtitution of the patient, and the manner of treating the diſeaſe.

THE moſt favourable ſymptoms are, after the fourth or fifth day, a gentle looſeneſs, with a warm, mild ſweat. Theſe, when continued for a conſiderable time, often carry off the fever,

ver, and ſhould never be imprudently ſtopped. Small miliary puſtules appearing between the petechiæ, or purple ſpots, are likewiſe favourable, as alſo hot ſcabby eruptions about the mouth and noſe. It is a good ſign when the pulſe riſes upon the uſe of wine, or other cordials, and the nervous ſymptoms abate; deafneſs coming on towards the decline of the fever, is likewiſe a favourable ſymptom, and ſo are abſceſſes in the groin, or parotid glands.

AMONGST the unfavourable ſymptoms may be reckoned an exceſſive looſeneſs, with a hard ſwelled belly. Large black or livid blotches breaking out upon the ſkin, are a proof of the putrid diſſolution of the blood, and ſhew the danger to be very great. Aphthæ in the mouth, and cold clammy ſweats, are unfavourable ſigns, as alſo blindneſs, change of the voice, a wild ſtaring of the eyes, difficulty of ſwallowing, an inability to put out the tongue, and a conſtant inclination to uncover the breaſt. When the ſweat and ſaliva are tinged with blood, and the urine is black, or depoſites a black ſooty ſediment, the patient is in great danger. Starting of the tendons, and fœtid, ichorous, involuntary ſtools, attended with coldneſs of the extremities, are generally the forerunners of death.

REGIMEN—— In the management of this diſeaſe we are to endeavour, as far as poſſible, to counteract the putrid tendency of the humours; to ſupport the patient's ſtrength and ſpirits;

ſpirits; and to aſſiſt nature in expelling the morbific matter, by gently promoting perſpiration and the other evacuations.

IT has been obſerved, that putrid fevers are often occaſioned by unwholeſome air, and of courſe they muſt be aggravated by it. Care muſt therefore be taken to prevent the air from ſtagnating in the patient's chamber, to keep it cool, and renew it frequently, by opening the doors or windows of ſome adjacent apartment. The breath and perſpiration of perſons in perfect health ſoon render the air of a ſmall apartment noxious; but this will ſooner happen from the perſpiration and breath of a perſon whoſe whole maſs of humours are in a putrid ſtate. Theſe fevers are often ſo heightened by the ſame infected air being breathed over and over, that the patient is in a manner ſuffocated by his own atmoſphere.

BESIDES the frequent admiſſion of freſh air, we would recommend the uſe of vinegar, verjuice, juice of lemon, Sevil orange, or any kind of vegetable acid that can be moſt readily obtained. Theſe ought frequently to be ſprinkled upon the floor, the bed, and every part of the room. They may alſo be evaporated with an hot iron, or by boiling, &c. The freſh ſkins of lemons or oranges ought likewiſe to be laid in different parts of the room, and they ſhould be frequently held to the patient's noſe. The uſe of acids in this manner would not only prove very refreſhing to the patient, but would tend

tend greatly to prevent the infection from ſpreading among thoſe who attend him. Strong ſmelled herbs, as rue, tanſy, roſemary, wormwood, &c. may likewiſe be laid in different parts of the houſe, and ſmelled to by thoſe who go near the patient.

THE patient muſt not only be kept cool, but likewiſe quiet and eaſy. The leaſt noiſe will affect his head, and the ſmalleſt fatigue will be apt to make him faint away.

NOTHING is of ſo great importance in this diſeaſe, as the liberal uſe of acids. Theſe are to be mixed with all the patient's food as well as drink. Orange, lemon, or vinegar whey, are all very proper, and may be drank in turns, according to the patient's inclination. Theſe may be rendered cordial by the addition of wine in ſuch quantity as the patient's ſtrength ſeems to require. When he is very low, he may drink negas, with only one half water, and ſharpened with the juice of orange or lemon. In ſome caſes a glaſs of clear wine may now and then be allowed. The moſt proper wine is Rheniſh; but if the belly be open, red Port or Claret is to be preferred.

WHEN the belly is bound, a tea-ſpoonful of the cream of tartar may be put into a cup of the patient's drink, as there is occaſion; or he may eat a few tamarinds, which will both quench his thirſt and keep his belly eaſy.

IF camomile-tea will ſit upon the ſtomach, it is a very proper drink in this diſeaſe. It may be be ſharpened by adding to every cup of the tea fifteen or twenty drops of the elixir of vitriol.

THE food muſt be light, as panada, groat-gruel, and ſuch like; to theſe a little wine may be added, if the patient be weak and low, and they ought all to be ſharpened with the juice of orange, or the jelly of currants, raſp-berries, &c. The patient ought likewiſe to eat freely of ripe fruits, either baked, roaſted, or raw, as roaſted apples, currant, or gooſeberry-tarts, preſerved cherries, plumbs, and ſuch like.

THE patient muſt never be long without nouriſhment. Taking a little food or drink frequently not only ſupports the ſpirits, but counteracts the putrid tendency of the humours; for which reaſon he ought conſtantly to be ſipping ſmall quantities of ſome of the acid liquors mentioned above, or any that may be more agreeable to his palate, or more readily obtained.

IF the patient be delirious, his feet and hands ought to be frequently fomented with ſtrong infuſions of camomile flowers. This, or an infuſion of the bark, to ſuch as can afford it, cannot fail to have a good effect. Fomentations of this kind not only relieve the head, by relaxing the veſſels in the extremities, but as their contents are abſorbed, and taken into the blood, they muſt by their antiſeptic qualities aſſiſt in preventing the putreſcency of the humours.

IF

If the patient be not able to put his feet and hands into the decoction, cloths dipt in it may be applied to them.

MEDICINE.—— If a vomit be taken at the very beginning of this fever, it will hardly fail to have a good effect; but if the fever has gone on for some days, and the symptoms are violent, vomits must not be taken without proper advice.

Bleeding is seldom necessary in putrid fevers. If there be signs of an inflammation, it may sometimes be permitted at the first onset; but the repetition of it often proves fatal.

Blistering plasters are never to be used unless in the greatest extremities. If the petechiæ or spots should suddenly disappear, the patient's pulse sink remarkably, and a delirium, with other bad symptoms, come on, blistering may be permited. In this case the blistering plasters are to be applied to the head, and the insides of the legs or thighs. But as they are sometimes apt to occasion a gangrene, we would rather recommend warm poultices or cataplasms to be applied to the feet, having recourse to blisters only in the utmost extremities.

A very ridiculous notion has long prevailed, of expelling the poisonous matter of malignant diseases by strong doses of cordial or alexipharmic medicines. In consequence of this notion the contrayerva root. the cordial confection, and

and the mithridate, &c. have been extolled as infallible remedies. There is reaſon to believe, that theſe oftener do harm than good. Where cordials are neceſſary, we know none that is ſuperior to good wine; and therefore again recommend it both as the ſafeſt and beſt. Wine, with other acid and antiſeptic medicines, are the only things to be relied on in the cure of malignant fevers.

We have already recommended acids in various forms, and ſhall only add one more, viz. camphorated vinegar. This is made by rubbing a dram of camphor with a ſmall quantity of ſpirits of wine in a mortar, till it becomes ſoft, then adding half an ounce of loaf-ſugar, and rubbing the whole together till perfectly united. Afterwards take an Engliſh pint of warm vinegar, and add it by little and little, ſtill continuing the trituration, till they be uniformly mixed. Let it ſtand to cool, and afterwards ſtrain it. This may be taken in the doſe of a table-ſpoonful or two every two or three hours, according as it agrees with the ſtomach. If it ſhould heat the patient, or occaſion a nauſea, it muſt be diſcontinued.

In the moſt dangerous ſpecies of this diſeaſe, when it is attended with purple, livid, or black ſpots, the jeſuites bark is the only medicine that can be depended upon. I have ſeen it, when joined with acids, almoſt perform wonders, even in caſes where the petechiæ had the moſt threatening aſpect. But, to anſwer this purpoſe, it muſt not only be given in large doſes, but duly perſiſted in.

THE beſt method for adminiſtering the bark is certainly in ſubſtance. An ounce of it in powder may be mixt with half an Engliſh pint of water, and the ſame quantity of red wine, and ſharpened with the elixir or ſpirit of vitriol, which will both make it ſit eaſier on the ſtomach, and render it more beneficial. Two or three ounces of the ſyrup of lemon may be added, and two table-ſpoonfuls of the mixture taken every two hours, or oftener, if the ſtomach will bear it.

THOSE who cannot take the bark in ſubſtance may infuſe it in wine, as recommended page 231.

IF there be a violent looſeneſs, the bark muſt be boiled in red wine with a little cinnamon, and ſharpened with the elixir of vitriol, as above. Nothing can be more beneficial in this kind of looſeneſs than plenty of acids, and ſuch things as promote the perſpiration.

IF the patient be troubled with vomiting, a dram of the ſalt of wormwood diſſolved in an ounce and half of freſh lemon-juice, and made into a draught with an ounce of ſimple cinnamon-water, or peppermint-water, and a bit of ſugar, may be given to the patient, and repeated as often as it is neceſſary.

IF ſwellings of the glands appear, their ſuppuration is to be promoted by the application of poultices, ripening cataplaſms, &c. And as ſoon

ſoon as there is any appearance of matter in them, they ought to be laid open, and the poultices continued.

I have known patients in the decline of this fever have large ulcerous ſores break out in various parts of the body, of a livid gangrenous appearance, and a moſt putrid cadaverous ſmell. Theſe gradually healed, and the patient recovered, by the plentiful uſe of jeſuites bark mixed in wine, and ſharpened with the ſpirits of vitriol.

ALL who would avoid this dreadful diſeaſe, ſhould ſtudy univerſal cleanlineſs, and ſhould live regularly, avoiding the extremes of too high or too low a diet with equal care.

INFECTION, above all things, is be avoided. No conſtitution is proof againſt it. I have known perſons ſeized with a putrid fever, by only making a ſingle viſit to a patient in it; others have caught it by going through a town where it prevailed; and ſome by attending the funerals of ſuch as died of it.

ANY one who is apprehenſive of having caught the infection, ought immediately to take a vomit, and to work it off by drinking plentifully of camomile tea. This may be repeated in a day or two, if the apprehenſions ſtill continue, or any unfavourable ſymptoms appear.

THE perſon ought likewiſe to take an infuſion of the bark and camomile flowers for his ordinary drink; and before he goes to bed, he may drink an Engliſh pint of pretty ſtrong ne-

gas,

gas, or a few glaſſes of generous wine. I have been frequently obliged to follow this courſe, when malignant fevers prevailed, and have likewiſe recommended it to others with conſtant ſucceſs.

PEOPLE generally fly to bleeding and purging as antidotes againſt infection; but theſe are ſo far from ſecuring them, that they often increaſe the danger.

PHYSICIANS, and ſuch as attend the ſick in putrid fevers, ought always to have a piece of ſpunge or a handkerchief dipt in vinegar, or juice of lemon, to hold at their noſe. They ought likewiſe to waſh their hands, and, if poſſible, to change their cloaths, before they viſit any other patient.

OF THE MILIARY FEVER.

THIS fever takes its name from the ſmall puſtules or bladders which appear on the ſkin, reſembling, in ſhape and ſize, the ſeeds of millet. The puſtules are either red or white, and ſometimes both are mixed together.

SOMETIMES the whole body is covered with puſtules; but they are generally more numerous where the ſweat is moſt abundant, as on the breaſt, the back, &c. A gentle ſweat, or moiſture on the ſkin, greatly promotes the eruption; but where the ſkin is dry, the eruption is both more painful and dangerous.

SOME-

SOMETIMES this is a primary diſeaſe; but it is much oftener only a ſymptom of ſome other malady, as the ſmall pox, meaſles, ardent, putrid, or nervous fever, &c. In all theſe caſes it is generally the effect of too hot a regimen or medicines.

THE miliary fever chiefly attacks the idle and the phlegmatic, or perſons of a relaxed habit. The young and the aged are more liable to it than thoſe in the vigour and prime of life. It is likewiſe more incident to women than men, eſpecially the delicate and the indolent, who, neglecting exerciſe, keep continually within doors, and live upon weak watery diet. Such females are extremely liable to be ſeized with this diſeaſe in childbed, and often loſe their lives by it.

CAUSES.—— The miliary fever is often occaſioned by violent paſſions or affections of the mind; as exceſſive grief, anxiety, thoughtfulneſs, &c. It may likewiſe be occaſioned by exceſſive watching, great evacuations, a weak watery diet, rainy ſeaſons, eating too freely of cold, watery, unripe fruits, as plumbs, cherries, cucumbers, melons, &c. Impure waters, or proviſions which have been ſpoiled by rainy ſeaſons, long keeping, &c. may likewiſe cauſe miliary fevers. They may alſo be occaſioned by the ſtoppage of any cuſtomary evacuation, as iſſues, ſetons, ulcers, the bleeding piles in men, or the menſtrual flux in women, &c.

THIS

THIS diſeaſe in childbed-women is ſometimes the effect of great coſtiveneſs during pregnancy; ſometimes it is occaſioned by their exceſſive uſe of green unripe fruits, and other unwholeſome things in which pregnant women are too apt to indulge But its moſt general cauſe is indolence. Such women as indulge an eaſy ſedentary life during pregnancy, and at the ſame time live groſs and full, can hardly eſcape this diſeaſe in childbed. Hence it proves extremely fatal to women of faſhion, and likewiſe to thoſe women in manufacturing towns, who, in order to aſſiſt their huſbands, ſit cloſe within doors for almoſt the whole of their time. But among women who are active and laborious, who live in the country, and take enough of exerciſe without doors, this diſeaſe is very little known.

SYMPTOMS.—— When this is a primary diſeaſe, it makes its attack, like moſt other eruptive fevers, with a ſlight ſhivering, which is ſucceeded by heat, loſs of ſtrength, faintiſhneſs, ſighing, a low quick pulſe, difficulty of breathing, with great anxiety and oppreſſion of the breaſt. The patient is reſtleſs, and ſometimes delirious; the tongue appears white, and the hands ſhake, with often a burning heat in the palms; and in childbed-women the milk generally goes away, and the other diſcharges ſtop.

THE patient feels an itching or pricking pain under the ſkin, after which innumerable ſmall pu-

puſtules of a red or white colour begin to appear. Upon this the ſymptoms generally abate, the pulſe becomes more full and ſoft, the ſkin grows moiſter, and the ſweat, as the diſeaſe advances, begins to have a peculiar fœtid ſmell; the great load on the breaſt and oppreſſion of the ſpirits generally go off, and the cuſtomary evacuations gradually return. About the ſixth or ſeventh day from the eruption, the puſtules begin to dry and fall off, which occaſions a very diſagreeable itching in the ſkin.

It is impoſſible to aſcertain the exact time when the puſtules will either appear or go off. They generally come out on the third or fourth day, when the eruption is critical; but, when ſymptomatical, they may appear at any time of the diſeaſe.

Sometimes the puſtules appear and vaniſh by turns. When that is the caſe, there is always danger; but when they ſtrike in all of a ſudden, and do not appear again, the danger is very great.

In childbed-women the puſtules are commonly at firſt filled with clear water, afterwards they grow yellowiſh. Sometimes they are interſperſed with puſtules of a red colour. When theſe only appear, the diſeaſe goes by the name of a *raſh*.

REGIMEN.—— In all eruptive fevers, of whatever kind, the chief point is to prevent the ſudden ſtriking in of the puſtules. For this purpoſe the patient muſt be kept in ſuch a temperature,

rature, as neither to push out the eruption too fast, nor to cause it retreat prematurely. The diet and drink ought therefore to be in a moderate degree nourishing and cordial; but neither strong nor heating. The patient's chamber ought neither to be kept too hot nor cold; and he should not be too much covered with cloaths. Above all, the mind is to be kept easy and chearful. Nothing so certainly makes an eruption strike in as fear, or the apprehension of danger.

The food must be weak chicken-broth with bread, water-pap, with sago, and groat-gruel, &c.; to a gill of which may be added a spoonful or two of wine, as the patient's strength requires, with a few grains of salt and a little sugar. Good apples roasted or boiled, with other ripe fruits of an opening cooling nature, may be eat.

The drink must be suited to the state of the patient's strength and spirits. If these be pretty high, the drink ought to be weak; as water-gruel, balm-tea or the following decoction.

Take two ounces of the shavings of hartshorn, and the same quantity of sarsaparilla, boil them in two English quarts of water. To the strained decoction add a little white sugar, and let the patient take it for his ordinary drink.

When the patient's spirits are low, and the eruption does not rise sufficiently, his drink must be a little more generous; as wine-whey, or small negas, sharpened with the juice of orange

range or lemon, and made ſtronger or weaker as the circumſtances may require.

SOMETIMES the miliary fever approaches towards a putrid nature, in which caſe the patient's ſtrength muſt be ſupported with generous cordials, joined with acids; and if the degree of putreſcency be great, the jeſuites bark muſt be adminiſtered. If the head be much affected, the belly muſt be kept open by emolient clyſters.

IN the *commercium literarium* for the year 1735, we have the hiſtory of an epidemical miliary fever, which raged at Straſburg in the months of November, December, and January; from which we learn the neceſſity of a temperate regimen in this diſeaſe, and likewiſe that phyſicians are not always the firſt who diſcover the proper treatment of diſeaſes. "This fever made terrible havoc among men of robuſt conſtitutions, and all medicine proved in vain. They were ſeized in an inſtant with ſhivering, yawning, ſtretching, and pains in the back, ſucceeded by a moſt intenſe heat; at the ſame time there was great loſs of ſtrength and appetite. On the ſeventh or ninth day the miliary eruptions appeared or ſpots like flea-bites, with great anxiety, a delirium, reſtleſſneſs, and toſſing in bed. Bleeding was fatal. While matters were in this unhappy ſituation, a midwife, of her own accord, gave to a patient, in the height of the diſeaſe, a clyſter of rain-water and butter without ſalt, and for his ordinary drink a quart of ſpring-water, half a pint of generous wine, the juice of one lemon, and ſix ounces of the whiteſt ſugar gently boiled till a ſcum aroſe, and this with great ſucceſs; for the belly was ſoon looſened, the grievous ſymptoms vaniſhed, and the patient was reſtored to his ſenſes, and ſnatched from the jaws of death." This practice was imitated by others with the like happy effects.

MEDICINE.—— If the food and drink be properly regulated, there will be little occaſion for medicine in this diſeaſe. Should the eruption however not riſe, or the ſpirits flag, it will be neceſſary to ſupport the patient with cordials, and to apply bliſters. The moſt proper cordial in this caſe is good wine, which may either be taken in the patient's food or drink; and if there be any ſigns of putreſcency, which frequently happens, the bark and acids may be mixed with wine, as directed in the putrid fever.

SOME recommend bliſters through the whole courſe of the diſeaſe; and where nature flags, and the eruption comes and goes, it may be neceſſary to keep up a ſtimulus, by a continual ſucceſſion of ſmall bliſters; but we would not recommend above one at a time. If however the pulſe ſhould ſink remarkably, the puſtules ſtrike in, and the head be affected, it will be neceſſary to apply ſeveral bliſtering plaiſters to the moſt ſenſible parts, as the inſide of the legs and thighs, &c.

BLEED-

Bleeding is ſeldom neceſſary in this diſeaſe, and ſometimes it does much hurt, as it weakens the patient, and depreſſes his ſpirits. It is therefore never to be attempted unleſs by the advice of a phyſician. We mention this, becauſe it has been cuſtomary to treat this diſeaſe in childbed-women by bleeding, and other evacuations, as if it were highly inflammatory. But this practice is generally very unſafe. Patients in this ſituation bear evacuations very ill. And indeed the diſeaſe ſeems often to be more of a putrid than an inflammatory nature.

Tho' this fever be often occaſioned in childbed women by too hot a regimen, yet it would be dangerous to leave that off all of a ſudden, and have recourſe to a very cool regimen, and large evacuations. We have reaſon to believe, that ſupporting the patient's ſpirits, and promoting the natural evacuations, is here much ſafer than to have recourſe to artificial ones, as every thing that tends to depreſs the patient's ſpirits conſtantly increaſes the danger.

If this diſeaſe proves tedious, or the recovery ſlow, we would recommend the jeſuites bark, which may either be taken in ſubſtance, or infuſed in wine or water, as the patient inclines.

The miliary fever, like other eruptive diſeaſes, after it is gone, requires purging, which ſhould not be neglected as ſoon as the patient's ſtrength will permit.

To avoid this diſeaſe, a pure dry air, plenty of exerciſe and wholeſome food, are neceſſary. Pregnant women ſhould guard againſt coſtiveneſs, and take daily as much exerciſe as they can bear, avoiding all green traſhy fruits, and other unwholeſome things; and when in childbed, they ought ſtrictly to obſerve a cool regimen.

OF THE SMALL POX.

THIS diſeaſe is ſo general, that very few eſcape it at one time of life or another. It is the moſt contagious malady in theſe parts; and has, for upwards of a thouſand years, proved the ſcourge of Europe.

THE ſmall pox generally appear towards the ſpring. They are very frequent in ſummer, leſs ſo in autumn, and leaſt of all in winter. Children are moſt liable to this diſeaſe; and thoſe whoſe food is unwholeſome, who want proper exerciſe, and abound with groſs humours, run the greateſt hazard from it.

THE diſeaſe is diſtinguiſhed into the diſtinct and confluent kind; the latter of which is always attended with danger. There are likewiſe other diſtinctions of the ſmall pox; as the lymphatic, the cryſtalline, the bloody, &c.

CAUSES.—— The ſmall pox are commonly

monly caught by infection. Since the disease was brought into Europe, the infection has never been wholly extinguished; nor have any proper methods, so far as we know, ever been taken for that purpose; so that now it has become in a manner constitutional. Children who have over-heated themselves by running, wrestling, &c. or adults after a debauch, are very apt to be seized with this disease.

SYMPTOMS. --- This disease is so generally known, that a minute description of it is unnecessary. Children commonly look a little dull, seem listless and drowsy for a few days before the more violent symptoms of the small pox appear. They are likewise more inclined to drink than usual, have little appetite for solid food, complain of weariness, and, upon taking exercise, are apt to sweat. These are succeeded by slight fits of cold and heat in turns, which, as the time of the eruption approaches, become more violent, and are accompanied with pains of the head and loins, vomiting, &c. The pulse is quick, with a great heat of the skin, and restlessness. When the patient drops asleep, he wakes in a kind of horror, with a sudden start, which is a very common symptom of the approaching eruption; as are also convulsion-fits in very young children.

About the third or fourth day from the time of sickening, the small pox generally begin to appear; sometimes indeed they appear sooner, but that is no advantage. At first they very nearly

nearly resemble flea-bites, and are most early discovered on the face, arms and breast.

THE most favourable symptoms are a slow eruption, and an abatement of the ever as soon as the pustules appear. In a mild distinct kind of small pox the pustules seldom appear before the fourth day from the time of sickening, and they generally keep coming out gradually for several days after. Pustules which are distinct, with a florid red basis, and which fill with thick purulent matter, first of a whitish, and afterwards of a yellowish colour, are the best.

A livid brown colour of the pustules is an unfavourable symptom; as also when they are small and flat, with black specks in the middle. Pustules which contain a thin watery ichor are very bad. A great number of pox on the face is always a bad sign, especially if they be confluent, or run into one another.

BUT the most unfavourable symptom is the petechiæ, or purple, brown and black spots interspersed among the pustules. These are signs of a putrid dissolution of the blood, and show the danger to be very great. Bloody stools or urine, with a swelled belly, are bad symptoms; as is also a continual strangury. When the urine is very pale, and there is a violent throbbing of the arteries of the neck, it portends a delirium or convulsion fits. When the face does not swell, or falls before the pox come to maturity, it is a very bad sign. If the face begins to fall about the eleventh or twelfth day,

and

and the hands begin to ſwell, and afterwards the feet, the patient generally does well; but when theſe do not ſucceed, there is reaſon to apprehend danger. When the tongue is covered with a brown cruſt, it is an unfavourable ſymptom. Cold ſhivering fits coming on at the height of the diſeaſe, are likewiſe unfavourable. Grinding of the teeth, when it proceeds from an affection of the nervous ſyſtem, is a bad ſign; but ſometimes it is occaſioned by worms, or a diſordered ſtomach.

REGIMEN.—— When the firſt ſymptoms of the ſmall pox appear, people are ready to be alarmed, and often fly to the uſe of medicine, to the great danger of the patient's life. I have known children, to appeaſe the anxiety of their parents, bled, bliſtered, purged, and vomited, during the fever which preceeded the eruption of the ſmall pox, to ſuch a degree, that Nature was not only diſturbed in her operation, but rendered unable to ſupport the puſtules after they were out; ſo that the patient, exhauſted by mere evacuations, ſunk under the diſeaſe.

WHEN convulſions appear, they give a dreadful alarm. Immediately ſome noſtrum is applied, as if this were a primary diſeaſe; whereas it is only a ſymptom, and far from being an unfavourable one, of the approaching eruption. As the fits generally go off before the actual appearance of the ſmall pox, it is attributed to the

the medicine, which by this means acquires a reputation without any merit.

ALL that is, generally ſpeaking neceſſary during the eruptive fever, is to keep the patient within doors, and to allow him to drink freely of ſome weak diluting liquors; as balm-tea, barley-water, clear whey, gruels, &c. He ſhould neither be kept in too warm a room, nor confined to bed; but ſhould ſit up as much as he is able, and ſhould have his feet and legs frequently bathed in lukewarm water. His food, if he takes any, ought to be very light; and he ſhould be as little diſturbed with noiſe and company as poſſible.

MUCH miſchief is done at this period by confining the patient too ſoon to his bed, and plying him with warm cordials or ſudorific medicines. Every thing that heats and inflames the blood increaſes the fever, and puſhes out the puſtules too faſt. This has numberleſs ill effects. It not only increaſes the number of puſtules, but likewiſe tends to make them run into one another; and when they have been puſhed out with too great violence, they generally fall in before they come to maturity.

THE good women, as ſoon as they ſee the ſmall pox begin to appear, commonly ply their tender charge with cordials, ſaffron and marigold teas, wines, punch, and even brandy itſelf. All theſe are given with a view to throw out the eruption, as they pretend, from the heart. This, like moſt other popular miſtakes, is the abuſe

abuſe of a very juſt obſervation, *That when there is a moiſture on the ſkin, the pox riſe better, and the patient is eaſier than when it continues dry and parched.* But that is no reaſon for forcing the patient into a ſweat. Sweating never relieves unleſs where it comes ſpontaneouſly, or is the effect of drinking weak diluting liquors.

THE patient ought to have no more covering in bed than is neceſſary to prevent his catching cold, and he ſhould be frequently taken up, if it were only for a few minutes; this will both keep him cool, and prevent too great a flux of blood towards the head.

CHILDREN are often ſo peeviſh that they will not lie a-bed without a nurſe conſtantly by them. This, we have reaſon to believe, has many bad effects. Even the natural heat of the nurſe cannot fail to augment the fever of the child; but if ſhe too proves feveriſh, the danger muſt be increaſed. I have known a nurſe contract a malignant fever by lying in bed with a child the whole time of its being ill of a bad kind of ſmall pox.

LAYING ſeveral children who have the ſmall pox in the ſame bed, has many ill conſequences. They ought, if poſſible, never to be in the ſame chamber, as the perſpiration, the heat, and the ſmell, &c. all tend to augment the fever, and to heighten the diſeaſe. It is common among the poor to ſee two or three children lying in the ſame bed, with ſuch a load of puſtules that their very ſkins ſtick together. One can hardly view a ſcene of this kind without being ſickened by the ſight and ſmell. How much more muſt theſe affect the poor patients, many of whom periſh by this uſage?

This obſervation is likewiſe applicable to hoſpitals, workhouſes, &c. where numbers of children happen to have the ſmall pox at the ſame time. I have ſeen above forty children cooped up in one apartment all the while they had this diſeaſe, without any of them being admitted to breathe the freſh air. No one can be at a loſs to ſee the impropriety of ſuch conduct, which generally proceeds from a piece of ill judged œconomy, to ſave the trifling expence of a few nurſes. It ought to be a rule, not only in hoſpitals for the ſmall pox, but likewiſe for other diſeaſes, that no patient ſhould be within ſight or hearing of another. This is a matter to which too little regard is paid in moſt hoſpitals and infirmaries, where the ſick, the dying, and the dead are often to be ſeen in the ſame apartment.

A very dirty cuſtom prevails amongſt the lower ſort of people, of allowing children in the ſmall pox to keep on the ſame linen during the whole period of that loathſome diſeaſe. This is done leſt they ſhould catch cold, but it has many ill conſequences. The linen becomes hard by the moiſture which it abſorbs, and frets the tender ſkin. It likewiſe occaſions a bad ſmell, which is very pernicious both to the

the patient and thoſe about him; beſides the filth and ſordes which adhere to the linen being abſorbed, or taken up again into the body, greatly augment the diſeaſe.

A patient ſhould not be kept dirty in any diſeaſe, eſpecially in the ſmall pox. Cutaneous diſorders are often occaſioned by naſtineſs alone, and are always increaſed by it. Were the patient's linen to be changed every day it would greatly refreſh him. Care indeed is to be taken that the linen be thoroughly dry. It ought likewiſe to be warmed, and put on when the patient is moſt cool.

So ſtrong is the vulgar prejudice in this country, notwithſtanding all that has been ſaid againſt keeping children too warm in the ſmall pox, that numbers ſtill fall a ſacrifice to that error. I have ſeen poor women travelling in the depth of winter, and carrying their children along with them in the ſmall pox; and have frequently obſerved others begging by the wayſide, with infants in their arms covered with the puſtules; yet I could never learn that one of theſe children died by this ſort of treatment. We would not however propoſe this as an example worthy of imitation; we only mention it to ſhew, that the danger of expoſing children to the open air in this diſeaſe is not ſo great as people are apt to imagine.

Strong prejudices when got over, often produce the oppoſite extremes. We would therefore adviſe people, when they avoid one error, not

to

to run into another. Some celebrated inoculators order their patients to walk about all the while they are under the diseaie, as if nothing weie the matter. We should think it adviseable however to keep within doors, at least during the eruption, as cold air is apt to check the perspiration, and to prevent the pox from rising, or filling with matter. I do not remember ever to have seen large well filled pustules where the patient was exposed to the external air. In winter the air of this country is abundantly cool within doors, and in summer a patient may be kept more uniformly cool in the house than he can be out of it. For these and other reasons, we should think it right to confine the patient to the house while the eruption is out, but never to allow the heat of his chamber to be greater than is agreeable to a person in perfect health.

THE food in this disease ought to be very light, and of a cooling nature, as water pap, rice, or bread boiled with milk, good apples roasted or boiled with milk, and sweetened with a little sugar, or such like.

THE drink may be equal parts of milk and water, clear sweet whey, barley water, or thin gruel, &c. After the pox are full, butter-milk is an excellent drink, it being of an opening and cleansing nature.

MEDICINE.—— This disease is generally divided into four different periods, *viz.* the fever which preceeds the eruption, the eruption

tion itſelf, the ſuppuration, or maturation of the puſtules, and the ſecondary fever.

It has already been obſerved, that little more is neceſſary during the primary fever than to keep the patient cool and quiet, allowing him to drink diluting liquors, and bathing his feet frequently in warm water. Tho' this be generally the ſafeſt courſe that can be taken with infants, yet adults of a ſtrong conſtitution and plethoric habit ſometimes require bleeding. When a full pulſe, a dry ſkin, and other ſymptoms of inflammation, render this operation neceſſary, it ought to be performed; but, unleſs theſe ſymptoms are urgent, it is ſafer to truſt to fomentations; and, if the belly be bound, emollient clyſters may be thrown in.

If there be a great nauſea or vomiting, weak camomile tea or lukewarm water may be drank, in order to clean the ſtomach. At the beginning of a fever Nature generally attempts a diſcharge, either upwards or downwards, which, if promoted by gentle means, would tend greatly to abate the force or violence of the diſeaſe.

Tho' every method is to be taken during the primary fever, by a cool regimen, &c. to prevent too great an eruption; yet, after the puſtules have made their appearance, our buſineſs is to promote the ſuppuration, by gentle warmth, diluting drink, light food, and, if nature ſeems to flag, by generous cordials; but the latter ought never to be given unleſs where there

there is an abſolute neceſſity. When a low, creeping pulſe, faintiſhneſs, and great loſs of ſtrength, render cordials neceſſary, we would recommend good wine, which may be made into negas, with an equal quantity of water, and ſharpened with the juice of orange, the jelly of currants, or the like. Wine-whey ſharpened as above, is likewiſe a proper drink in this caſe; great care however muſt be taken not to overheat the patient by any of theſe things. This would retard inſtead of promoting the eruption.

SOMETIMES the riſing of the ſmall pox is prevented by the violence of the fever; in which caſe the cool regimen is ſtrictly to be obſerved. For example, the patient's chamber muſt be kept cool; he ought likewiſe frequently to be taken out of bed, and to be lightly covered with cloaths while in it.

EXCESSIVE reſtleſſneſs often prevents the riſing and filling of the ſmall pox. When that happens, gentle opiates are neceſſary. Theſe however ought always to be adminiſtred with the greateſt caution. To an infant, a tea-ſpoonful of the ſyrup of poppies may be given every five or ſix hours, till it has the deſired effect. An adult perſon will require a table-ſpoonful in order to anſwer the ſame purpoſe; and to others, the doſe muſt be proportioned to their age and the violence of the ſymptoms.

IF the patient be troubled with a ſtrangury, or ſuppreſſion of urine, which often happens in the

the ſmall pox, he ſhould be frequently taken out of bed, and, if he be able, ſhould walk a-croſs the room with his feet bare. When he cannot do this, he may be frequently ſet on his knees in bed, and ſhould endeavour to paſs his urine as often as he can. When theſe do not ſucceed, a tea-ſpoonful of the ſweet ſpirits of nitre may be occaſionally mixed in his drink. Nothing more certainly relieves the patient, or is more beneficial in the ſmall pox, than a plentiful diſcharge of urine.

If the mouth be foul, and the tongue dry and chapped, it ought to be frequently waſhed, and the throat gargled with warm water and honey, ſharpened with a little vinegar or currant jelly.

During the riſing of the ſmall pox, it frequently happens that the patient is eight or ten days without a ſtool. This not only tends to heat and inflame the blood, but the fœces, by lodging ſo long in the body, become acrid and even putrid; from whence bad conſequences muſt enſue. It will therefore be proper, when the belly is bound, to throw in an emollient clyſter every ſecond or third day, through the whole courſe of the diſeaſe. This will greatly cool and relieve the patient.

When petechiæ, or purple, black, or livid ſpots appear among the ſmall pox, the jeſuits bark muſt immediately be adminiſtred in as large doſes as the patient's ſtomach can bear. For a child, two drams of the bark in powder may be mixed in three

three ounces of common water, one ounce of ſimple cinnamon-water, and two ounces of the ſyrup of orange or lemon. This may be ſharpened with the ſpirits of vitriol, and a table ſpoonful of it given every hour. If it be given to an adult in the ſame form, he may take at leaſt three or four ſpoonfuls every hour. This medicine ought not to be trifled with, but muſt be thrown in as faſt as the ſtomach can bear; in which caſe it will often produce very happy effects. I have frequently ſeen the petechiæ diſappear, and ſmall pox, which had a very threatening aſpect, riſe and fill with laudable matter, by the uſe of the jeſuits bark and acids.

The patient's drink ought likewiſe in this caſe to be acidulated with the ſpirits of vitriol, vinegar, juice of lemon, jelly of currants, or ſuch like. His food muſt conſiſt of apples roaſted or boiled, preſerved cherries, plumbs, and other ſharp fruits.

Camomile tea, if the patient's ſtomach will bear it, is likewiſe a very proper drink in this caſe. It may be ſharpened with any of the acids mentioned above, and drank at pleaſure. When the pulſe and ſpirits are low, red wine negas, or pretty ſtrong wine-whey, ſharpened with the juice of lemon, muſt be given for the patient's ordinary drink.

The bark and acids are not only neceſſary when the petechiæ or putrid ſymptoms appear, but likewiſe in the lymphatic or cryſtalline ſmall

ſmall pox, where the matter is thin, and not duly prepared. The jeſuits bark ſeems poſſeſſed of a ſingular power to aſſiſt Nature in preparing laudable pus, or what is called good matter; conſequently it muſt be very beneficial, both in this and other diſeaſes whoſe criſis depends on a ſuppuration. I have often obſerved where the ſmall pox were flat, and the matter contained in them quite clear and tranſparent, and where they had the appearance of running into one another, that the uſe of a few drams of the jeſuits bark, acidulated as above, not only promoted the ſuppuration, but changed the colour and conſiſtence of the matter, and produced the moſt happy effects.

When the eruption ſubſides ſuddenly, or, as the good women term it, when the ſmall pox ſtrike in, before they have arrived at maturity, the danger is very great. This is often the effect of a hot regimen or medicines which at the beginning puſh out the matter before it has been properly prepared. When this happens, bliſtering plaſters mutt be immediately applied to the wriſts and ancles, and the patient's ſpirits ſupported with cordials.

Sometimes bleeding has a ſurpriſing effect in raiſing the puſtules after they have ſubſided; but it requires ſkill to know when this is proper, or to what length the patient can bear it. Sharp cataplaſms however may be applied to the feet and hands, as they tend to promote the

 ſwelling

ſwelling of theſe parts, and by that means to draw the humour towards the extremities.

THE moſt dangerous period of the diſeaſe is what we call the ſecondary fever. This generally comes on when the ſmall pox begin to turn on the face, and moſt of thoſe who die of the ſmall pox are carried off by this fever.

NATURE generally attempts, at the turn of the ſmall pox, to relieve the patient by looſe ſtools. Her endeavours this way are by no means to be counteracted, but promoted, and the patient at the ſame time ſupported by things of a light but nouriſhing nature. Patients have often been remarkably relieved at this time by a few looſe ſtools, either brought on by nature or procured by art. That ſhould encourage us to endeavour to aſſiſt Nature in this way, eſpecially if the ſymptoms be threatening, and the belly continues bound.

IF at the approach of the ſecondary fever the pulſe be very quick, hard, and ſtrong, the heat intenſe, and the breathing laborious, with other ſymptoms of an inflammation of the breaſt, the patient muſt immediately be bled, otherwiſe a fatal peripneumony will enſue. The quantity of blood to be let muſt be regulated by the patient's ſtrength, age, and the urgency of the ſymptoms.

BUT, in the ſecondary fever, if the patient be faintiſh, the puſtules become pale and ſhrink, and if there be great coldneſs of the extremities, bliſtering plaſters muſt be applied, and the patient muſt be ſupported with generous

generous wine. Wine and even ſpirits have ſometimes been given in ſuch deſperate caſes with amazing ſucceſs.

As the ſecondary fever is in great meaſure, if not wholely, owing to the abſorption of the matter, it would ſeem highly conſonant to reaſon, that the puſtules, as ſoon as they come to maturity, ſhould be opened. That is every day practiced in other phlegmons which tend to ſuppuration; and there ſeems to be no reaſon why it ſhould be leſs proper here. On the contrary, we have reaſon to believe, that by this means the ſecondary fever might always be leſſened, and often wholely prevented.

The puſtules ſhould be opened when they begin to turn of a yellow colour. Very little art is neceſſary for this operation. They may either be opened with a pair of ſciſſars or a needle, and the matter abſorbed by a wet ſpunge or a little lint. As the puſtules are generally firſt ripe on the face, it will be proper to begin with opening theſe, and the others in courſe as they become ripe. The puſtules generally fill again, a ſecond or even a third time, &c.; for which cauſe the operation muſt be repeated, or rather continued ſo long as there is any conſiderable appearance of matter in the puſtules.

We have reaſon to believe, that this operation, rational as it is, has been neglected from a piece of miſtaken tenderneſs in parents. They believe, that it muſt give great pain to the poor

poor child; and therefore would rather ſee it die than have it thus tortured. This notion however is entirely without foundation. It is only the ſcarf-ſkin that is cut, which, upon the top of the puſtules, by the time they are ripe, becomes quite inſenſible. I have frequently opened the puſtules when the patients did not ſee me, without their being in the leaſt ſenſible of it; but ſuppoſe it were attended with a little pain, that is nothing in compariſon to the advantages which ariſe from it.

OPENING the puſtules not only prevents the abſorption of the matter into the blood, but likewiſe takes off the tenſion of the ſkin, and by that means greatly relieves the patient. It likewiſe prevents the pitting, which is a matter of no ſmall importance. Acrid matter, by lodging long in the puſtules, cannot fail to corrode the tender ſkin; by which many a handſome face becomes ſo deformed as hardly to bear a reſemblance to the human figure.

IT is always neceſſary, after the ſmall pox are gone off, to purge the patient. If however the belly has been open through the whole courſe of the diſeaſe, or if butter-milk and other things of an opening nature have been given after the height of the ſmall pox, purging becomes leſs neceſſary; but it ought never wholely to be neglected.

FOR very young children an infuſion of ſenna and prunes, with a little rhubarb, may be ſweetened with manna or coarſe ſugar, and given

ven in ſmall quantities till it operates. Thoſe who are farther advanced muſt take medicines of a ſharper nature. For example, a child of four or five years of age may take ten grains of fine rhubarb in powder over night, and the ſame quantity of jalap in powder next morning, with two or three grains of calomel, mixed in currant-jelly, or made into a bolus with a little honey. He ought to keep the houſe all day, and to drink nothing that is cold. The doſe may be repeated three or four times, five or ſix days intervening betwixt each doſe. For children further advanced, and adults, the doſe muſt be increaſed in proportion to the age and conſtitution.

When impoſthumes happen after the ſmall pox, which is not ſeldom the caſe, they are to be brought to ſuppuration as ſoon as poſſible, by means of ripening poultices; and, when they have been opened, or break of their own accord, the patient muſt be purged.

When a cough, a difficulty of breathing, or other ſymptoms of a conſumption, ſucceed to the ſmall pox, the patient muſt be ſent to a well aired place, and put upon a courſe of aſſes milk, with ſuch exerciſe as he can bear. For further directions in this caſe, ſee the article Conſumptions.

Tho' no diſeaſe, after it is formed, baffles the powers of medicine more than the ſmall pox, yet more may be done before hand to render this diſeaſe favourable than any one we know, as almoſt all the danger from it may be prevented by inoculation. This ſalutary invention has been known in Europe about half a century, but, like moſt other uſeful diſcoveries, it has met with great oppoſition. It muſt however be aknowledged, to the honour of this country, that inoculation has met with a more favourable reception here than by any of our neighbours. It is ſtill however far from being general, which we have reaſon to fear will ever be the caſe, ſo long as the practice continues in the hands of the Faculty.

No diſcovery can ever be of general utility while the practice of it is kept in the hands of a few. Had the inoculation of the ſmall pox been introduced as a faſhion, and not as a medical diſcovery, and had it been practiced by the ſame kind of operators here as it is in thoſe countries from whence we had it, it had long ago been univerſal. The fears, the jealouſies, the prejudices, and the oppoſite intereſts of the Faculty, are, and ever will be the moſt effectual obſtacles to the progreſs of any ſalutary diſcovery. Hence it is that the practice of inoculation never became, in any meaſure, general, even in England, till taken up by men not bred to phyſic. Theſe have not only rendered the practice more extenſive, but likewiſe more ſafe, and, by acting under leſs reſtraint than the regular practitioners, have taught them that the patient's greateſt danger aroſe, not from the want of care, but from the exceſs of it.

THEY

THEY know very little of the matter, who impute the ſucceſs of modern inoculators to any ſuperior ſkill, either in preparing the patient or communicating the diſeaſe. Some operators indeed, from a ſordid deſire of ingroſſing the whole practice to themſelves, pretend to have extraordinary ſecrets or noſtrums in preparing perſons for inoculation, which never fail of ſucceſs. But this is only a pretence calculated to blind the ignorant and inattentive. Common ſenſe and prudence alone are ſufficient both in the choice of the ſubject and management of the operation. Whoever is poſſeſſed of theſe may perform this office for his children whenever he finds it convenient, provided they be in a proper ſtate of health; and may reſt aſſured that he will ſucceed as well as the moſt celebrated inoculator.

THIS ſentiment is not the reſult of theory, but of obſervation. Tho' few phyſicians have had more opportunities of trying inoculation in all its different forms, ſo little appears to me to depend on theſe, generally reckoned important circumſtances, of preparing the body, communicating the infection by this or the other method, &c. that for ſeveral years paſt I have cauſed the parents or nurſes perform the whole themſelves, and have found that method followed with equal ſucceſs, while it is free from many inconveniencies that attend the other.

A critical ſituation, too often to be met with, firſt put me upon trying this method. A gentleman

man who had loſt all his children except one ſon by the natural ſmall pox, was determined to have him inoculated. He told me his intention, and deſired I would perſuade the mother and grandmother, &c. of its propriety. But that was impoſſible. They were not to be perſuaded, and either could not get the better of their fears, or were determined againſt conviction. It was always a point with me, not to perform the operation without the conſent of parties concerned. I therefore adviſed the father, after giving his ſon a doſe or two of rhubarb, to go to a patient who had the ſmall pox of a good kind, to open two or three of the puſtules, taking up the matter with a little cotton, and as ſoon as he came home to take his ſon into a private room, and give his arm a ſlight ſcratch with a pin, as if it had been by accident, afterwards to rub the place well with the cotton, and take no further notice of it. All this he punctually performed; and at the uſual period the ſmall pox made their appearance, which were of an exceeding good kind, and ſo mild as not to confine the boy an hour to his bed. None of the other relations knew but the diſeaſe had come in the natural way till the patient was well.

We do not propoſe this as the only method in which the ſmall pox can be communicated. It appears from experience, that this may be done various ways with equal ſucceſs. In Turkey, from whence we learned the practice, the women

women communicate the diſeaſe to children, by opening a bit of the ſkin with a needle, and putting into the wound a little matter taken from a ripe puſtule. On the coaſt of Barbary they paſs a thread wet with the matter thro' the ſkin, between the thumb and fore-finger; and in Europe inoculation is generally performed by making a ſmall inciſion thro' the cuticle of the arm or leg with a lancet, and laying a bit of thread wet with the matter upon the wound, which is covered with a piece of ſticking plaſter, and kept on for two or three days.

Some of the people in England who make a trade of inoculation, only open one of the ripe puſtules with a lancet, and while it is wet with the matter make a ſlight inciſion in the arm of the perſon to whom they want to communicate the diſeaſe; afterwards they cloſe up the wound, and leave it without any other dreſſing. This ſeems to be no real improvement. It frequently fails to communicate the diſeaſe, and is far leſs certain than when a ſcratch with a pin or a needle is made, and a bit of thread wet with the matter kept on the wound for ſome days by a ſticking plaſter.

Indeed, if the matter be applied long enough to the ſkin, there is no occaſion for any wound at all. Let a bit of thread, about half an inch long, wet with the matter, be applied to the arm, midway between the ſhoulder and elbow, and covered with a piece of the common black ſticking plaſter, and kept on for eight or ten days. This will ſeldom fail to communicate the diſeaſe. We mention this method becauſe many people are afraid of a wound; and doubtleſs the more eaſily the operation can be performed, it has the greater chance to become general. Some people imagine, that the diſcharge from a wound leſſens the eruption; but there is not much ſtreſs to be laid upon this notion: Beſides, deep wounds often ulcerate, and become troubleſome.

We do not find that inoculation is at all conſidered as a medical operation in thoſe countries from whence we learned it. In Turkey it is performed by the women, and in the Eaſt Indies by the Brachmins or Prieſts. In this country the cuſtom is ſtill in its infancy; we make no doubt however but it will become ſo familiar, that parents will think no more of inoculating their own children than at preſent they do of giving them a doſe of phyſic.

No ſet of men have it ſo much in their power to render the practice of inoculation general as the clergy, the greateſt oppoſition to it ſtill ariſing from ſome ſcruples of conſcience, which they alone can remove. We would recommend it to them not only to endeavour to remove the religious objections which weak minds may have to this ſalutary practice, but to enjoin it as a duty, and to point out the danger of neglecting to make uſe of a mean which Providence has put in our power for ſaving the

lives

lives of our offspring. Surely ſuch parents as wilfully neglect the means of ſaving their children alive, are as guilty as thoſe who put them to death. We wiſh this matter were duly weighed. No one is more ready to make allowance for human weakneſs and religious prejudices, yet I cannot help recommending it, in the warmeſt manner, to parents to conſider how great an injury they do their children, by neglecting to give them this diſeaſe in the early period of life.

THE numerous advantages attending inoculation of the ſmall pox, have been pretty fully pointed out by the learned Dr M'Kenzie in his hiſtory of health: "Many and great, ſays this humane author, are the dangers attending the natural infection, from all which the inoculation is quite ſecure. The natural infection may invade weak or diſtempered bodies, by no means diſpoſed for its kindly reception. It may attack them at a ſeaſon of the year either violently hot or intenſely cold. It may be communicated from a ſort of ſmall pox impregnated with the utmoſt virulence. It may lay hold upon people unexpectedly, when a dangerous ſort is imprudently imported into a maritime place. It may ſurpriſe us ſoon after exceſſes committed in luxury, intemperance or lewdneſs. It may likewiſe ſeize on the innocent after indiſpenſible watchings, hard labour, or neceſſary journies. And is it a trivial advantage, that all theſe unhappy circumſtances can be prevented ed by inoculation? By inoculation numbers are ſaved from deformity as well as from death. In the natural ſmall pox, how often are the fineſt features, and the moſt beautiful complexions miſerably disfigured? Whereas inoculation rarely leaves any ugly marks or ſcars, even where the number of puſtules on the face have been very conſiderable, and the ſymptoms by no means favourable. And many other grievous complaints, that are frequently ſubſequent to the natural ſort, ſeldom follow the artificial. Does not inoculation alſo prevent thoſe inexpreſſible terrors that perpetually haraſs perſons who never had this diſeaſe, inſomuch that when the ſmall pox is epidemical, intire villages are depopulated, markets ruined, and the face of diſtreſs ſpread over the whole country? From this terror it ariſes, that juſtice is frequently poſtponed, or diſcouraged at ſeſſions or aſſizes where the ſmall pox rages. Witneſſes and juries dare not appear; and, by reaſon of the neceſſary abſence of ſome gentlemen our honourable and uſeful judges are not attended with that reverence and ſplendor due to their office and merit. Does not inoculation in like manner prevent our brave ſailors from being ſeized with this diſtemper on ſhipboard, where they muſt quickly ſpread the infection among ſuch of the crew who never had it before, and where they have ſcarce any chance to eſcape, being half-ſtifled with the cloſeneſs of their cabins, and but very indifferently nurſed?

ſed? Laſtly, With regard to the ſoldiery, the miſeries attending theſe poor creatures, when attacked by the ſmall pox on a march, is inconceivable, without attendance, without lodgings, without any accommodations; ſo that one of three commonly periſhes."

We ſhall only add, that ſuch as have not had the ſmall pox in the early period of life, are not only rendered unhappy, but likewiſe, in a great meaſure, unfit for ſuſtaining many of the moſt uſeful and important offices. Few people would chuſe even to hire a ſervant who had not had the ſmall pox, far leſs to purchaſe a ſlave who had the chance of dying of this diſeaſe. How could a phyſician or a ſurgeon, who had never had the ſmall pox himſelf, attend others under that malady? Thus, beſides, the continual fears and anxiety which haunt thoſe perſons who have not had the ſmall pox, we might ſhew numberleſs inconveniencies which ariſe from it. For example,

How deplorable is the ſituation of females, who arrive at mature age without having had the ſmall pox! A woman with child ſeldom ſurvives this diſeaſe: And if an infant happens to be ſeized with the ſmall pox upon the mother's breaſt who has not had the diſeaſe herſelf, the ſcene muſt be diſtreſſing! If ſhe continues to ſuckle the child, it is at the peril of her own life; and if ſhe weans it, in all probability it will periſh. How often is the affectionate mother forced to leave her houſe, and abandon

abandon her children, at the very time when her care is moſt neceſſary? But ſhould parental affection get the better of her fears, the conſequences will often prove fatal. I have known the tender mother and her infant-child laid in the ſame grave, both untimely victims to this dreadful malady. But theſe are ſcenes too ſhocking even to mention. Let parents who run away with their children to avoid the ſmall pox, or who refuſe to inoculate them in infancy, conſider to what deplorable ſituations they may be reduced by this miſtaken tenderneſs.

As the ſmall pox has now become a conſtitutional diſeaſe in moſt parts of the known world, no other choice remains but to render the malady as mild as poſſible; that is the only manner of extirpation now left in our power; and, tho' it may ſeem paradoxical, this artificial method of planting the diſeaſe, could it be rendered univerſal, would amount to nearly the ſame thing as rooting it out. It is a matter of ſmall conſequence, whether a diſeaſe be entirely extirpated, or rendered ſo mild as neither to deſtroy life nor hurt the conſtitution; but that this may be done by inoculation, does not now admit of a doubt. The numbers who die under inoculation hardly deſerve to be named. In the natural way, one in four or five generally die; but by inoculation not one of a thouſand. Nay ſome can boaſt of having inoculated ten

ten thousand without the loss of a single patient.

I have often wished to see some plan established for rendering this salutary practice universal; but am afraid I shall never be so happy. The difficulties indeed are many; yet the thing is by no means impracticable. The aim is great; no less than saving the lives of one fourth of mankind. What ought not to be attempted in order to accomplish such an end?

THE first step towards rendering the practice universal, must be to remove the religious prejudices against it. This, as already observed, can only be done by the clergy. They must not only recommend it as a duty to others, but likewise practice it on their own children. Example will ever have more influence than precept.

THE next thing requisite is to put it in the power of all. For this purpose we would recommend it to the Faculty to inoculate the children of the poor *gratis*. It is hard that those who are certainly the most useful part of mankind should, by their poverty, be excluded from such a benefit.

SHOULD this fail, it is surely in the power of any State to render the practice general, at least as far as their dominion extends. We do not mean, that it ought to be inforced by a law: That, there is reason to believe, would rather tend to obstruct its progress. The way to promote it it would be to employ a ſufficient number of operators at the public expence to inoculate the children of the poor. This would only be neceſſary till the practice became general; afterwards cuſtom, the ſtrongeſt of all laws, would oblige every one to inoculate their children to prevent reflections.

It may be objected to this ſcheme, that the poor would refuſe to employ the inoculators: That is eaſily removed. A ſmall premium to enable mothers to attend their children while under the diſeaſe, would be a ſufficient inducement; beſides, the ſucceſs attending the operation would ſoon baniſh all objections to it. Even conſiderations of profit would induce the poor to embrace this plan. They often bring up their children to the age of ten or twelve, and when they come to be uſeful, they are ſnatched away by this malady, to the great loſs of their parents and detriment of the public.

The Britiſh legiſlature has, of late years, ſhown great attention to the preſervation of infant-lives, by ſupporting the foundling-hoſpital, &c. But we will venture to ſay, if one tenth part of the ſums laid out in ſupporting that inſtitution, had been beſtowed towards promoting the practice of inoculation of the ſmall pox among the poor, that not only more uſeful lives had been ſaved, but the practice ere now rendered quite univerſal in this iſland. It is not to be imagined what effect example and a little

little money will have upon the poor; yet, if left to themſelves, they will go on for ever in the old way, without thinking of any improvement. We only mean this as a hint to the humane and public-ſpirited. Should ſuch a ſcheme be ever put in practice, a proper plan might eaſily be laid down for the execution of it.

As all public plans are very difficult to bring about, and often, by the ſelfiſh views or miſconduct of thoſe intruſted with the execution of them, fail of anſwering the noble purpoſes for which they were deſigned: We ſhall therefore point out ſome other methods by which the benefits of inoculation may be extended to the poor.

There is no doubt but inoculators will be daily more numerous. We would therefore have every pariſh in Britain to allow one of them a ſmall annual ſalary for inoculating all the children of the pariſh at a proper age. Tho' ſome refractory perſons might for a while object to this method, they would ſoon be obliged to comply with it, or run the hazard of being reckoned the murderers of their own children.

Two things chiefly operate to prevent the progreſs of inoculation. The one is a wiſh to put the evil day as far off as poſſible. This is a principle in our nature; and as inoculation ſeems rather to be anticipating a future evil, it is no wonder mankind are ſo averſe from it. But this objection is ſufficiently anſwered by the ſucceſs. Who in his ſenſes would not prefer a leſſer evil to-day to a greater to-morrow, provided it were equally certain?

The other obſtacle is the fear of reflections. This has very great weight with the bulk of mankind. Should the child die, they think the world would look down upon them. This they cannot bear. Here lies the difficulty which pinches, and till that be removed, inoculation will make but ſmall progreſs. Nothing can remove it but cuſtom. Make the practice faſhionable, and all objections at once vaniſh. It is faſhion alone that has led the multitude ſince the beginning of the world, and will lead them to the end. We muſt therefore call upon the more enlightened part of mankind to ſet a pattern to the reſt. Their example, tho' it may for ſome time meet with oppoſition, muſt at length infallibly prevail.

I am aware of an objection to this practice from the expence with which it may be attended; this is eaſily obviated. We do not mean that every pariſh ought to employ a Sutton or a Dimſdale as inoculators. Theſe have, by their ſucceſs, already recommended themſelves to crowned heads, and are beyond the vulgar reach; but have not others an equal chance to ſucceed? They certianly have. Let them make the ſame trial, and the difficulties will ſoon vaniſh. There is not a pariſh, and hardly a village in Britain, deſtitute of ſome perſon who can bleed. But this is a far more difficult

ficult operation, and requires both more ſkill and time than inoculation.

The perſons to whom we would chiefly recommend the performance of this operation are the clergy. Moſt of them know ſomething of medicine. Almoſt all of them bleed, and can order a purge, which are all the qualifications neceſſary for the practice of inoculation. The Prieſts among the leſs enlightened Indians perform this office, and why ſhould a Chriſtian teacher think himſelf above it? Surely the bodies of men, as well as their ſouls, merit a part of the paſtor's care; at leaſt the greateſt Teacher who ever appeared among men ſeems to have thought ſo.

Should all other methods fail, we would recommend it to parents to perform the operation themſelves Let them take any method of communicating the diſeaſe they pleaſe, provided the ſubject be healthy, and of a proper age; and we may venture to warrant their ſucceſs. I have known many inſtances of parents performing the operation, and never ſo much as heard of one bad conſequence. A planter in one of the Weſt India iſlands is ſaid to have inoculated, with his own hand, in one year, three hundred of his ſlaves, who, notwithſtanding the warmth of the climate, and other unfavourable circumſtances, all did well. Common mechanics have often, to my knowledge, performed the operation with as good ſucceſs as phyſicians. We do not however mean to diſcourage

thoſe

thofe who have it in their power from employing people of ſkill to inoculate their children, and attend them while under the diſeaſe, but only to ſhew, that where ſuch cannot be had, the operation ought not upon that account to be neglected.

INSTEAD of multiplying arguments to this effect, I ſhall juſt beg leave to mention the method which I took with my own child, an only ſon. After giving him two gentle purges, I ordered the nurſe to take a bit of thread which had been previouſly wet with freſh matter from a pock, and to lay it upon his arm, covering it with a piece of ſticking plaſter. This ſtaid on ſix or ſeven days, till it was rubbed off by accident. At the uſual time the ſmall pox made their appearance, and were exceedingly favourable. Sure this, which is all that is neceſſary, may be done without any ſkill in medicine.

THE beſt ſeaſon of the year for inoculation is towards the end of the ſpring, and in the beginning of ſummer. It may however be done at any time of the year, if circumſtances render it neceſſary.

THE moſt proper age for inoculation is betwixt two and five. Many diſagreeable circumſtances attend inoculating children upon the breaſt, which we have not time to enumerate. Neither ſhould the operation be too long delayed. When the fibres begin to grow rigid, and children make uſe of groſſer food, the ſmall pox become more dangerous.

CHILDREN

CHILDREN who have conſtitutional diſeaſes, muſt nevertheleſs be inoculated. It will often mend the habit of body; but ought to be performed at a time when they are moſt healthy. Accidental diſeaſes ſhould always be removed before inoculation.

THE moſt healthy ſtate is always to be choſen, as that muſt be the beſt preparation. The next ſtep is to regulate the diet for ſome time before the diſeaſe is communicated. In children great alteration in diet is ſeldom neceſſary, their food being commonly of the moſt ſimple and wholeſome kind; as milk, water-pap, ſmall broths, bread, light pudding, mild roots, and white meats.

CHILDREN however who have been accuſtomed to a hotter diet, who are of a groſs habit, or abound with bad humours, ought to be put upon a ſpare diet before they be inoculated. Their food ſhould be of a light cooling nature; and their drink whey, butter-milk, and ſuch like.

WE would recommend no other medicinal preparation but two or three mild purges, which ought to be ſuited to the age and ſtrength of the patient. It is no doubt poſſible by purgative and mercurial medicines, to leſſen the eruption; but it very ſeldom happens, that the eruption in this way proves too great; and we have always obſerved, that thoſe children who had a pretty free eruption, and where the pox filled well, enjoyed the beſt health afterwards.

THE

The regimen during the diſeaſe muſt be the ſame as under the natural ſmall pox. The patient muſt be kept cool, his diet muſt be light, and his drink weak and diluting, &c. Should any bad ſymptoms appear, which ſeldom happens, they muſt be treated in the ſame way as directed in the natural ſmall pox. Purging is not leſs neceſſary after the ſmall pox by inoculation, than in the natural way, and ought by no means to be neglected.

OF THE MEASLES.

The meaſles appeared about the ſame time with the ſmall pox, and are nearly related to that diſeaſe. They both came from the Eaſt, are both infectious, and ſeldom attack people more than once. The meaſles are moſt common in the ſpring-ſeaſon, and generally diſappear in ſummer. The diſeaſe itſelf, when properly managed, is ſeldom dangerous; but its conſequences are often fatal.

CAUSE.—— This diſeaſe, like the ſmall pox, proceeds from infection, and is more or leſs dangerous according to the conſtitution of the patient, the ſeaſon of the year, the climate, &c.

SYMPTOMS.—— The meaſles, like other fevers, are preceded by alternate fits of heat and cold, ſickneſs, and loſs of appetite. The tongue is white, but generally moiſt. There is is a ſhort cough, a heavineſs of the head and eyes, drowſineſs, and running of the noſe. Sometimes indeed the cough does not come before the eruption The eye-lids frequently ſwell ſo as to occaſion blindneſs. The patient generally complains of his throat; and vomiting or looſeneſs often precedes the eruption. The ſtools in children are commonly greeniſh; they complain of an itching of the ſkin, and are remarkably peeviſh. Bleeding at the noſe is common, both before and in the progreſs of the diſeaſe.

About the fourth day, ſmall ſpots, reſembling flea-bites, appear, firſt upon the face, then upon the breaſt, and afterwards on the extremities: Theſe may be diſtinguiſhed from the ſmall pox by their ſcarcely riſing above the ſkin. The fever, cough, and difficulty of breathing, inſtead of being removed by the eruption, as in the ſmall pox, are rather increaſed; but the vomiting generally ceaſes.

About the ſixth day, the meaſles begin to grow dry on the face, and afterwards upon the body; ſo that by the ninth day they entirely diſappear. The fever however and difficulty of breathing often continue, eſpecially if the patient has been kept upon too hot a regimen. Petechiæ, or purple ſpots, may likewiſe be occaſioned by this error.

A violent looſeneſs ſometimes ſucceeds the meaſles; in which caſe the patient's life is in imminent danger.

Such as die of the meafles generally expire about the ninth day, and are evidently carried off by a peripneumony, or inflammation of the lungs.

The moft favourable fymptoms are a moderate loofenefs, gentle fweats, and a plentiful difcharge of urine.

When the eruption fuddenly falls in, and the patient is feized with a delirium, he is in the greateft danger. If the meafles turn of a pale colour, it is an unfavourable fymptom, as are alfo great weaknefs, vomiting, reftlefsnefs, and difficulty of fwallowing. Purple or black fpots appearing among the meafles, are very unfavourable. When a continual cough, with hoarfenefs, fucceeds the difeafe, there is reafon to fufpect an approaching confumption of the lungs.

Our bufinefs in this difeafe is to affift Nature, if her efforts be too languid, in throwing out the morbid matter, by proper cordials; but when they are too violent, they muft be reftrained by evacuations, and cool diluting liquors, &c. We ought likewife to endeavour to appeafe the moft urgent fymptoms, as the cough, reftleffnefs, and difficulty of breathing.

REGIMEN.—— The regimen in this difeafe fhould be of the fame kind with that recommended in the fmall pox, viz. cooling and diluting. Acids however do not anfwer fo well here as in the fmall pox, as they tend to exafperate the cough. Small beer likewife, tho' a good

good drink in the ſmall pox, is here improper. The moſt ſuitable liquors are decoctions of liquorice with marſh mallow roots and ſarſaparilla, infuſions of linſeed, or of the flowers of elder with milk, clarified whey, barley-water, and ſuch like. Theſe, if the belly be bound, may be ſweetened with honey; or, if that ſhould diſagree with the ſtomach, a little manna may occaſionally be added to them.

MEDICINE.—— The meaſles being an inflammatory diſeaſe, without any critical diſcharge of matter, as in the ſmall pox, bleeding is commonly neceſſary, eſpecially when the fever runs high, with difficulty of breathing, and great oppreſſion of the breaſt. But if the diſeaſe be of a mild kind, bleeding may be omitted.

BATHING the feet and legs in lukewarm water both tends to abate the violence of the fever, and to promote the eruption.

THE patient is often greatly relieved by vomiting. When there is a tendency this way, it ought not to be ſtopped, but encouraged by drinking lukewarm water, or weak camomile tea.

WHEN the cough is very troubleſome, with dryneſs of the throat, and difficulty of breathing, it will greatly relieve the patient if he holds his head over the ſteam of warm water, and draws the ſteam into his lungs.

HE may likewiſe lick a little ſperma ceti and

ſugar-candy pounded together; or take now and then a ſpoonful of the oil of ſweet almonds, with ſugar candy diſſolved in it. Theſe will ſoften the throat, and relieve the tickling cough.

In caſe the meaſles ſhould ſuddenly diſappear, it will be neceſſary to purſue the ſame method which we have recommended when the ſmall pox fall in. The patient muſt be ſupported with wine and cordials. Bliſtering plaſters muſt be applied to the extremities, and the body rubbed all over with warm flannels. Warm poultices may likewiſe be applied to the feet and palms of the hands.

When purple or black ſpots appear, the patient's drink ſhould be ſharpened with ſpirits of vitriol; and if the putrid ſymptoms run high, the jeſuits bark muſt be adminiſtered in the ſame manner as directed in the ſmall pox.

Opiates are ſometimes neceſſary, but ſhould never be given except in caſe of extreme reſtleſſneſs, a violent looſeneſs, or when the cough is very troubleſome. For children, the ſyrup of poppies is ſufficient. A tea ſpoonful or two may be occaſionally given, according to the patient's age, or the violence of the ſymptoms.

After the meaſles are gone off, purging is abſolutely neceſſary. This may be conducted in the ſame manner as directed in the ſmall pox.

If a violent looſeneſs ſucceeds the meaſles, it may be checked by taking for ſome days a gentle doſe

dose of rhubarb in the morning, and an opiate over night; but if these do not remove it, bleeding will seldom fail to have that effect.

PATIENTS recovering after the measles should be very careful what they eat or drink. Their food, for some time, should be light, and in small quantities, and their drink diluting, and rather of an opening nature; as butter-milk, whey, and such like. They ought also to beware of exposing themselves to the cold air, lest a suffocating catarrh, an asthma, or a consumption of the lungs should ensue.

SHOULD a cough, with difficulty of breathing, and other symptoms of a consumption, remain after the measles, we would recommend small quantities of blood to be frequently let at proper intervals, as the patient's strength and constitution will bear. He ought likewise to drink asses milk, to remove to a free air, if necessary, and to ride daily on horseback. He must keep close to a diet consisting of milk and vegetables; and lastly, if these do not succeed, let him remove to a warmer climate.

OF THE SCARLET FEVER.

THE scarlet fever is so called from the colour of the patient's skin, which appears as if it were tinged with red wine. It happens at any season of the year, but is most common in the

the latter end of ſummer; at which time it often ſeizes whole families, eſpecially children.

It begins with coldneſs and ſhivering, as in other fevers, without any violent ſickneſs. Afterwards the ſkin is covered with red ſpots, which are broader, more florid, and leſs uniform than the meaſles. They continue two or three days, and then diſappear; after which the cuticle, or ſcarf-ſkin falls off.

There is ſeldom any occaſion for medicine in this diſeaſe. The patient ought however to keep within doors, to abſtain from fleſh, ſtrong liquors, and cordials, and to take plenty of cool diluting drink. If the fever be high, the belly muſt be kept gently open by emollient clyſters, or ſmall doſes of nitre and rhubarb. A ſcruple of the former, with five grains of the latter, may be taken thrice a-day, or oftener if neceſſary.

Children and young perſons are ſometimes ſeized, at the beginning of this diſeaſe, with a kind of ſtupor and epileptic fits. In this caſe the feet and legs ſhould be bathed with warm water, a large bliſtering plaſter applied to the neck, and a doſe of the ſyrup of poppies given every night till the patient recovers.

After the fever is gone off, the patient ought to be purged once or twice.

OF

OF THE ERYSIPELAS, OR ST ANTHONY's FIRE.

THIS diſeaſe, which in many parts of Britain is called *the roſe*, attacks perſons at all periods of life, but is moſt common between the age of thirty and forty. Perſons of a ſanguine or plethoric habit, are moſt liable to it. It often attacks young people, and pregnant women; and ſuch as have once been afflicted with it are very liable to have it again. Sometimes it is a primary diſeaſe, and at other times only a ſymptom of ſome other malady. Every part of the body is liable to be attacked by an eryſipelas, but it moſt frequently ſeizes the legs or face, eſpecially the latter. It prevails moſt in autumn, or when hot weather is ſucceeded by cold and wet.

CAUSES.—— The eryſipelas is frequently occaſioned by violent paſſions or affections of the mind; as fear, anger, &c. It is likewiſe occaſioned by cold. When the body has been heated to a great degree, and is immediately expoſed to the cold air, ſo that the perſpiration is ſuddenly checked, an eryſipelas will often enſue. It may alſo be occaſioned by exceſs of ſtrong liquor, by continuing too long in a warm bath, or by any thing that overheats the blood. If any of the natural evacuations be obſtructed, or in too ſmall quantity, it may cauſe an eryſipelas. The ſame effect will follow from the ſtoppage

ſtoppage of artificial evacuations; as iſſues, ſetons, or the like.

SYMPTOMS.—— The eryſipelas attacks with a violent ſhaking, heat, thirſt, loſs of ſtrength, pain in the head and back, reſtleſſneſs, and a quick pulſe; to which may be added vomiting, and ſometimes a delirium. On the ſecond, third, or fourth day, the part ſwells, becomes red and ſmall puſtules appear; at which time the fever generally abates.

WHEN the eryſipelas ſeizes the foot, the parts contiguous ſwell, the ſkin ſhines; and, if the pain be violent, it will aſcend to the leg, and will not bear to be touched.

WHEN it attacks the face, it ſwells, appears red, and the ſkin is covered with ſmall puſtules filled with clear water. One or both eyes are generally cloſed with the ſwelling; and there is a difficulty of breathing. If the mouth and noſtrils be very dry, and the patient drowſy, there is reaſon to ſuſpect an inflammation of the brain.

IF the eryſipelas affects the breaſt, it ſwells, and becomes exceedingly hard, with great pain, and is apt to ſuppurate. There is a violent pain in the arm-pit on the ſide affected, where an abſceſs is often formed.

THERE is a kind of eryſipelas, which in ſome parts of Britain goes by the name of the *ring-worm*. It frequently attacks children about the region of the navel, where it ſurrounds the body like a girdle, and is not without danger.

THE

THE event of this diſeaſe depends greatly upon the conſtitution of the patient. It is ſeldom dangerous; yet I have known it prove fatal to people in the decline of life, who were of a ſcorbutic habit, or whoſe humours were vitiated by irregular living, or unwholeſome diet.

IF in a day or two the ſwelling ſubſides, the heat and pain ceaſe, the roſy colour turns yellow, and the cuticle breaks and falls off in ſcales, the danger is over.

WHEN the eryſipelas is large, deep, and affects a very ſenſible part of the body, the danger is great. If the red colour changes into black or blue, it will end in a mortification. Sometimes the inflammation cannot be diſcuſſed, but comes to a ſuppuration; in which caſe fiſtulas, a gangrene or mortification, generally enſue. Where the conſtitution was bad, I have frequently ſeen the leg ſwell to a prodigious ſize, and the cure prove extremely difficult.

SUCH as die of this diſeaſe are moſtly carried off by the fever, which is attended with difficulty of breathing, ſometimes with a delirium and great drowſineſs. They generally die about the ſeventh or eight day.

REGIMEN.——In this diſeaſe the patient muſt neither be kept too hot nor cold, as either of theſe extremes will tend to make the diſeaſe retreat, which is always to be guarded againſt. When the diſeaſe is mild, it will be ſufficient to keep

keep the patient within doors, without confining him to his bed, and to promote the perſpiration by diluting liquors, &c.

THE diet ought to be very ſpare, and of a moderately cooling and moiſtening quality; as groat-gruel, panado, ſmall chicken or barley broth, with cooling herbs and fruits, &c. avoiding fleſh, fiſh, ſtrong drink, ſpices, pickles, and all other things that may heat and inflame the blood; the drink may be barley water, an infuſion of elder flowers, common whey, and ſuch like.

BUT if the pulſe be low, and the ſpirits ſunk, the patient muſt be ſupported with ſmall negas, and other things of a cordial nature. His food may be ſago gruel with a little wine, and nouriſhing broths, taken in ſmall quantities, and often repeated. Great care however muſt be had not to overheat him.

MEDICINE.—— In this diſeaſe much miſchief is often done by medicine, eſpecially by external applications. People, when they ſee an inflammation, immediately think of ſome external applications. Theſe indeed are neceſſary in large phlegmons; but in an eryſipelas the ſafer courſe is to apply nothing. Almoſt all ointments, ſalves and plaſters, are of a greaſy nature, and tend rather to obſtruct and repel than promote any diſcharge from the part. At the beginning of this diſeaſe it is neither ſafe to promote a ſuppuration, nor to repel the matter too quickly. The eryſipelas in many reſpects reſembles

resembles the gout, and is to be treated with the greatest caution. Fine wool, or very soft flannel, are the safest applications to the part. These not only defend it from the external air, but likewise promote the perspiration, which has a great tendency to carry off the disease.

It is a common thing to bleed in the erysipelas; but this likewise requires caution. If however the fever be high, the pulse hard and strong, and the patient vigorous, it will be proper to bleed; but the quantity must be regulated by these circumstances, and the operation repeated or not as the symptoms may require. If the patient has been accustomed to strong liquors, and the disease attacks his head, bleeding is absolutely necessary.

Bathing the feet and legs frequently in lukewarm water, when the disease attacks the face or brain, has an excellent effect. It tends to draw the humours from the head towards the inferior extremities, and seldom fails to relieve the patient. When bathing proves ineffectual, poultices, or sharp sinapisms, may be applied to the soles of the feet for the same purpose.

In cases where bleeding is requisite, it is likewise necessary to keep the belly gently open. This may be effected by emollient clysters, or small doses of nitre and rhubarb, such as are prescribed in the foregoing disease. Some indeed recommend very large doses of nitre in this case; but nitre seldom sits easy on the stomach when taken in large quantities. It is however one of the beſt medicines in this caſe, and when the fever and inflammation run high, half a dram of it may be taken in the patient's ordinary drink, three or four times a-day.

THE ſaline julep, as it is called, is likewiſe a very proper medicine in the eryſipelatous fever. It may be made by diſſolving two drams of ſalt of wormwood, or ſalt of tartar, in three ounces of freſh lemon-juice, to which may be added two ounces of common water and an ounce or two of pepper-mint water, with as much white ſugar as will render it agreeable. Of this two table-ſpoonfuls may be taken every two or three hours.

WHEN the eryſipelas leaves the extremities, and ſeizes the head, ſo as to occaſion a delirium or ſtupor, it is abſolutely neceſſary to open the belly. If clyſters and mild purgatives fail to have that effect, ſtronger ones muſt be given. Bliſtering plaſters muſt likewiſe be applied to the neck, or behind the ears, and ſharp cataplaſms laid to the ſoles of the feet.

WHEN the eryſipelas cannot be diſcuſſed, and the pain lies deep, and ſeems to reach to the membrane which covers the bones, and the part has a tendency to ulcerate, it will then be proper to promote ſuppuration, which may be done by the application of ripening poultices with ſaffron, warm fomentations, and ſuch like.

WHEN the black, livid, or blue colour of the part ſhews a tendency to mortification, the jeſuits bark muſt be adminiſtered. It may be taken

taken along with acids, as recommended in the ſmall pox, or in any other form more agreeable to the patient. It muſt not however be trifled with, as the patient's life is at ſtake. Half a dram may be taken every two hours, or oftener, if the ſymptoms be threatening, and cloths dipped in warm camphorated ſpirits of wine, or the tincture of myrrh and aloes, may be applied to the part, and frequently renewed.

IN what is commonly called the ſcorbutic eryſipelas, which continues for a conſiderable time, it will only be neceſſary to give gentle laxatives, and ſuch things as purify the blood. Medicines which promote the perſpiration are likewiſe proper. Thus, after the inflammation has been checked by opening medicines, a decoction of the ſudorific woods, as ſaſſafras and guaiacum, with liquorice-root, may be drank, and afterwards a courſe of bitters, which will both ſtrengthen the ſtomach and purify the blood.

SUCH as are liable to frequent attacks of the eryſipelas ought carefully to guard againſt all violent paſſions; to abſtain from ſtrong liquors, and all fat, viſcid, and highly nouriſhing food. They ſhould take abundance of exerciſe, carefully avoiding the extremes of heat or cold. Their food ſhould conſiſt chiefly of milk, and ſuch fruits, herbs, and roots, as are of a cooling quality; and their drink ought to be ſmall beer, whey, butter milk, and ſuch like.

like. They ſhould never ſuffer themſelves to be too long coſtive. If that cannot be prevented by diet alone, it will be proper to take frequently a gentle doſe of rhubarb and cream of tartar, the lenitive electuary, or ſome other mild purgative.

OF THE INFLAMMATION OF THE BRAIN.

THIS is ſometimes a primary diſeaſe, but oftener only a ſymptom of ſome other malady; as the inflammatory, eruptive, or ſpotted fever, &c. It is very common however as a primary diſeaſe in warm climates, and is moſt incident to perſons about the prime or vigour of life. The paſſionate, the ſtudious, and thoſe whoſe nervous ſyſtem is weak, are very liable to it.

CAUSES.—— This diſeaſe is often occaſioned by night-watching, eſpecially when joined with hard ſtudy: It likewiſe proceeds from hard drinking, from anger, grief, or anxiety. It may alſo be occaſioned by a ſedentary life, or the ſtoppage of uſual evacuations; as the bleeding piles in men, the cuſtomary diſcharges of women, &c. Such as imprudently expoſe themſelves to the heat of the ſun, eſpecially by ſleeping without doors in a hot ſeaſon, with their heads uncovered, are often ſuddenly ſeized with

with an inflammation of the brain, ſo as to awake quite delirious. When repellents are imprudently uſed in an eryſipelas, an inflammation of the brain is often the conſequence. It may likewiſe be occaſioned by external injuries, as blows or bruiſes upon the head, &c.

SYMPTOMS.—— The ſymptoms which precede a true inflammation of the brain are, pain of the head, redneſs of the eyes, a violent fluſhing of the face, diſturbed ſleep, or a total want of it, great dryneſs of the ſkin, coſtiveneſs, a retention of urine, a ſmall dropping of blood from the noſe, ſinging of the ears, and extreme ſenſibility of the nervous ſyſtem.

WHEN the inflammation is formed, the ſymptoms in general are ſimilar to thoſe of the inflammatory fever. The pulſe indeed is often weak, irregular, and trembling; but ſometimes it is hard and contracted. When the brain itſelf is inflamed, the pulſe is always ſoft and low; but when the inflammation only affects the integuments of the brain, it is hard. A remarkable quickneſs of hearing is a common ſymptom of this diſeaſe; but that ſeldom continues long. Another uſual ſymptom is a great throbbing or pulſation in the arteries of the neck and temples. The tongue is often black and dry; yet the patient ſeldom complains of thirſt, and even refuſes drink. The mind chiefly runs after ſuch objects as have before made a deep impreſſion upon it; and ſometimes, from a ſullen a ſullen ſilence, the patient becomes all of a ſudden quite outrageous.

A conſtant trembling and ſtarting of the tendons, is an unfavourable ſymptom, as alſo a ſuppreſſion of urine; a total want of ſleep; a conſtant ſpitting; a grinding of the teeth, which muſt be conſidered as a kind of convulſion. When this diſeaſe ſucceeds an inflammation of the lungs, of the inteſtines, or of the throat, &c. it is owing to a tranſlation of the morbific matter from theſe parts to the brain, and generally proves fatal. Hence we learn the neceſſity of proper evacuations, and the danger of repellents in all inflammatory diſeaſes.

The favourable ſymptoms are, a free perſpiration or ſweating, a copious diſcharge of blood from the noſe, the bleeding piles, a plentiful diſcharge of urine which lets fall a copious ſediment. Sometimes the diſeaſe is carried off by a looſeneſs, and in women by an exceſſive flow of the *menſes*.

As this diſeaſe often proves fatal in a few days, it requires the moſt ſpeedy applications. When it is prolonged, or improperly treated, it ſometimes ends in madneſs, or a kind of ſtupidity, which continues for life.

In the cure, two things are chiefly to be attended to, viz. to leſſen the quantity of blood in the brain, and to retard the circulation towards the head.

REGIMEN.—— The patient ought to be kept very quiet. Company, noiſe, and every thing

thing that affects the ſenſes, or diſturbs the imagination, increaſes the diſeaſe. Even too much light is hurtful; for which reaſon the patient's chamber ought be a little darkened, and he ſhould neither be kept too hot nor cold. It is not however neceſſary to exclude the company of an agreeable friend, as this has a tendency to ſooth and quiet the mind. Neither ſhould the patient be kept too much in the dark, leſt it ſhould occaſion a gloomy melancholy, which is too often the conſequence of this diſeaſe.

THE patient muſt, as far as poſſible, be ſoothed and humoured in every thing. Contradiction will ruffle his mind, and increaſe his malady. Even when he calls for things which are not to be obtained, or which might prove hurtful, he is not to be poſitively denied them, but rather put off with the promiſe of having them as ſoon as they can be obtained, or by ſome other excuſe. A little of any thing that the mind is ſet upon, tho' not quite proper, will hurt the patient leſs than a poſitive refuſal. In a word, whatever the patient is fond of, or uſed to be delighted with when in health, may here be tried, as pleaſing ſtories, ſoft muſic, or whatever has a tendency to ſooth the paſſions, and compoſe the mind. Boerhaave propoſes ſeveral mechanical experiments for this purpoſe; as the ſoft noiſe of water diſtilling by drops into a baſon, and the patient trying to reckon them, &c. Any uniform ſound, it low and continued,

tinued, has a tendency to procure ſleep, and conſequently may be of ſervice.

THE aliment ought to be light of farinaceous ſubſtances; as panado, and water-gruel ſharpened with jelly of currants, or juice of lemons, ripe fruits roaſted or boiled, jellies, preſerves, &c. The drink ſmall, diluting, and cooling; as whey, barley-water, or decoctions of barley, and tamarinds which latter not only renders the liquor more palatable, but likewiſe more beneficial, as they are of an opening cooling nature.

MEDICINES.—— In an inflammation of the brain, nothing more certainly relieves the patient than a free diſcharge of blood from the noſe. When this comes of its own accord, it is by no means to be ſtopped, but promoted, by applying cloths dipped in warm water to the part. When bleeding at the noſe does not happen ſpontaneouſly, it may be provoked by putting a ſtraw, or any other ſharp body up the noſtril.

BLEEDING in the temporal arteries greatly relieves the head; but as this operation cannot be generally performed, we would recommend in its ſtead bleeding in the jugular veins. When the patient's pulſe and ſpirits are ſo low, that he cannot bear bleeding with the lancet, leeches may be applied to the temples. Theſe not only draw off the blood more gradually, but by being applied nearer to the part affected, generally give more immediate relief.

A

A difcharge of blood from the hæmorrhoidal veins is likewife of great fervice, and ought by all means to be promoted. If the patient has been fubject to the bleeding piles, and that difcharge has been ftopped, every method muft be tried to reftore it; as the application of leeches to the parts, fitting over the fteams of warm water, fharp clyfters or fuppofitories made of honey, aloes, and rock-falt.

If the inflammation of the brain be occafioned by the ftoppage of any evacuation, either natural or artificial, as the menfes, iffues, fetons, or fuch like, all means muft be ufed to reftore it as foon as poffible, or to fubftitute fome other in its ftead.

If the patient be coftive, his belly muft be kept open by emollient clyfters, or gentle purgatives; as manna, rhubarb, cream of tartar, or fuch like. Thefe may either be given feparately or together in fmall dofes, and repeated as there may be occafion.

Small quantities of nitre ought frequently to be mixed with the patient's drink. Two drams, or more, if the cafe be dangerous, may be ufed every twenty-four hours.

The head fhould be fhaven, and frequently rubbed with vinegar and rofe-water a little warm. Cloths dipped in it may likewife be applied to the temples.

If the difeafe proves obftinate, and does not yield to thefe medicines, it will be neceffary to apply a bliftering plafter to the whole head.

OF THE INFLAMMATION OF THE EYES.

THIS diſeaſe may be occaſioned by external injuries; as ſtrokes, duſt thrown into the eyes, &c. It is often cauſed by the ſtoppage of cuſtomary evacuations; as the healing of old ſores, drying up of iſſues, or the like. Nothing more certainly brings on an inflammation of the eyes than the ſuppreſſing of gentle morning ſweats, or the ſweating of the feet. Long expoſure to the night-air, eſpecially in cold northerly wind, or whatever ſuddenly checks the perſpiration, eſpecially after the body has been much heated, is very apt to cauſe an inflammation of the eyes. Viewing ſnow or other white bodies for a long time, or looking ſtedfaſtly at the ſun, a clear fire, or any bright object, will likewiſe occaſion this malady. A ſudden tranſition from darkneſs to very bright light will often have the ſame effect.

NOTHING more certainly occaſions an inflammation of the eyes than night-watching, eſpecially reading or writing by candle-light. Drinking ſpirituous liquors and exceſs of venery, are very hurtful to the eyes. The acrid fumes of metals, and of ſeveral kinds of feuel, are likewiſe very pernicious. Sometimes an inflammation of the eyes proceeds from a venereal taint, and often from a ſcrophulous or gouty habit. It may likewiſe be occaſioned by hairs in in the eye lids turning inwards, and hurting the eyes. Sometimes the diſeaſe is epidemic, eſpecially after wet ſeaſons; and I have frequently known it prove infectious, particularly to thoſe who lived in the ſame houſe with the patient. It may be occaſioned by moiſt air, or living in low, damp houſes, eſpecially where people are not accuſtomed to ſuch ſituations. In children, it often proceeds from imprudently drying up of ſcabbed heads, a running behind the ears, or any other diſcharge of the ſame nature. Inflammations of the eyes often ſucceed the ſmall pox or meaſles, eſpecially in children of a ſcrophulous habit.

SYMPTOMS.—— An inflammation of the eyes is attended with acute pain, heat, redneſs, and ſwelling. The patient is not able to bear the light, and ſometimes he feels a pricking pain, as if his eyes were pierced with a thorn. Sometimes he imagines his eyes are full of motes, or thinks he ſees flies dancing before him. The eyes are filled with a ſcalding rheum, which ruſhes forth in great quantities whenever the patient attempts to look up. The pulſe is generally quick and hard, with ſome degree of fever. When the diſeaſe is violent, the neighbouring parts ſwell, and there is a throbbing or pulſation in the temporal arteries, &c.

A ſlight inflammation of the eyes, eſpecially from an external cauſe, is eaſily cured; but when the diſeaſe is violent, and continues long, it it leaves ſpecks upon the eyes, or dimneſs of ſight, and ſometimes total blindneſs.

If the patient be ſeized with a looſeneſs, it has a good effect; and when the inflammation paſſes from one eye to another, as it were by infection, it is no unfavourable ſymptom. When the diſeaſe is accompanied with a violent pain of the head, and continues long, the patient is in great danger of loſing his ſight.

REGIMEN.—— The diet, unleſs in ſcrophulous caſes, can hardly be too ſpare, eſpecially at the beginning. The patient muſt abſtain from every thing of a heating nature. His food muſt conſiſt chiefly of mild vegetables, weak broths, and gruels. His drink may be barley-water, balm-tea, common whey, and ſuch like.

The patient's chamber muſt be darkened, or his eyes ſhaded by a green cover, ſo as to exclude the light, but not to preſs upon the eyes. He ſhould not look at a candle, the fire, or any luminous object; and ought to avoid all ſmoak, as the fumes of tobacco, or any thing that may cauſe coughing, ſneezing, or vomiting. He ſhould be kept quiet, avoiding all violent efforts, either of body or mind, and encouraging ſleep as much as poſſible.

MEDICINE.—— This is one of thoſe diſeaſes wherein great hurt is done by external applications. Almoſt every perſon pretends to be poſſeſſed of a remedy for the cure of ſore eyes. Theſe remedies generally conſiſt of eye-waters and ointments, with other external applications,

plications All which do mifchief twenty times for once they do good. People ought therefore to be very cautious how they ufe fuch things, as the very preffure upon the eyes often increafes the malady.

BLEEDING, in a violent inflammation of the eyes, is always neceffary. This fhould be performed as near the part affected as poffible. An adult may lofe ten or twelve ounces of blood from the jugular vein, and the operation may be repeated according to the urgency of the fymptoms. If it be not however convenient to bleed in the neck, the fame quantity may be let from the arm, or any other part of the body.

LEECHES are often applied to the temples, or under the eyes, with good effect. The wounds muft be fuffered to bleed for fome hours, and if the bleeding ftop foon, it may be promoted by the application of cloths dipt in warm water. In obftinate cafes, it will be neceffary to repeat this operation feveral times.

OPENING and diluting medicines are by no means to be neglected. The patient may take a fmall dofe of Glauber's falts and cream of tartar, every fecond or third day, or a decoction of tamarinds with fenna. If thefe be not agreeable, gentle dofes of rhubarb and nitre, a little of the lenitive electuary, or any other mild purgative, will anfwer the fame end. The patient at the fame time muft drink freely of water-gruel, tea, or any other weak diluting liquor.

liquor. He ought likewiſe to take, at bed-time, a large draught of very weak wine-whey, in order to promote perſpiration. His feet and legs muſt frequently be bathed in lukewarm water, and his head ſhaved twice or thrice a-week, and afterwards waſhed in cold water. This has often a remarkably good effect.

After theſe evacuations have been continued for ſome time, if the inflammation does not yield to them, bliſtering plaſters muſt be applied behind the ears, to the temples, or upon the neck, and kept open for ſome time by the mild bliſtering ointment. I never knew theſe, if long enough kept open, fail to remove the moſt obſtinate inflammation of the eyes; but, for this purpoſe, it is often neceſſary to continue the diſcharge for ſeveral weeks.

When the diſeaſe has been of long ſtanding, I have ſeen very extraordinary effects from a ſeton in the neck, or betwixt the ſhoulders, eſpecially the latter. It ſhould be put upwards and downwards, or in the direction of the ſpine, and in the middle between the ſhoulder-blades. It may be dreſſed twice a-day with yellow baſilicon. I have known patients, who had been blind for ſeveral months, recover ſight by means of a ſeton betwixt the ſhoulders. When the ſeton is put a-croſs the neck, it ſoon wears out, and is both more painful and troubleſome than between the ſhoulders; beſides, it leaves a diſagreeable mark, and does not diſcharge ſo freely.

When

WHEN the heat and pain of the eyes is very great, a soft poultice of bread and milk, with plenty of sweet oil or fresh butter, may be applied to them, at least all night; and they may be bathed with lukewarm milk and water every morning.

IF the patient cannot sleep, which is sometimes the case, he must take ten or twelve drops of laudanum, or two spoonfuls of the syrup of poppies, over night, more or less according to his age, or the violence of the symptoms.

AFTER the inflammation is gone off, if the eyes still remain weak and tender, they may be bathed every night and morning with cold water and a little brandy, six parts of the former to one of the latter. A method should be contrived by which the eye can be quite immersed in the brandy and water, where it should be kept for some minutes. I have generally found this as good a strengthener of the eyes as any of the most celebrated collyriums.

WHEN an inflammation of the eyes proceeds from a scrophulous habit, it generally proves very obstinate. In this case the patient's diet must not be too low, and he may be allowed to drink small negas, or now and then a glass of wine. The most proper medicine is the jesuits bark, which may either be given in substance, or prepared in the following manner:

TAKE an ounce of jesuits bark in powder, with two drams of Winter's bark, and boil them in an English quart of water to a pint; when it has boiled nearly long enough, add half an ounce of liquorice root sliced. Let the liquor be strained. Two, three, or four table-spoonfuls, according to the age of the patient, may be taken three or four times a-day. It is impossible to say how long this medicine should be continued, as the cure is sooner performed in some than others; but in general it requires a considerable time to produce any lasting effects.

Dr Cheyne says, 'That æthiops mineral never fails in inflammations of the eyes, even scrophulous ones, if given in a sufficient dose, and persisted in for a sufficient time.' Both this and other mercurial preparations, are no doubt proper when the disease proves obstinate; more especially when there is reason to suspect, that it may proceed from a venereal taint; but as these medicines can never be safely administered unless under the direction of a physician, we shall omit specifying their particular doses, &c.

It will be proper frequently to look into the eyes, to see if any hairs be turned inwards, or pressing upon them, in order that they may be cut off without delay.

Such as are liable to frequent returns of this disease, ought constantly to have an issue in one or both arms. Bleeding or purging in the spring and autumn, will be very beneficial to such persons. They ought likewise to live regularly,

gularly, avoiding ſtrong liquor, and every thing of a heating quality. Above all, let them avoid the night-air and late ſtudies.

OF THE QUINSEY, OR INFLAMMATION OF THE THROAT.

THIS diſeaſe is very common in Britain, and is frequently attended with great danger. It prevails in the winter and ſpring, and is moſt fatal to young people of a ſanguine or plethoric habit.

CAUSES.—— In general it proceeds from the ſame cauſes as other inflammatory fevers, viz. an obſtructed perſpiration, or whatever heats or inflames the blood. An inflammation of the throat is often occaſioned by omitting ſome part of the covering uſually worn about the neck, by drinking cold liquor when the body is warm, by riding or walking againſt a cold northerly wind, or any thing that greatly cools the throat, and parts adjacent. It may likewiſe proceed from the neglect of bleeding, purging, or any cuſtomary evacuation.

SINGING, ſpeaking loud and long, or whatever ſtrains the throat, may likewiſe cauſe an inflammation of that organ. I have often known the quinſey prove fatal to jovial companions, after ſitting long in a warm room, drinking hot liquors and ſinging with vehemence; eſpecially when they were ſo imprudent as afterwards to go abroad in the cold night-air. Sitting with wet feet, or keeping on wet cloaths, are very apt to occasion this malady. It is likewise frequently occasioned by continuing long in a moist place, sleeping in a damp bed, sitting in a room that has been newly plastered, &c. I know people who never fail to complain of their throat after sitting but a very short while in a room that has been lately washed.

ACRID or irritating food may likewise inflame the throat, and occasion a quinsey. It may also proceed from bones, pins, or other sharp substances sticking in the throat, or from the caustic fumes of metals or minerals, as arsenic, antimony, &c. taken in by the breath. This disease is sometimes epidemic and infectious.

SYMPTOMS.—— The inflammation of the throat is evident from inspection, the parts appearing red and swelled; besides, the patient complains of pain in swallowing any thing. His pulse is quick and hard, with other symptoms of a fever. If blood be let, it is generally covered with a tough coat of a whitish colour, and the patient spits a tough phlegm. As the swelling and inflammation increase, the breathing and swallowing become the more difficult, the pain affects the ears; the eyes generally appear red, and the face swells. The patient is often obliged to keep himself in an erect posture, being in danger of suffocation; there is a constant nausea, naufea, or inclination to vomit, and the drink, inftead of paffing into the ftomach, is often returned by the nofe. The patient is frequently ftarved at laft, merely from an inability of fwallowing any kind of nourifhment. When the breathing is performed with a hiffing noife, and the pulfe begins to intermit, death is at hand.

As feveral of the organs neceffary for life are affected by this difeafe, it can never be without danger; no time therefore fhould be loft in attempting to remove it, as a little delay often renders it incurable.

WHEN the breathing is laborious, with ftraitnefs of the breaft and anxiety, the danger is great. Tho' the pain of fwallowing be very great, yet while the patient breathes eafy, there is not fo much danger. An external fwelling is no unfavourable fymptom; but if it fuddenly falls, and the morbific matter is thrown upon the breaft, the danger is very great. When a quinfey is the confequence of fome other difeafe, which has already weakened the patient, his fituation is dangerous. A frothing at the mouth, with a fwelled tongue, a pale, ghaftly countenance, and coldnefs of the extremities, are fatal fymptoms.

REGIMEN.—— The regimen in this difeafe is in all refpects the fame as in the pleurify or peripneumony. The food muft be light, and in fmall quantity, and the drink plentiful, weak, and diluting, mixed with acids.

IT

It is highly neceſſary in this diſeaſe, that the patient be kept eaſy and quiet. Violent paſſions of the mind, or great efforts of the body, may prove fatal. He ſhould not even attempt to ſpeak but in a low voice. Such a degree of warmth as to promote a conſtant gentle ſweat is proper. When the patient is in bed, his head ought to be raiſed a little higher than uſual.

It is peculiarly neceſſary that the throat be kept warm; for which purpoſe ſeveral folds of ſoft flannel may be wrapt round the neck: That alone will often remove a ſlight complaint of the throat, eſpecially if applied in due time. We cannot here omit obſerving the propriety of a cuſtom which prevails amongſt the peaſants of this country. When they feel any uneaſineſs of the throat, they wrap a ſtocking about it all night. So effectual is this remedy, that in many places it paſſes for a charm, and the ſtocking is applied with particular ceremonies: The cuſtom however is undoubtedly a good one, and ſhould never be neglected. When the throat has been thus wrapt up all night, it muſt not be expoſed to the cold air through the day, but a handkerchief, or a piece of flannel, kept about it till the inflammation be gone.

The jelly of black currants is a medicine very much in eſteem for complaints of the throat; and indeed the whole *materia medica* cannot afford a better. It ſhould be almoſt conſtantly kept in the mouth, and ſwallowed down leiſurely.

ly. It may likewiſe be mixed in the patient's drink, or taken any other way. When it cannot be obtained, the red currant jelly or the mulberry may be uſed in its ſtead.

GARGLES for the throat are likewiſe very beneficial. They may be made by adding to half an Engliſh pint of the pectoral decoction mentioned page 186. two or three ſpoonfuls of honey, and the ſame quantity of currant jelly. This may be uſed three or four times a-day; and if the patient be troubled with tough viſcid phlegm, the gargle may be made more ſharp and cleanſing, by adding to it a tea ſpoonful of the ſpirits of *ſal ammoniac.* Some recommend gargles made of a decoction of the leaves or bark of the blackberry-buſh; but where the jelly can be had, theſe are unneceſſary.

THERE is no diſeaſe wherein the benefits of bathing the feet and legs in lukewarm water are more apparent: That practice ought therefore never to be neglected. If people were careful to keep warm, to wrap up their throats with flannel, to bathe their feet and legs in warm water, and to uſe a ſpare diet, with diluting liquors, at the beginning of this diſeaſe, it would ſeldom proceed to any great height, or be attended with any danger; but when theſe precautions are neglected, and the diſeaſe becomes violent, more powerful medicines are neceſſary.

MEDICINE.—— An inflammation of the throat being one of the moſt acute and dangerous

gerous diſtempers, which ſometimes takes off the patient in a few hours, the moſt early remedies are with the greateſt care and diligence to be adminiſtered. In the very firſt attack, therefore, when it is violent, it will be proper to bleed in the arm or rather in the jugular vein, and to repeat the operation if the ſymptoms require.

THE belly ſhould likewiſe be gently opened. This may either be done by giving the patient for his ordinary drink a decoction of figs and tamarinds, or ſmall doſes of rhubarb and nitre, as recommended page 292. Theſe may be increaſed according to the age of the patient, and repeated till they have the deſired effect.

I have often known very good effects from a bit of *ſal prunel*, or purified nitre, held in the mouth, and ſwallowed down as it melted. This promotes the diſcharge of *ſaliva*, by which means it anſwers the end of a gargle, while at the ſame it cools the blood, by promoting the diſcharge of urine, &c.

THE throat ought likewiſe to be rubbed twice or thrice a-day with a little of the volatile liniment. This may be made by taking an ounce of oil of ſweet almonds, and half an ounce of ſpirit of hartſhorn, and ſhaking them together in a vial till they be united. I do not remember ever to have ſeen this fail to produce ſome good effects. The throat ſhould be carefully covered with wool or flannel, to prevent the cold from penetrating the ſkin, as this application

plication renders it very tender. Many other external applications are recommended in this diſeaſe, as a ſwallow's neſt, poultices made of the fungus called Jews ears, &c. But as we do not look upon any of theſe to be preferable to a common poultice of bread and milk, we ſhall take no further notice of them.

Blistering upon the neck or behind the ears in violent inflammations of the throat, is very beneficial. After the plaſters are taken off, the parts ought to be kept running by the application of ſharp ointment, till the inflammation is gone; otherwiſe, upon their drying up, the patient will be in danger of a relapſe.

When the patient has been treated as above, a ſuppuration ſeldom happens. This however is ſometimes the caſe in ſpite of all our endeavours to prevent it. When the inflammation and ſwelling continue, and it is evident that a ſuppuration will enſue, it ought to be promoted by drawing the ſteam of warm water into the throat through a tunnel, or the like. Soft poultices ought likewiſe to be applied outwardly, and the patient may keep a roaſted fig conſtantly in his mouth.

It ſometimes happens, before the tumour breaks, that the ſwelling is ſo great, as entirely to prevent any thing from getting down into the ſtomach. In this caſe the patient muſt inevitably periſh, unleſs he can be ſupported in ſome other way. This can only be done by nouriſhing clyſters of broth, or gruel with milk,

milk, &c. Patients have often been ſupported by theſe for ſeveral days, till the tumor has broke; and afterwards they have recovered.

Not only the paſſage of the food, but the breathing is often prevented by the tumor. In this caſe nothing can ſave the patient's life, but opening the *trachea* or wind-pipe. That has been ſo often done with ſucceſs, that no perſon, in ſuch deſperate circumſtances, ought to heſitate a moment about the operation; but as it can only be performed by a ſurgeon, it is not neceſſary here to give any directions about it.

When a difficulty of ſwallowing is not attended with an acute pain or inflammation, it is generally owing to an obſtruction of the glands about the throat, and only requires that the part be kept warm, and the throat frequently gargled with ſomewhat that may gently ſtimulate the glands, as a decoction of figs with vinegar and honey; to which may be added a little muſtard, or a ſmall quantity of ſpirits. But this kind of gargle is never to be uſed where there are ſigns of an inflammation. This ſpecies of *angina* has various names among the common people, as the *pap of the throat*, the falling down of the *almonds of the ears*, &c. Accordingly to remove it, they pull the patient up by the hair of the head, and thruſt their fingers under his jaws, &c.; all which practices are at beſt uſeleſs, and often hurtful.

Those who are ſubject to inflammations of the

the throat, in order to prevent too great a fulneſs of blood and other humours, ought to live temperately. Such as do not chuſe to obſerve this rule, muſt have frequent recourſe to purging and other evacuations, to diſcharge the ſuperfluous humours. They ought likewiſe to beware of catching cold, and ſhould abſtain from aliment and medicines of an aſtringent or ſtimulating nature.

VIOLENT exerciſe, by increaſing the motion and force of the blood, is apt to occaſion an inflammation of the throat, eſpecially if cold liquor be drank immediately after it, or the body ſuffered ſuddenly to cool. Thoſe who would avoid this diſeaſe ought therefore, after ſpeaking aloud, ſinging, running, drinking warm liquor, or doing any thing that may ſtrain the throat, or increaſe the circulation of the blood towards it, to take care to cool gradually, and to wrap plenty of coverings about their necks, &c.

I have often known perſons who had been ſubject to ſore throats, kept entirely free from that complaint by only wearing a ribband, or a bit of flannel, conſtantly about their necks, or by wearing a pair of thicker ſhoes, &c. Theſe may ſeem trifling, but they have great effect. There is danger indeed in leaving them off after perſons have been accuſtomed to them; but ſurely the inconveniency of uſing ſuch things for life is not to be compared with the danger which may attend the neglect of them.

OF THE MALIGNANT QUINSEY, OR PUTRID, ULCEROUS SORE THROAT.

THIS kind of quinſey is but little known in the northern parts of Britain, tho', for ſome time paſt, it has been very fatal in the more ſouthern counties. Children are more ſubject to it than adults, females than males, and the delicate than thoſe who are hardy and robuſt. It prevails moſt in autumn, or after a long courſe of damp, or ſultry weather.

CAUSE.—— This is evidently a contageous diſtemper, and is generally communicated by infection. Whole families, and even entire villages often receive the infection from one perſon. This ought to put people upon their guard againſt going near ſuch patients as labour under the diſorder; as by that means they endanger not only their own lives, but likewiſe thoſe of their friends and connections.

SYMPTOMS.—— It begins with alternate fits of ſhivering and heat. The pulſe is quick, but low and unequal, and generally continues ſo through the whole courſe of the diſeaſe. The patient complains greatly of weakneſs and oppreſſion of the breaſt; his ſpirits are low, and he is apt to faint away when ſet upright; he is troubled with a nauſea, and often with a vomiting or purging. The two latter are moſt common in children. The eyes appear

appear red and watery, and the face ſwells. The urine is at firſt pale and crude; but, as the diſeaſe advances, it turns more of a yellowiſh colour. The tongue is white, and generally moiſt, which diſtinguiſhes this from an inflammatory diſeaſe. Upon looking into the throat it appears ſwelled, and of a florid red colour. Pale or aſh coloured ſpots, however are here and there interſperſed, and ſometimes one broad patch or ſpot, of an irregular figure, and pale white colour, ſurrounded with florid red, only appears. Theſe whitiſh ſpots or ſloughs cover ſo many ulcers underneath.

An efflorеſcence, or eruption upon the neck, arms, breaſt, and fingers, about the ſecond or third day, is a common ſymptom of this diſeaſe. When it appears, the purging and vomiting generally ceaſe.

There is often a ſlight degree of delirium, and the face frequently appears blotted, and the inſide of the noſtrils red and inflamed. The patient complains of a diſagreeable putrid ſmell, and his breath is very offenſive.

The putrid, ulcerous ſore throat may be diſtinguiſhed from the inflammatory by the vomiting and looſeneſs with which it is generally uſhered in; by the foul ulcers in the throat covered with a white or livid coat; and by the exceſſive weakneſs of the patient; with other ſymptoms of a putrid fever.

Unfavourable ſymptoms are, an obſtinate purging, extreme weakneſs, dimneſs of the ſight,

ſight, a livid or black colour of the ſpots, and frequent ſhiverings, with a weak, fluttering pulſe. If the eruption upon the ſkin ſuddenly diſappears, or becomes of a livid colour, with a diſcharge of blood from the noſe or mouth, the danger is very great.

If a gentle ſweat breaks out about the third or fourth day, and continues with a ſlow, firm, and equal pulſe; if the ſloughs caſt off in a kindly manner, and appear clean and florid at the bottom; and if the breathing be ſoft and free, with a lively colour of the eyes, there is reaſon to hope for a ſalutary criſis.

REGIMEN.—— The patient muſt be kept quiet, and, for the moſt part, in bed, as he will be apt to faint when taken out of it. His food muſt be nouriſhing and reſtorative; as ſago-gruel with red wine, jellies, broths, &c. His drink ought to be generous, and of an antiſeptic quality; as red wine negas, white wine whey, and ſuch like.

MEDICINE.—— The medicine in this kind of quinſey is entirely different from that which is proper in the inflammatory. All evacuations, as bleeding, purging, &c. which weaken the patient, muſt be avoided. Cooling medicines, as nitre, and cream of tartar, are likewiſe hurtful. Strengthening cordials alone can be uſed with ſafety; and theſe ought never to be neglected.

If, at the beginning, there be a great nauſea, or inclination to vomit, the patient muſt drink

an

an infuſion of green tea, camomile flowers, or *carduus benedictus*, in order to clean the ſtomach. If theſe be not ſufficient, he may take a few grains of the powder of ipecacoanha, or any other gentle vomit.

IF the diſeaſe be mild, the throat may be gargled with an infuſion of ſage and roſe leaves, to a gill of which may be added a ſpoonful or two of honey, and as much vinegar as will make it agreeably ſharp; but, when the ſymptoms are urgent, the ſloughs large and thick, and the breath very offenſive, the following gargle may be uſed.

To ſix or ſeven ounces of the pectoral decoction, when boiling, add half an ounce of contrayerva root; let it boil for ſome time, and afterwards ſtrain the liquor; to which add two ounces of white wine vinegar, an ounce of fine honey, and an ounce of the tincture of myrrh. This ought not only to be uſed as a gargle, but a little of it ſhould frequently be injected with a ſyringe to clean the mouth, before the patient takes any meat or drink. This method is peculiarly neceſſary for children, who cannot uſe a gargle.

IT will be of great benefit if the patient frequently receives into his mouth, through an inverted funnel, the ſteams of warm vinegar, myrrh, and honey.

WHEN the putrid ſymptoms run high, and the diſeaſe is attended with danger, the only medicine that can be depended upon is the jeſuits

ſuits bark. It may be taken in ſubſtance, if the patient's ſtomach will bear it. If not, an ounce of bark groſsly powdered, with two drams of Virginian ſnake root, may be boiled in an English pint and half of water, to half a pint; to which a tea-ſpoonful of the elixir of vitriol may be added, and an ordinary tea cupful of it taken every three or four hours. Bliſtering plaſters are very beneficial in this diſeaſe, eſpecially when the patient's pulſe and ſpirits are low. They may be applied to the throat, behind the ears, or upon the back-part of the neck.

SHOULD the vomiting prove troubleſome, it will be proper to give the patient two table-ſpoonfuls of the ſaline julep, recommended page 298. every two hours, or oftner, if neceſſary. Tea made of mint and a little cinnamon, will likewiſe be a proper drink, eſpecially if an equal quantity of red wine be mixed with it.

IN caſe of a violent looſeneſs, the ſize of a nutmeg of *diaſcordium*, or the japonic confection, may be taken two or three times a-day, or oftener if neceſſary; and the patient's drink muſt be red wine negas.

IF a diſcharge of blood from the noſe happens, the ſteams of warm vinegar may be received up the noſtrils frequently; and the drink may be ſharpened with ſpirits of vitriol, or tincture of roſes.

IN caſe of a ſtrangury, the belly muſt be fomented

mented with warm water, and emollient clysters given three or four times a-day.

AFTER the violence of the diſeaſe is over, the belly ſhould be opened with mild purgatives; as manna, ſenna, rhubarb, or the like.

IF great weakneſs and dejection of ſpirits, or night-ſweats, with other ſymptoms of a conſumption, ſhould remain after this diſeaſe, we would recommend it to the patient to continue the uſe of the jeſuits bark, with the elixir of vitriol, and to take frequently a glaſs of generous wine. Theſe, together with a milk-diet, and riding on horſeback, are the moſt likely means for recovering his ſtrength.

OF COLDS.

IT has already been obſerved, that colds are the effect of an obſtructed perſpiration; the common cauſes of which we have likewiſe endeavoured to point out, and ſhall not here repeat them. Neither ſhall we ſpend time in enumerating all the various ſymptoms of colds, as they are pretty generally known. It may not however be amiſs to obſerve, that almoſt every cold is a kind of fever, and only differs in degree from ſome of thoſe which have already been treated of.

NO age, ſex, nor conſtitution is exempted from this diſeaſe; neither is it in the power of medicine to prevent it. The inhabitants of every

very climate are liable to catch cold, nor can even the greateſt circumſpection defend them againſt its attacks. Indeed, if the human body could be kept conſtantly in an uniform degree of warmth, ſuch a thing as catching cold would be impoſſible: But as that cannot be effected by any means, the perſpiration muſt be liable to many changes. Such changes however, when ſmall, do not affect the health; but, when exceſſive, they muſt prove hurtful. Hence the great ſecret of preventing colds, lies in avoiding, as far as poſſible, all extremes either of heat or cold.

WHEN oppreſſion of the breaſt, a ſtuffing of the noſe, unuſual wearineſs, or a pain of the head, &c. give ground to believe that the perſpiration is obſtructed, or, in other words, that the perſon has caught cold, he ought immediately to leſſen his diet, at leaſt the uſual quantity of his ſolid food, and to abſtain from all ſtrong liquors. Inſtead of fleſh, fiſh, eggs, milk, and other nouriſhing diet, he may eat light bread-pudding, veal or chicken broth, paps or gruels, and ſuch like. His drink may be water-gruel ſweetened with a little honey; an infuſion of balm, or linſeed ſharpened with the juice of orange or lemon; a decoction of barley and liquorice with tamarinds, or any other cool, diluting acid liquor.

ABOVE all, his ſupper ſhould be light; as ſmall poſſet, or water-gruel ſweetened with honey, and a little toaſted bread in it. If honey ſhould

ſhould diſagree with the ſtomach, the gruel may be ſweetened with treacle or coarſe ſugar, and ſharpened with the jelly of currants. Thoſe who have been accuſtomed to generous liquors may take white wine whey inſtead of gruel, which may be ſweetened as above.

THE patient ought to ly longer than uſual a-bed, and to encourage a gentle ſweat, which is eaſily brought on towards morning, by drinking tea, or any kind of warm diluting liquor. I have often known this practice, in a day or two, carry off a cold, which, in all probability, had it been neglected, would have coſt the patient his life, or have confined him for ſome months to his bed. Would people ſacrifice a little time to eaſe and warmth, and practice a moderate degree of abſtinence when the firſt ſymptoms of a cold appear, we have reaſon to believe, that moſt of the bad effects which flow from an obſtructed perſpiration, might be prevented. But, after the diſeaſe has gathered ſtrength by delay, all attempts to remove it often prove in vain. A pleuriſy, a peripneumony, or a fatal conſumption of the lungs, are the common effects of colds that have either been totally neglected, or treated improperly.

MANY attempt to cure a cold, by getting drunk. But this, to ſay no worſe of it, is a very hazardous and fool hardy experiment. No doubt it may ſometimes ſucceed, by ſuddenly reſtoring the perſpiration; but when there is any degree of inflammation, which is frequently the caſe, ſtrong liquors, inſtead of removing the malady, will increaſe it. By this means a common cold is often converted into an inflammatory fever.

WHEN thoſe who labour for their daily bread have the misfortune to catch cold, they grudge to loſe a day or two, in order to keep themſelves warm, and take a little medicine, by which means the diſorder is often ſo aggravated as to confine them for a long while, or even to render them ever after unable to ſuſtain hard labour. Such of the labouring poor as can afford to take care of themſelves, are often too hardy to do it; they affect to deſpiſe colds, and as long as they can crawl about, ſcorn to be confined by what they call a *common cold.* Hence it comes to paſs, that colds deſtroy ſuch numbers of mankind. Like an enemy deſpiſed, they gather ſtrength from delay, till, at length, they become invincible. We often ſee this verified in travellers, who, rather than loſe a day in the proſecution of their buſineſs, throw away their lives, by purſuing their journey with this diſeaſe upon them, even in the coldeſt ſeaſon.

BUT colds may be too much as well as too little indulged. When a perſon, for a ſlight cold, ſhuts himſelf up in a warm room, and drinks great quantities of warm liquor, it may bring on ſuch a general relaxation of the ſolids as will not be eaſily removed. It will therefore

be

be proper, when the diſeaſe will permit, and the weather is mild, to join to the regimen mentioned above, gentle exerciſe; as walking, riding on horſeback, or in a machine, &c. An obſtinate cold, which no medicine can remove, will yield to a proper courſe of exerciſe when duly perſiſted in.

Bathing the feet and legs every night in warm water has a great tendency to reſtore the perſpiration. But care muſt be taken that the water be not too warm, otherwiſe it will do hurt. It ſhould never be warmer than new milk, and the patient ſhould go immediately to bed after uſing it. Bathing the feet in warm water, lying in bed, and drinking warm water-gruel, or other weak liquors, will ſooner take off a ſpaſm, and reſtore the perſpiration, than all the hot ſudorific medicines in the world. This is all that is neceſſary for removing a common cold; and if this courſe be taken at the beginning, and purſued for a few days, it will ſeldom fail.

But when the ſymptoms do not yield to abſtinence, warmth, and diluting liquors, there is reaſon to fear the approach of ſome other diſeaſe, as an inflammation of the breaſt, an ardent fever, &c. If the pulſe therefore be hard and frequent, the ſkin hot and dry, and the patient complains of his head and breaſt, &c. it will be neceſſary to bleed, and to give the cooling opening powders mentioned page 292. every three or four hours, till they give a ſtool.

It

It will likewiſe be proper to put a bliſtering plaſter on the back, to give two table-ſpoonfuls of the ſaline mixture ordered page 298. every three hours, and, in ſhort, to treat the patient in all reſpects as for a ſlight fever. I have often ſeen this courſe, when obſerved at the beginning, remove the complaint in two or three days, when the patient had all the ſymptoms of an approaching ardent fever, or an inflammation of the breaſt.

OF COUGHS.

A cough is generally the effect of a cold, which has either been improperly treated, or intirely neglected. When it proves obſtinate, there is always reaſon to fear the conſequences, as this ſhews a weak ſtate of the lungs, and is often the forerunner of a conſumption.

If the cough be violent, and the patient young and ſtrong, with a hard quick pulſe, bleeding will be neceſſary, to leſſen the quantity of the humours, and prevent a rupture of the blood veſſels of the lungs, &c.; but in weak and relaxed habits, bleeding rather prolongs the diſeaſe. When the patient ſpits freely, bleeding is unneceſſary, and ſometimes hurtful, as it tends to leſſen that diſcharge

When the cough is not attended with a fever, and the ſpittle is viſcid and tough, ſharp pectoral medicines are to be adminiſtered; as gum

gum ammoniac, ſquills, &c. The ſolution of gum ammoniac may be prepared as directed page 198. and two table-ſpoonfuls of it taken three or four times a day, more or leſs, according to the age and conſtitution of the patient. Squills may be given various ways; Two ounces of the vinegar, the oxymel, or the ſyrup, may be mixed with the ſame quantity of ſpirituous cinnamon water, to which may be added an ounce of common water, and an ounce of balſamic ſyrup. Two table-ſpoonfuls of this mixture may be taken three or four times a-day.

A ſyrup made of equal parts of lemon-juice, honey and ſugar-candy, is likewiſe very proper in this kind of cough. A table-ſpoonful of it may be taken at pleaſure.

WHEN the defluxion is ſharp and thin, theſe medicines rather do hurt. In this caſe gentle opiates, oils, and mucilages are proper. A cup of the infuſion of wild poppy leaves, with marſh mallow roots, or the flowers of coltsfoot, may be taken frequently; or a tea ſpoonful of the paregoric elixir may be put into the patient's drink twice a day. He may likewiſe take an emulſion made of an ounce and half of olive-oil, ſix ounces of water, one ounce of pectoral ſyrup, and a tea-ſpoonful of ſpirits of hartſhorn. Theſe muſt be well ſhaken together, and two table ſpoonfuls of the mixture taken every three or four hours. Fuller's Spaniſh infuſion is alſo a very proper medicine in this caſe, and may be taken, if the above ſhould diſagree

disagree with the patient's stomach. It is made by infusing in an English quart of boiling water, two drams of salt of tartar, half a dram of saffron cut into small pieces, and an ounce of Spanish juice likewise cut small. These must stand in a close vessel for twenty-four hours, in a gentle degree of warmth. Afterwards let the infusion be strained, and a tea-cupful of it taken three or four times a-day.

WHEN a cough is occasioned by acrid humours tickling the throat and *fauces*, the patient should keep some soft pectoral lozenges almost constantly in his mouth; as the Pontefract liquorice cakes, barley-sugar, the Spanish juice, &c. These blunt the acrimony of the humours, and by taking off their stimulating quality, help to appease the cough.

IN obstinate coughs, proceeding from a flux of humours upon the lungs, it will often be necessary, besides expectorating medicines, to have recourse to issues, setons, or some other drain. In this case I have always observed the most happy effects from a Burgundy-pitch plaster applied between the shoulders. I have ordered this simple remedy in the most obstinate coughs, in a great number of cases, and in many different constitutions, without ever knowing it fail, unless where there were evident signs of an ulcer in the lungs. About the bulk of a nutmeg of Burgundy-pitch may be spread thin upon a piece of soft leather, about the size of the hand, and laid between the shoulder-blades. It may be taken off

and

and wiped every three or four days, and ought to be renewed once a fortnight or three weeks. This is indeed a cheap and ſimple medicine, and conſequently apt to be deſpiſed; but we will venture to affirm, that the whole *materia medica* does not afford an application more efficacious in almoſt every kind of cough. It has not indeed an immediate effect; but, if continued long enough, it will ſucceed where moſt other medicines fail.

The only inconveniency attending this plaſter is the itching, which it occaſions in the part to which it is applied; but ſurely this may be diſpenſed with, conſidering the advantage which the patient may expect to reap from the application; beſides, when the itching becomes very uneaſy, the plaſter may be taken off, and the part rubbed with a dry cloth, or waſhed with a little warm milk and water. Some caution indeed is neceſſary in diſcontinuing the uſe of ſuch a plaſter; this however may be ſafely done by making it ſmaller by degrees, and at length quitting it altogether in a warm ſeaſon.

But coughs proceed from many other cauſes beſides defluxions upon the lungs. In theſe caſes the cure is not to be attempted by pectoral medicines. Thus, in a cough proceeding from a foulneſs and debility of the ſtomach, ſyrups, oils, mucilages, and all kind of balſamic medicines do hurt. This cough may be known from one that is owing to a fault in the lungs by this

this mark, that in the latter the patient coughs whenever he inſpires, or draws in his breath fully; but in the former that does not happen.

THE cure of this cough depends chiefly upon cleanſing and ſtrengthening the ſtomach; for which purpoſe gentle vomits and bitter purgatives are moſt proper. Thus, after a vomit or two, the ſacred tincture, as it is called, may be taken for a conſiderable time in the doſe of a table-ſpoonful or two twice a-day, or as often as it is found neceſſary to keep the belly gently open. People may make this tincture themſelves, by infuſing an ounce of *hiera picra* in an Engliſh pint of white wine, letting it ſtand a few days, and then ſtraining it off for uſe.

IN coughs which proceed from a debility of the ſtomach, the jeſuits bark is likewiſe of conſiderable uſe. It may either be chewed, taken in powder, or made into a tincture along with other ſtomachic bitters.

A *nervous cough* can only be removed by change of air, and proper exerciſe; to which may be added the uſe of gentle opiates. A tea-ſpoonful of the paregoric elixir, or two of the ſaponaceous pills may be taken twice a-day. If theſe prove too weak, ten, fifteen, or twenty drops of liquid laudanum, more or leſs, as circumſtances require, may be taken at bed-time, or when the cough is moſt troubleſome. Putting the feet and hands in warm water will often appeaſe the violence of a nervous cough.

WHEN a cough is only the ſymptom of ſome other

other malady, it is in vain to attempt to remove it without firſt curing the diſeaſe from which it proceeds. Thus, when a cough is occaſioned by the cutting of teeth; keeping the belly open, ſcarifying the gums, or whatever facilitates the teething, likewiſe appeaſes the cough. In like manner, when worms occaſion a cough, ſuch medicines as remove theſe will generally cure the cough; as bitter purgatives, oily clyſters, and ſuch like.

WOMEN, during the laſt months of pregnancy, are often greatly afflicted with a cough, which is, generally relieved by bleeding, and keeping the belly open. They ought to avoid all flatulent food, and to wear a looſe eaſy dreſs.

A cough is not only a ſymptom, but is often likewiſe the forerunner of diſeaſes. Thus, the gout is frequently uſhered in by a very troubleſome cough, which affects the patient for ſome days before the coming on of the fit. A paroxyſm of the gout generally removes this cough, which ſhould therefore be promoted, by keeping the extremities warm, drinking warm liquors, and bathing the feet and legs frequently in lukewarm water.

Of the CHIN-COUGH.

THIS cough ſeldom affects adults, but is often epidemical among children. Such children as live upon thin watery diet, who breathe unwholesome air, and have too little exercise, are most liable to this disease, and generally suffer most from it.

THE chin cough is so well known, even to nurses, that no description of it is necessary. Whatever hurts the digestion, obstructs the perspiration, or relaxes the solids, predisposes to this disease: Consequently its cure must depend upon cleaning and strengthening the stomach, bracing the solids, and, at the same time, promoting perspiration, and the different secretions.

THE diet in this disease must be light, and of easy digestion; for children, good bread made into pap or pudding, chicken-broth, with other light spoon meats, are proper; but those who are farther advanced may be allowed sago-gruel, and if the fever be not high, a little boiled chicken, or other white meats. The drink may be penny royal tea, sweetened with honey or sugar candy, small wine whey; or, if the patient be weak, he may sometimes be allowed a little negas.

THE most effectual remedy in this disease is change of air. This often removes the malady even when the change seems to be from a purer to a less wholesome air. This may in some measure depend on the patient's being removed from the place where the infection prevails. Most of the diseases of children are infectious; nor is it at all uncommon to find the chin-cough prevailing

prevailing in one town or village, when another, at a very ſmall diſtance, is quite free from it. But, whatever be the cauſe, we are ſure of the fact. No time ought therefore to be loſt in removing the patient at ſome diſtance from the place where he caught the diſeaſe, and, if poſſible, into a more pure and dry air.

When the diſeaſe proves violent, and the patient is in danger of being ſuffocated by the cough, he ought to be bled, eſpecially if there be a fever with a hard full pulſe. But as the chief intention of bleeding is to prevent a rupture of the blood-veſſels of the lungs, and to render it more ſafe to give vomits, it will ſeldom be neceſſary to repeat the operation; yet if there be ſymptoms of an inflammation of the lungs, a ſecond, or even a third bleeding may be requiſite.

It is a favourable ſymptom when the patient vomits after the fit. This cleans the ſtomach, and greatly relieves the cough. It will therefore be proper to promote this diſcharge, either by camomile tea or lukewarm water; and when theſe are not ſufficient, ſmall doſes of ipecacoanha may be given. A child of three or four years of age may take five or ſix grains; and to others, leſs or more muſt be given according to their age and ſtrength.

It is very difficult to make children drink after a vomit. I have often ſeen them happily deceived, by infuſing a ſcruple or half a dram of the powder of ipecacoanha in a tea-

pot,

pot, with half an Engliſh pint of boiling water. If this be diſguiſed with a few drops of milk and a little ſugar, they will imagine it tea, and drink it very greedily. A ſmall tea-cupful of this may be given every quarter of an hour, or rather every ten minutes, till it operates. When they begin to puke, there will be no occaſion for drinking any more, as the water already on their ſtomach will be ſufficient.

Vomits not only clean the ſtomach, which in this diſeaſe is generally loaded with viſcid phlegm, but they likewiſe promote the perſpiration and other ſecretions; and ought therefore to be repeated according to the obſtinacy of the diſeaſe. They ſhould not however be too ſtrong; gentle vomits frequently repeated are both leſs dangerous, and more beneficial than ſtrong ones.

As the patient is generally coſtive, it will be proper to keep his belly gently open. The beſt medicines for this purpoſe are rhubarb and its preparations, or the ſacred tincture, if the patient can be brought to take it. Of this a tea-ſpoonful or two may be given to a young child twice or thrice a day, as there is occaſion. To ſuch as are farther advanced, the doſe muſt be proportionally increaſed, and repeated till it has the deſired effect Thoſe who cannot be brought to take the bitter tincture, may have an infuſion of ſenna and prunes, ſweetened with manna, coarſe ſugar, or honey; or a few grains of of rhubarb mixed with a ſpoonful or two of ſyrup, or currant jelly, ſo as to diſguiſe the taſte. Moſt children are fond of ſyrups and jellies, and ſeldom refuſe even a bitter medicine when mixed with them.

MANY people believe that oily, pectoral, and balſamic medicines poſſeſs wonderful virtues for the cure of the chin cough, and accordingly exhibite them plentifully to patients of every age and conſtitution, without conſidering that every thing of this nature muſt load the ſtomach, hurt the digeſtion, and of courſe aggravate the diſorder.

THE *miliepedes*, or woodlice, are greatly recommended for the cure of a chin cough. Thoſe who chuſe to make uſe of theſe inſects, may infuſe two ounces of them bruiſed in an Engliſh pint of ſmall white-wine for one night. Afterwards the liquor may be ſtrained thro' a cloth, and a table-ſpoonful of it given to the patient three or four times a day.

OPIATES are ſometimes neceſſary to allay the violence of the cough. For this purpoſe a little of the ſyrup of poppies, or ten, fifteen, or twenty drops, according to the age of the patient, of the paregoric elixir, may be taken in a cup of hyſop or penny royal tea, three or four times a day. An adult may take a table ſpoonful of the ſyrup, or a tea ſpoonful of the elixir.

THE garlic ointment is a well known remedy in North Britain for the chin-cough. It is made by by beating in a mortar garlic with an equal quantity of hogs lard, butter, or oil. With this the ſoles of the feet may be rubbed twice or thrice a-day, or it may be ſpread thin upon a rag, and applied as a plaſter. It ſhould be renewed every night and morning at leaſt, as the garlic ſoon loſes its virtue. This is an exceeding good medicine both in the chin-cough, and in moſt other coughs of an obſtinate nature. It ought not however to be uſed when the patient is very hot or feveriſh, leſt it increaſe theſe ſymptoms.

THE feet ſhould be bathed once every two or three days in warm water; and the Burgundy pitch plaſter, mentioned in page 334. may be applied betwixt the ſhoulders. But when the diſeaſe proves very violent, it will be neceſſary, inſtead of it, to apply a bliſtering plaſter, and to keep the part open for ſome time with iſſue-ointment.

WHEN the diſeaſe is prolonged, and the patient is free of a fever, the jeſuits bark, and other bitters, are the moſt proper medicines. The bark may either be taken in ſubſtance, or in a decoction or infuſion, as is moſt agreeable to the patient. For a child, ten, fifteen, or twenty grains may be given for a doſe, according to the age of the patient. For an adult, half a dram or two ſcruples will be proper. Some give the extract of the bark with cantharides; but to manage this requires ſome ſkill and attention. It is more ſafe to give a few grains of caſtor along with the bark. A child of ſix or ſeven years of age may take ſeven or eight grains of caſtor, with fifteen grains of powdered bark, for a doſe. This may be made into a mixture with two or three ounces of any ſimple diſtilled water, and a little ſyrup, and taken three or four times a-day.

INFLAMMATION OF THE STOMACH.

THIS is a dangerous diſeaſe, and requires the moſt ſpeedy aſſiſtance, as it frequently ends in a ſuppuration; and ſometimes in a mortification, which is certain death.

CAUSES.——It may proceed from any of the cauſes which produce an inflammatory fever; as cold liquor drank while the body is warm, an obſtructed perſpiration, the ſudden ſtriking in of any eruption, &c. It may likewiſe proceed from the acrimony of the bile, or from acrid and ſtimulating ſubſtances taken into the ſtomach; as ſtrong vomits or purges, corroſive poiſons, and ſuch like. When the gout has been repelled from the extremities, either by cold or improper applications, it often occaſions an inflammation of the ſtomach. Hard or indigeſtable ſubſtances taken into the ſtomach, as bones, the ſhells of nuts, &c. have likewiſe that effect.

SYMPTOMS.—— It is attended with a fixed pain and burning heat in the ſtomach; great reſtleſſneſs and anxiety; a ſmall, quick, hard

hard pulſe; vomiting, or, at leaſt, a nauſea and ſickneſs; exceſſive thirſt; coldneſs of the extremities; difficulty of breathing; cold clammy ſweats; and ſometimes convulſions and fainting fits. The ſtomach is ſwelled, and often feels hard to the touch. One of the moſt certain ſigns of this diſeaſe is the ſenſe of pain, which the patient feels upon taking any kind of food or drink, eſpecially if too hot or cold, into his ſtomach.

When the patient vomits every thing he eats or drinks, is extremely reſtleſs, has a hiccup, with an intermitting pulſe, and frequent fainting fits, the danger is very great.

REGIMEN.—— The patient muſt, with the greateſt care, avoid all acrimonious, heating, and irritating food and drink. His weakneſs may deceive the by-ſtanders, and induce them to give him wines, ſpirits, or other cordials; but all theſe increaſe the diſeaſe, and often occaſion ſudden death. The inclination to vomit may likewiſe impoſe on the attendants, and make them think a vomit neceſſary; but that too is almoſt certain death.

The food muſt be light, thin, cool, and eaſy of digeſtion. It muſt be given in ſmall quantities, and ſhould neither be quite cold nor too hot. Thin gruel made of barley or oatmeal, light toaſted bread diſſolved in boiling water, or very weak chicken broth, are the moſt proper. The drink ſhould be clear whey, barley-water,

water, or decoctions of emollient vegetables; as liquorice and marsh-mallow roots, &c.

MEDICINE.—— Bleeding in this disease is absolutely necessary, and is almost the only medicine that can be depended on. When the disease proves obstinate, it will often be necessary to repeat this operation several times, nor must the low state of the pulse deter us from doing so. The pulse in this case generally rises upon bleeding, and so long as that happens the operation is safe.

FREQUENT fomentations with warm water, or a decoction of emollient vegetables, are likewise beneficial. Flannel cloths dipped in these must be applied to the region of the stomach, and removed as they turn cool. They must neither be applied too warm, nor suffered to continue till they become quite cold, as either of these extremes would aggravate the disease.

THE feet and legs ought likewise to be frequently bathed in lukewarm water, and warm bricks or poultices may be applied to the soles of the feet.

THE only internal medicines which we shall venture to recommend in this disease, are mild clysters. These may be made of warm water, or thin water-gruel, and if the patient be costive, a little sweet oil, honey or manna, may be added. Clysters answer the purpose of an internal fomentation, while they keep the belly open, and at the same time nourish the patient, who is often, in this disease, unable to retain

 any

any thing upon his ſtomach. For theſe reaſons they muſt not be neglected, as the patient's life may depend on the application of them.

OF THE ILIAC PASSION.

THIS is one of the moſt painful and dangerous diſeaſes that mankind are liable to. It proceeds from the ſame *cauſes* as the inflammation of the ſtomach; to which may be added coſtiveneſs, worms, eating unripe fruits, or great quantities of nuts, drinking hard windy malt liquors, as ſtale beer, bottled ale, or ſour wine, cyder, &c. It may likewiſe be occaſioned by a rupture, by ſcirrhous tumours of the inteſtines, or by their oppoſite ſides growing together.

THE *ſymptoms* here are nearly the ſame as in the foregoing diſeaſe; only the pain, if poſſible, is more acute, and is ſituate lower down about the region of the navel. The vomiting is likewiſe more violent, and ſometimes even the excrements, together with the clyſters and ſuppoſitories, are diſcharged by the mouth. The patient is continually belching up wind, and has often an obſtruction of his urine.

WHILE the pain ſhifts, and the vomiting only returns at certain intervals, and while the clyſters paſs downwards, there is ground to hope; but when the clyſters and *fæces* are vomited, and the patient is exceeding weak, with a low a low fluttering pulſe, a pale countenance, and a diſagreeable or ſtinking breath, there is great reaſon to fear, that the conſequences will prove fatal. Clammy ſweats, black fœtid ſtools, with a ſmall intermitting pulſe, and a total ceſſation of pain, are the ſigns of a gangrene, and approaching death.

REGIMEN.—— The regimen in this diſeaſe is in general the ſame as in an inflammation of the ſtomach. The patient muſt be kept quiet, avoiding cold, and all violent paſſions of the mind. His food muſt be thin, weak, and given in ſmall quantities: his drink weak and diluting; as clear whey, barley water, and ſuch like.

MEDICINE.—— Bleeding in this, as well as in the inflammation of the ſtomach, is the remedy moſt to be depended on. It ſhould be performed as ſoon as the ſymptoms appear, and muſt be repeated according to the ſtrength of the patient, and the violence of the ſymptoms.

A bliſtering plaſter applied immediately over the part where the moſt violent pain is, has often a very good effect. Even clyſters, which before had no effect, will operate when the bliſter begins to riſe.

Fomentations and laxative clyſters are by no means to be omitted. The patient's feet and legs ſhould frequently be bathed in warm water; and cloths dipped in it applied to his belly. Bladders filled with warm water may

may likewiſe be applied to the region of the navel, and warm bricks, or bottles filled with warm water, to the ſoles of the feet. The clyſters may be made of barley-water or thin gruel, and ſoftened with plenty of ſweet oil or freſh butter. Theſe may be adminiſtered every two or three hours, or oftner, if the patient continues coſtive.

If common clyſters have not the deſired effect, we would recommend the ſmoke of tobacco. It may be blown into the bowels throw an inverted pipe. This may be repeated after ſome time, unleſs the effect of the firſt renders it unneceſſary.

If the diſeaſe does not yield to clyſters and fomentations, recourſe muſt be had to pretty ſtrong purgatives; but as theſe by irritating the bowels often increaſe their contraction, and by that means fruſtrate their own intention, it will be neceſſary to join them with opiates; theſe, by allaying the pain, and relaxing the ſpaſmodic contractions of the guts, greatly aſſiſt the operation of purgatives in this caſe.

What often anſwers the purpoſe of purging very well, is a ſolution of the bitter purging ſalts. Two ounces of theſe may be diſſolved in an Engliſh pint of warm water, or thin gruel, and two or three table-ſpoonfuls given every half hour till it operates. At the ſame time fifteen, twenty, or twenty five drops of laudanum may be given in a glaſs of pepper mint or ſimple cinna-

cinnamon water, to appeaſe the irritation and prevent the vomiting, &c.

Acids have often a very happy effect in ſtaying the vomiting, and appeaſing the other violent ſymptoms of this diſeaſe. It will therefore be of uſe to ſharpen the patient's drink with cream of tartar, juice of lemon ; or, when theſe cannot be obtained, a little vinegar may be added to it.

But it often happens that no liquid whatever will ſtay on the ſtomach. In this caſe the patient muſt take purgative pills. I have generally found the following anſwer very well. Take jalap in powder, and vitriolated tartar, each half a dram, opium one grain, Caſtile ſoap as much as will make the maſs fit for pills. Theſe muſt be taken at one doſe, and if they do not operate in ſix or ſeven hours, the doſe may be repeated.

If a ſtool cannot be procured by any of the above means, it will be neceſſary to immerſe the patient in warm water up to the breaſt. I have often ſeen this ſucceed when other means proved in vain. The patient muſt continue in the water as long as he can eaſily bear it without fainting, and if one immerſion does not ſucceed, it may be repeated after ſome time, when the patient's ſtrength and ſpirits are recruited. It is more ſafe for him to go frequently into the bath than to continue too long at a time;

time; and it is often neceſſary to repeat it ſeveral times before it has the deſired effect.

It has ſometimes happened, after all other means of procuring a ſtool had been tried in vain, that this was brought about by immerſing the patient's lower extremities in cold water, making him walk upon a wet pavement, and daſhing his legs and thighs with the cold water, &c. This method, when others fail, at leaſt merits a trial. It is indeed attended with ſome danger; but a doubtful remedy is better than none.

In deſperate caſes it is common to give quickſilver. This may be taken to the quantity of ſeveral ounces, or even a pound, but ſhould not exceed that. When there are evident marks of an inflammation, or any reaſon to ſuſpect a mortification of the guts, this medicine ought not to be tried. In that caſe it will only haſten the patient's death. But when the obſtruction is occaſioned by any cauſe that can be removed by force, quickſilver is not only a proper medicine, but the beſt that can be applied, as it is the fitteſt body we know for making its way through the inteſtinal canal.

If the diſeaſe proceeds from a rupture, the patient muſt be laid with his head very low, and the inteſtines returned by gentle preſſure with the hand. If this, with fomentations and clyſters, ſhould not ſucceed, recourſe muſt be had to a ſurgical operation, which may give the patient relief.

Such

SUCH as would avoid this excruciating and dangerous diſeaſe, muſt take care never to be too long without a ſtool. Some who have died of it have had ſeveral pounds of hard, dry *fæces* taken out of their guts. They ſhould likewiſe beware of eating too freely of ſour or unripe fruits, or drinking ſtale windy liqours, pricked wines, or the like. I have often known it brought on by living too much on baked fruits, which are ſeldom good. It likewiſe proceeds frequently from cold caught by wet cloaths, &c. but eſpecially from wet feet.

OF THE COLIC.

THE colic has great affinity, both in its ſymptoms and method of cure, with the two preceeding diſeaſes. It is generally attended with coſtiveneſs and acute pain of the bowels; and requires diluting diet, evacuations, fomentations, &c.

COLICS are variouſly denominated according to their cauſes, as the *flatulent*, the *bilious*, the *hyſteric*, the *nervous*, &c. As each of theſe requires a particular treatment, we ſhall point out their moſt general ſymptoms, and the means to be uſed for their relief.

THE *flatulent*, or wind colic, is generally occaſioned by an indiſcreet uſe of unripe fruits, meats of hard digeſtion, windy vegetables, fermented liquors, and ſuch like. It may likewiſe

wiſe proceed from an obſtructed perſpiration, or catching cold. Delicate people, whoſe digeſtive powers are weak and debilitated, are moſt liable to this kind of colic.

THE flatulent colic may either affect the ſtomach or inteſtines. It is attended with a painful ſtretching of the ſtomach, or that part of the bowels where it is lodged. The patient feels a rumbling in his guts, and is generally relieved by a diſcharge of wind either upwards or downwards. The pain is ſeldom confined to any particular part, as the vapour wanders from one diviſion of the bowels to another, till ſuch time as it finds a vent.

WHEN the diſeaſe proceeds from windy liquor, eating green fruit, ſour herbs, or the like, the beſt medicine is to take immediately a dram of brandy, gin, or any good ſpirits, and to apply warm cloths to the ſtomach and bowels. The patient ſhould likewiſe ſit with his feet upon a warm hearth ſtone, or apply warm bricks to them; and he may drink camomile tea, or water-gruel with as much pepper in it as to render it moderately warm.

THIS is the only colic wherein ardent ſpirits, ſpiceries, or any thing of a hot nature, may be ventured upon. Nor indeed are they to be uſed here unleſs at the very beginning, before there be any ſymptoms of inflammation. We have reaſon to believe, that a colic occaſioned by wind or flatulent food might always be cured by ſpirits and warm liquors, if they were taken imme-

immediately upon perceiving the firſt uneaſineſs; but when the pain has continued for a conſiderable time, and there is reaſon to fear an inflammation of the bowels is already begun, all hot things are to be avoided, and the patient is to be treated in the ſame manner as for the iliac paſſion.

SEVERAL kinds of food, as honey, eggs, &c. occaſion colics in ſome particular conſtitutions. I have generally found, the beſt cure for theſe colics was to drink plentifully of ſmall diluting liquors, as water-gruel, ſmall poſſet, toaſt and water, &c.

COLICS which proceed from exceſs and indigeſtions, generally cure themſelves, by occaſioning vomiting or purging. Theſe diſcharges are by no means to be ſtopped, but promoted by drinking plenty of warm water, or weak poſſet. When their violence is over, the patient may take a doſe of rhubarb, or any other gentle purge, to carry off the dregs of his debauch.

COLICS which are occaſioned by wet feet, or catching cold, may generally be removed at the beginning, by bathing the feet and legs in warm water, and drinking ſuch warm diluting liquors as will promote the perſpiration, as weak wine-whey, or water-gruel with a ſmall quantity of ſpirits in it.

THESE flatulent colics, which prevail ſo much in the country, might generally be prevented if people were careful to change their cloaths when they get wet. They ought likewiſe to take a dram, or to drink ſome warm liquor after eating any kind of green traſh. We do not mean to recommend the practice of dram-drinking, but in this caſe ardent liquors prove a real medicine, and indeed the beſt that can be applied.

THE *bilious* colic is attended with very acute pain about the region of the navel. The patient complains of great thirſt, and is generally coſtive. He vomits a hot, bitter, yellow-coloured bile, which being diſcharged, ſeems to afford ſome relief, but is quickly followed by the ſame violent pain as before. As the diſtemper advances, the propenſity to vomit increaſes, in ſo much that ſometimes it becomes almoſt continual, and the proper motion of the inteſtines is ſo far perverted, that there are all the ſymptoms of an impending iliac paſſion.

IF the patient be young and ſtrong, and the pulſe full and frequent, it will be proper to bleed, after which clyſters may be adminiſtered. Clear whey or gruel, ſharpened with the juice of lemon, or cream of tartar, muſt be drank freely. Small chicken broth, with a little manna diſſolved in it, or a ſlight decoction of tamarinds, are likewiſe very proper, or any other thin, acid, opening liquor.

BESIDES bleeding and plentiful dilution, it will be neceſſary to foment the belly with cloths dipped in warm water, and if this ſhould not ſucceed, the patient muſt be ſet in a warm bath up to the middle.

MILD

Mild purgatives are here likewiſe neceſſary, as the lenitive electuary, manna, cream of tartar, or, what will anſwer very well, the bitter purging ſalts. Theſe may be diſſolved in water, and given in the ſame manner as directed page 348. If theſe medicines will not ſtay on the ſtomach, it will be neceſſary to join an opiate with them.

Such as are liable to frequent returns of the bilious colic ſhould uſe fleſh ſparingly, and live chiefly upon a light vegetable diet. They ſhould likewiſe take frequently a doſe of cream of tartar with tamarinds, or any other cool acid purge.

The *hyſteric* colic bears a great reſemblance to the bilious. It is attended with acute pains about the region of the ſtomach, vomiting, &c. But what the patient vomits in this caſe is commonly of a greeniſh colour. There is a great ſinking of the ſpirits, with dejection of mind and difficulty of breathing, which are the characteriſtic ſymptoms of this diſorder. Sometimes it is accompanied with the jaundice, but this generally goes off of its own accord in a few days.

In this colic all evacuations, as bleeding, purging, vomiting, &c. do hurt. Every thing that weakens the patient, or ſinks the ſpirits, is to be avoided. If however the vomiting ſhould prove violent, weak camomile tea, or ſmall poſſet, may be drank to cleanſe the ſtomach. Afterwards the patient may take fifteen, twenty, or twenty five drops of liquid laudanum in a glaſs

glaſs of cinnamon-water. This may be repeated every ten or twelve hours till the ſymptoms abate.

THE patient may likewiſe take four or five of the fœtid pills three times a-day, and drink a cup of penny royal tea after them. If aſafœtida ſhould diſagree with the ſtomach, which is ſometimes the caſe, a tea-ſpoonful of the tincture of caſtor in a cup of penny-royal-tea, or thirty or forty drops of the balſam of Peru dropped upon a bit of loaf ſugar, may be taken in its ſtead. The anti-hyſteric plaſter may alſo be applied to the region of the navel, which has often a good effect.

THE *nervous* colic prevails moſt among miners, ſmelters of lead, plumbers, the makers of white lead, &c. It is very difficult to cure, and often ends in a palſy.

No diſeaſe of the bowels is attended with more excruciating pain than this. Nor is it ſoon at an end. I have known it continue eight or ten days with very little intermiſſion, the belly all the while continuing bound in ſpite of medicine, yet at length yield, and the patient recover.

THE general treatment of this diſeaſe is ſo nearly the ſame with that of the iliac paſſion, or inflammation of the guts that we ſhall not inſiſt upon it. The belly is to be opened by mild purgatives given in ſmall doſes, and frequently repeated, and their operation muſt be aſſiſted by ſoft oily clyſters, fomentations, &c.

THE

The Barbadoes tar is ſaid to be a proper medicine in this diſeaſe. It may be taken to the quantity of two drams three times a-day, or oftener if the ſtomach will bear it. This tar, mixed with an equal quantity of ſtrong rum, is likewiſe proper for rubbing the ſpine, in caſe any tingling, or other ſymptoms of a palſy are felt. When this tar cannot be obtained, the back may be rubbed with ſtrong ſpirits, or a little of the oil of nutmegs or roſemary.

If the patient remains weak and languid after this diſeaſe, he muſt take exerciſe on horſeback, and uſe an infuſion of the jeſuits bark in wine. When the diſeaſe ends in a palſy, the bath-waters are found to be extremely proper.

To avoid this colic, people muſt ſhun all ſour fruits, acid and auſtere liquors, &c. Thoſe who work in lead ought never to go to their buſineſs faſting, and their food ſhould be oily or fat. They may take a glaſs of ſalad oil, with a little brandy or rum every morning, but ſhould never take ſpirits alone. Liquid aliment is beſt for them; as fat broths, &c.; but low living is bad. They ſhould now and then go a little out of the tainted air; and ſhould, at leaſt, take phyſic every ſpring and fall.

Sundry other kinds of this diſeaſe might be mentioned, but too many diſtinctions would tend only to perplex and bewilder the reader. Theſe already mentioned are the moſt material, and ſhould indeed be attended to, as their treatment is very different. But even thoſe who

who are not in a condition to diſtinguiſh very accurately in theſe matters, may nevertheleſs be of great ſervice to patients in colics, by only obſerving the following general rules : Firſt, To bathe the patient's feet and legs in warm water, and next to apply bladders filled with warm water, or cloths dipped in it, to his ſtomach and bowels. Afterwards, To make him drink freely of weak diluting warm liquors. And, laſtly, To give him an emollient clyſter every two or three hours.

INFLAMMATION OF THE KIDNEYS.

CAUSES.—— This diſeaſe may proceed from any of thoſe cauſes which produce an inflammatory fever. It is likewiſe occaſioned by wounds, or bruiſes of the kidneys, and by ſmall ſtones or gravel lodging within them. It may alſo proceed from ſtrong diuretic medicines; as ſpirits of turpentine, tincture of cantharides, &c. Violent motion; as hard riding or walking, eſpecially in hot weather, or whatever drives the blood forcibly into the kidneys, may occaſion this malady. It may likewiſe proceed from lying too ſoft, or too much on the back, or from involuntary contractions, or ſpaſms in the urinary veſſels, &c.

SYMPTOMS.—— There is a ſharp pain about the region of the kidneys, with ſome degree of fever, and a ſtupor, or dull pain in the thigh

thigh of the affected ſide. The urine is at firſt clear, and afterwards of a rediſh colour; but in the worſt kind of the diſeaſe it generally continues pale, is paſſed with difficulty, and commonly in ſmall quantities at a time. The patient feels great uneaſineſs when he endeavours to walk or ſit upright. He lies with more eaſe on the affected ſide than on the ſound; and has generally a nauſea or vomiting, reſembling that which happens in the colic.

THIS diſeaſe however may be diſtinguiſhed from the colic by the pain being ſeated farther back, and by the difficulty of paſſing urine, which is a conſtant ſymptom of this diſeaſe, but does not always happen in the other.

REGIMEN.—— Every thing of a heating or ſtimulating nature is to be avoided. The food muſt be thin and light; as water-pap, ſmall broths, with mild vegetables, and the like. Emollient and ſoft liquors muſt be plentifully drank; as clear whey, or balm-tea ſweetened with honey, decoctions of marſh mallow roots, with barley and liquorice, &c. The patient, notwithſtanding the vomiting, muſt conſtantly keep ſipping ſmall quantities of theſe or other diluting liquors. Nothing ſo ſafely and certainly abates the inflammation, and expels the obſtructing cauſe, as copious dilution. The patient muſt be kept eaſy, quiet, and free from cold, ſo long as any ſymptoms of inflammation appear.

MEDICINE.—— Bleeding is here very neceſſary, eſpecially at the beginning. Ten or twelve

twelve ounces may be let from the arm or foot with a lancet, and if the pain and inflammation continue, the operation may be repeated in twenty-four hours, eſpecially if the patient be of a full habit. Leeches may likewiſe be applied to the hæmorrhoidal veins, as a diſcharge from theſe will greatly relieve the patient.

Cloths dipped in warm water, or bladders filled with it, muſt be applied to the part affected, and renewed as they grow cool. If the bladders be filled with a decoction of mallows and camomile flowers, to which a little ſaffron is added, and mixed with about a third part of new milk, it will be ſtill more beneficial.

Emollient clyſters are likewiſe frequently to be adminiſtered; and if theſe no do not open the belly, a little honey or manna may be added to them.

The ſame courſe is to be followed where gravel or a ſtone is lodged in the kidney; but when the gravel or ſtone is ſeparated from the kidney, and lodges in any of the urinary paſſages, it will be proper, beſides the fomentations, to rub the part with a little ſweet oil, and to give gentle diuretics; as juniper water ſweetned with the ſyrup of marſh mallows, or a tea ſpoonful of the ſweet ſpirits of nitre, now and then in a cup of the patient's drink. He ought likewiſe to take exerciſe on horſeback, or in a coach, &c.

When the diſeaſe is protracted beyond the ſeventh or eighth day, and the patient complains of of a ſtupor, and heavineſs of the part, has frequent returns of chillneſs, ſhivering, &c. there is reaſon to ſuſpect, that matter is forming in the kidney, aud that an abſceſs or ulcer will enſue.

When matter in the urine ſhews, that an ulcer is already formed in the kidney, the patient muſt be careful to abſtain from all acrid, ſour, and ſalted proviſions; and muſt live chiefly upon mild mucilaginous herbs and fruits, together with the broth of young animals, made with barley and common pot herbs, &c. His drink may be whey, and butter milk that is not ſour. The latter is reckoned a ſpecific remedy in ulcers of the kidneys. To anſwer this character however it muſt be drank for a conſiderable time. Chalybeat waters have likewiſe been found beneficial in this diſeaſe. This medicine is eaſily obtained, as it is found in every part of Great Britain. It muſt likewiſe be uſed for a conſiderable time, in order to produce any ſalutary effects.

Those who are liable to frequent returns of inflammation, or obſtruction of the kidneys, muſt abſtain from wines, eſpecially ſuch as abound with tartar; and their food muſt be light, and of eaſy digeſtion. They ſhould uſe moderate exerciſe, and ſhould not lie too hot, nor too much on their back.

INFLAMMATION OF THE BLADDER.

The inflammation of the bladder proceeds, in a great meaſure, from the ſame cauſes as that of the kidneys. It is known by an acute pain towards the bottom of the belly, and difficulty of paſſing urine, with ſome degree of fever, a conſtant inclination to go to ſtool, and a perpetual deſire to make water.

This diſeaſe muſt be treated on the ſame principles as the immediately preceeding. The diet muſt be light and thin, and the drink cooling and diluting. Bleeding is very proper at the beginning, and in rubuſt conſtitutions, it will often be neceſſary to repeat it. The bottom of the belly muſt be frequently fomented with warm water, or a decoction of mild vegetables; and emollient clyſters muſt frequently be adminiſtered, &c.

The patient ſhould abſtain from every thing that is of a hot, acrid, and ſtimulating nature; and ſhould live entirely upon ſmall broths, gruels, or mild vegetables.

A ſtoppage of urine may proceed from other cauſes beſides an inflammation of the bladder; as a ſwelling of the hæmorrhoidal veins, hard *fæces* lodged in the *rectum*; a ſtone in the bladder, excreſcences in the urinary paſſages, a palſy of the bladder, hyſteric affections, &c. Each of theſe requires a particular treatment, which does not fall under our conſideration here. We ſhall

ſhall only obſerve,that in all of them a mild and gentle treatment is the ſafeſt, as ſtrong diuretic medicines, or things of an irritating nature, generally increaſe the danger. Some perſons have killed themſelves by introducing probes into the urinary paſſages, to remove, as they thought, ſomewhat that obſtructed the paſſage of the urine; and others have brought on a violent inflammation of the bladder, by uſing ſtrong diuretics for that purpoſe.

INFLAMMATION OF THE LIVER.

THE liver is leſs ſubject to inflammation than any of the other viſcera, as in it the circulation is ſlower; but when an inflammation does happen, it is with difficulty removed, and often ends in a ſuppuration or ſchirrus.

CAUSES.—— Beſides the common cauſes of inflammation, we may here reckon the following, viz exceſſive fatneſs, a ſchirrus of the liver itſelf, violent ſhocks from ſtrong vomits when the liver was before unſound, an aduſt or atrabilarian ſtate of the blood, any thing that ſuddenly cools the liver after it has been greatly heated, ſtones obſtructing the courſe of the bile, drinking ſtrong wines or ſpiritous liquors, uſing hot ſpicy aliment, obſtinate hypochondriacal diſtempers, &c.

SYMPTOMS.—— This diſeaſe is known by a painful tenſion of the right ſide under the

the falſe ribs, attended with ſome degree of fever, a ſenſe of weight, or fulneſs of the part, difficulty of breathing, loathing of food, great thirſt, with a pale or yellowiſh colour of the ſkin and eyes.

THE *ſymptoms* here are various, according to the degree of inflammation, and likewiſe according to the particular part of the liver where the inflammation happens. Sometimes the pain is ſo inconſiderable, that an inflammation is not ſo much as ſuſpected; but when it happens in the upper or convex part of the liver, the pain is more acute, the pulſe quicker, and the patient is often troubled with a dry cough, a hiccup, and a pain extending to the ſhoulder, with difficulty of lying on the left ſide, &c.

THIS diſeaſe may be diſtinguiſhed from the pleuriſy by the pain being leſs violent, ſeated under the falſe ribs, the pulſe not ſo hard, and by the difficulty of lying on the left ſide. It may be diſtinguiſhed from the hyſteric and hypochondriac diſorders by ſome degree of fever, with which it is always attended.

THIS diſeaſe, if properly treated. is ſeldom mortal. A conſtant hiccupping, violent fever, and exceſſive thirſt, are very bad ſymptoms. If it ends in a ſuppuration, and the matter cannot be brought to diſcharge itſelf outwardly, the danger is great. When a ſchirrus of the liver enſues, the patient, if he obſerves a proper regimen, may live a number of years tolerably eaſy; but if he indulges in animal

food

food and ſtrong liquors, or takes medicines of an acrid or irritating nature, the ſchirrus will be converted into a cancer, which muſt infallibly prove fatal.

REGIMEN.—— The ſame regimen is to be obſerved in this as in other inflammatory diſorders. All hot things are to be carefully avoided, and cool reſolving liquors, as whey, barley-water, &c. drank freely. The food muſt be light and thin, and the body, as well as the mind, muſt be kept eaſy and quiet.

MEDICINE.—— Bleeding is proper at the beginning of this diſeaſe, and it will often be neceſſary, even though the pulſe ſhould not feel hard, to repeat the operation. The belly muſt be kept gently open; but all violent purgatives are to be avoided. A decoction of tamarinds, with a little honey or manna, will anſwer this purpoſe very well. The ſide affected muſt be frequently fomented with warm water, in the manner directed in the foregoing diſeaſes. Mild laxative clyſters ſhould be frequently adminiſtered; and if the pain ſhould notwithſtanding continue violent, a bliſtering plaſter may be applied over the part affected.

MEDICINES which promote the ſecretion of urine have a very good effect here. For this purpoſe half a dram of purified nitre, or half a tea-ſpoonful of the ſweet ſpirits of nitre, may be taken in a cup of the patient's drink three or four times a-day.

WHEN there is an inclination to ſweat, it ought

ought to be promoted, but not by warm ſudorifics. The only thing to be uſed for that purpoſe is plenty of diluting liquor drank about the warmth of the human blood. Indeed the patient in this caſe, as well as in all other to ical inflammations, ought to drink nothing that is colder than the blood.

If the ſtools ſhould be looſe, and even ſtreaked with blood, nothing muſt be given to ſtop them, unleſs they be ſo frequent as to weaken the patient. Looſe ſtools often prove critical, and carry off the diſeaſe.

If the diſorder, in ſpite of all endeavours to the contrary, ſhould end in a ſchirrus, the patient muſt be careful to regulate his diet, &c. in ſuch a manner as not to aggravate the diſeaſe. He muſt not indulge in fleſh, fiſh, ſtrong liquors, or any poignant or ſalted proviſions; but muſt, for the moſt part, live on mild vegetables, as fruits and roots, taking gentle exerciſe, and drinking whey, barley-water, or butter milk. If he takes any thing ſtronger, it ſhould be fine mild ale, which is much more ſafe than wines or ſpirits.

We ſhall take no notice of inflammations of the other viſcera. They muſt all be treated upon the ſame principles as thoſe already mentioned. The great rule with reſpect to all of them, is to avoid every thing that is ſtrong, or of a heating nature, to apply warm fomentations to the part affected, and to ſupply the patient

tient with plenty of weak, warm, diluting drink.

OF THE CHOLERA MORBUS, OR VOMITING AND LOOSENESS.

THIS is a violent purging and vomiting, attended with gripes, and a conſtant deſire to go to ſtool. It comes on ſuddenly, and is moſt common in autumn. There is hardly any diſeaſe that kills more quickly than this, when proper means are not uſed in due time for removing it.

CAUSES.—— It is occaſioned by a redundancy and putrid acrimony of the bile; by food that eaſily turns rancid or ſour on the ſtomach; as butter, fat pork, ſweet meats, cucumbers, melons, cherries, &c. It is ſometimes the effect of ſtrong acrid purges or vomits; or of poiſonous ſubſtances taken into the ſtomach. It may likewiſe proceed from violent paſſions of the mind; as fear, anger, &c.

SYMPTOMS.—— It is generally preceeded by a *cardialgia*, or heart burn, ſour belchings, and flatulences, with pain of the ſtomach and inteſtines. To theſe ſucceed exceſſive vomiting, and purging of green, yellow, or blackiſh-coloured bile, with a diſtention of the ſtomach, and violent griping pains. There is likewiſe a great thirſt, with a very quick unequal pulſe, and

and often a fixed acute pain about the region of the navel. As the diſeaſe advances, the pulſe often ſinks ſo low as to become quite imperceptible, the extremities grow cold, or cramped, and covered with a clammy ſweat, the urine is obſtructed, and there is a palpitation of the heart. Violent hiccupping, fainting, and convulſions are the ſigns of approaching death.

MEDICINE.—— At the beginning of this diſeaſe the efforts of nature to expel the offending cauſe muſt be aſſiſted, by promoting the purging and vomiting. For this purpoſe the patient muſt drink plenty of diluting liquors; as whey, butter milk, warm water, thin water gruel, ſmall poſſet, or, what is perhaps preferable to any of them, very weak chicken-broth. This ſhould not only be drank freely, to promote the vomiting, but a clyſter of it given every hour, in order to promote the purging.

AFTER theſe evacuations have been continued for ſome time, a decoction of toaſted oat-bread may be drank to ſtop the vomiting. The bread ſhould be toaſted till it is of a brown colour, but not burned, and afterwards boiled in ſpring water. If oat bread cannot be had, wheat bread, or oat meal well toaſted, may be uſed in its ſtead. If this does not put a ſtop to the vomiting, the ſaline mixture may be taken, as directed page 298.

THE vomiting and purging however ought never to be ſtopped too ſoon. So long as theſe

dif-

diſcharges do not weaken the patient they are ſalutary, and may be allowed to go on, or rather ought to be promoted. But when the patient is much exhauſted by the evacuations, or has a ſmall intermitting pulſe, coldneſs of the extremities, with other ſymptoms of weakneſs, recourſe muſt immediately be had to opiates, and generous cordial medicines. Ten or fifteen drops of liquid laudanum in half a glaſs of ſtrong cinnamon water, may be taken every four or five hours, till the violent ſymptoms be removed. Warm negas, or ſtrong wine-whey, may likewiſe be taken to ſupport the patient's ſpirits, and promote the perſpiration. His legs may be rubbed with flannel-cloths, or wrapped in warm blankets, and warm bricks applied to the ſoles of his feet.

WHEN the violence of the diſeaſe is over, to prevent a relapſe, it will be neceſſary, for ſome time, to continue the uſe of ſmall doſes of laudanum. Ten or twelve drops may be taken in a glaſs of wine, at leaſt twice a-day, for eight or ten days. The patient's food ought to be nouriſhing, but taken in ſmall quantities, and he ſhould uſe moderate exerciſe. As the ſtomach and inteſtines are generally much weakened, an infuſion of the bark, or other bitters, in ſmall wine may be drank for ſome time.

THO' phyſicians are ſeldom called in due time in this diſeaſe, they ought not however to deſpair of relieving the patient even in the moſt deſperate circumſtances. Of this I lately ſaw a very ſtriking inſtance in an old man and his ſon, who had been both ſeized with it about the middle of the night. I did not ſee them till next morning, when they had much more the appearance of dead than of living men. No pulſe could be felt; the extremities were quite cold, and rigid; the countenance was ghaſtly, and the ſtrength quite exhauſted. Yet from this deplorable condition they were both recovered by the uſe of opiates and cordial medicines, with the regimen mentioned above.

OF A DIARRHOEA, OR LOOSENESS.

A looſeneſs, in many caſes, is not to be conſidered as a diſeaſe, but rather as a ſalutary evacuation. It never ought to be ſtopped unleſs when it continues too long, or evidently weakens the patient. As this however ſometimes happens, we ſhall point out the moſt common cauſes of a looſeneſs, with the method of treatment proper in each caſe.

WHEN a looſeneſs is occaſioned by catching cold, or an obſtructed perſpiration, the patient ought to keep warm, to drink freely of weak diluting liquors, to bathe his feet and legs frequently in lukewarm water, to wear flannel next his ſkin, and to take every other method to reſtore the perſpiration.

IN

In a looſeneſs which proceeds from exceſs or repletion, a vomit is the proper medicine. Vomits not only clean the ſtomach, but promote all the ſecretions, which renders them of great importance in carrying off a debauch. Half a dram of ipecacoanha in powder will anſwer the purpoſe very well. A day or two after the vomit, the ſame quantity of rhubarb may be taken, and repeated two or three times, if the looſeneſs continues. The patient ought to live upon light vegetable food of eaſy digeſtion, and to drink whey, thin gruel, or barley water.

A looſeneſs occaſioned by the obſtruction of any cuſtomary evacuation, as the bleeding piles in men the monthly diſcharges in women, &c. generally requires bleeding. If that does not ſucceed, other evacuations, as iſſues, ſetons, &c. may be ſubſtituted in the room of thoſe which are obſtructed. At the ſame time, every method is to be taken to reſtore the uſual diſcharges, as not only the cure of the diſeaſe, but the patient's life may depend on this.

A periodical looſeneſs ought never to be ſtopped. It is always an effort of nature to carry off ſome offending matter, which, if retained in the body, might produce fatal diſeaſes. Children are very liable to this kind of looſeneſs, eſpecially while teething. It is however ſo far from being hurtful to them, that ſuch children generally get their teeth with leaſt trouble. If theſe looſe ſtools ſhould at any time prove ſour

or

or griping, a tea-ſpoonful of magneſia alba, with four or five grains of rhubarb, may be given to the child in a little pap or any other food. This, if repeated three or four times, will generally correct the acidity, and carry off the griping ſtools.

A diarrhœa or looſeneſs which proceeds from violent paſſions or affections of the mind, muſt be treated with the greateſt caution. Vomits in this caſe are highly improper. Nor are purges ſafe, unleſs they be very mild, and given in ſmall quantities. Opiates, and other antiſpaſmodic medicines are moſt proper. Ten or twelve drops of liquid laudanum may be taken in a cup of valerian or penny-royal tea, every eight or ten hours, till the ſymptoms abate. Eaſe, cheerfulneſs, and tranquillity of mind, are here of the greateſt importance.

WHEN a looſeneſs proceeds from acrid or poiſonous ſubſtances taken into the ſtomach, the patient muſt drink large quantities of diluting liquors, with oil or fat broths, to promote vomiting and purging. Afterwards, if the bowels are inflamed, bleeding will be neceſſary. Small doſes of laudanum may likewiſe be taken to remove the ſpaſms and the irritation of the bowels.

WHEN gouty matter, repelled from the extremities, occaſions a looſeneſs, it is by no means to be ſtopped, but promoted by gentle doſes of rhubarb, or other mild purgatives. The gouty matter is likewiſe to be ſollicited to the extre-

extremities by warm fomentations, and cataplasms. And the perspiration ought to be promoted by warm diluting liquors; as wine-whey with spirits of harshorn, or a few drops of liquid laudanum in it.

WHEN a looseness proceeds from worms, such medicines ought to be used as kill or carry off these vermin; as powder of tin, with purges of rhubarb and calomel, &c. The proper doses of these medicines will be pointed out when we come to treat of diseases occasioned by worms.

A looseness is often occasioned by bad water. When this is the case, the disease generally proves epidemical. When there is reason to believe, that this or any other disease proceeds from the use of unwholesome water, it ought immediately to be changed, or, if that cannot be done, it may be corrected by mixing with it quicklime, chalk, or the like.

IN people whose stomachs are weak, violent exercise immediately after meals will occasion a looseness. Tho' the cure of this is obvious, yet it will be proper, besides avoiding violent exercise, to use such medicines as tend to brace and strengthen the stomach, as infusions of the bark, with other bitter and astringent medicines, in white wine. The person ought likewise to take frequently a glass or two of old red port, or good claret.

PERSONS who, from a peculiar weakness, or too great an irritability of the bowels, are liable

able to frequent returns of this diſeaſe, ſhould live temperately, avoiding crude ſummer fruits, all unwholeſome food, and meats of hard digeſtion. They ought likewiſe to beware of cold, moiſture, or whatever may obſtruct the perſpiration, and ſhould wear flannel next their ſkin. All violent paſſions of the mind. as fear, anger, &c. are likewiſe carefully to be avoided.

OF THE DYSENTERY, OR BLOODY-FLUX.

THIS diſeaſe prevails in the ſpring and autumn. It is very infectious and often epidemical. Thoſe perſons are moſt liable to it who are much expoſed to the night air, or who live in places where the air is confined and unwholeſome. Hence it often proves fatal in camps, on ſhipboard, in jails, hoſpitals, and ſuch like places.

CAUSES.—— This diſeaſe may be occaſioned by any thing that obſtructs the perſpiration or renders the humors putrid; as damp beds, wet cloaths, unwholeſome diet, air, &c. But it is moſt frequently communicated by infection. This ought to make people extremely cautious in going near ſuch perſons as labour under the diſeaſe. Even the ſmell of the patient's excrements has been known to communicate the infection.

SYMPTOMS.—— It is known by a flux of the belly attended with violent pain of the bowels, a conſtant inclination to go to ſtool, and

and generally leſs or more of blood in the ſtools. It begins, like other fevers, with chillneſs, loſs of ſtrength, a quick pulſe, great thirſt, and an inclination to vomit. The ſtools are at firſt greaſy or frothy, afterwards they are ſtreaked with blood, and, at laſt, have frequently the appearance of pure blood, mixed with ſmall filaments, or bits of ſkin, which is part of the internal coat of the inteſtines abraded by the acrimony of the *fæces*. Sometimes however there is no blood in the ſtools thro' the whole courſe of the diſeaſe. When the patient goes to ſtool, he feels a bearing down, as if the whole bowels were falling out, and ſometimes a part of the inteſtine is actually protruded, which proves exceeding troubleſome, eſpecially in children.

THIS diſeaſe may be diſtinguiſhed from the diarrhœa or looſeneſs, by the acute pain of the bowels, and the blood which generally appears in the ſtools. It may be diſtinguiſhed from the *cholera morbus* by its not being attended with ſuch violent and frequent fits of vomiting, &c.

WHEN the dyſentery attacks the old, the delicate, or ſuch as have been waſted by ſcorbutic, conſumptive, or other lingering diſeaſes, it generally proves fatal. Vomiting and hiccuping are bad ſigns, as they ſhew an inflammation of the ſtomach. When the ſtools have an exceeding diſagreeable ſmell, are green, black, or mixed with ſmall glandular ſubſtances, or bits of ſkin, the danger is great. It is an unfavourable ſymptom

tom when clyſters are immediately returned; but ſtill more ſo, when the paſſage is ſo obſtinately ſhut, that they cannot be injected. A weak pulſe, coldneſs of the extremities, with difficulty of ſwallowing, and convulſions, are ſigns of approaching death.

REGIMEN.—— Nothing is of more importance in this diſeaſe than cleanlineſs. It contributes greatly to the recovery of the patient, and no leſs to the ſafety of ſuch as attend him. In all contagious diſeaſes the danger is increaſed, and the infection ſpread, by the neglect of cleanlineſs; but in none more than in this. Every thing about the patient ſhould be frequently changed. The excrements ſhould never be ſuffered to continue in his chamber, but removed immediately, and buried under ground. A conſtant ſtream of freſh air ſhould be admitted into the chamber; and it ought frequently to be ſprinkled with vinegar, juice of lemon, or ſome other ſtrong acid.

THE patient muſt not be diſcouraged, but his ſpirits kept up in hopes of a cure. Nothing tends more to render any putrid diſeaſe mortal than the fears and apprehenſions of the ſick. All diſeaſes of this nature have a tendency to ſink and depreſs the ſpirits, and when that is increaſed by fears and alarms from thoſe whom the patient believes to be perſons of ſkill, it cannot fail to have the worſt effects.

A flannel veſt worn next the ſkin has often a very good effect in a dyſentery. This promotes

promotes the perſpiration without greatly heating the body. Great caution however is neceſſary in leaving it off. I have often known a dyſentery brought on by imprudently throwing off a flannel veſt before the ſeaſon was ſufficiently hot. For whatever purpoſe this piece of dreſs be worn, it ſhould never be left off but in a warm ſeaſon.

In this diſeaſe the greateſt attention muſt be paid to the patient's diet. Fleſh, fiſh, and every thing that has a tendency to turn putrid or rancid on the ſtomach, muſt be abſtained from. Apples boiled in milk, water pap, and plain light pudding, with broth made of the gelatinous parts of animals, may be eat. Jelly broth not only anſwers the purpoſe of food, but likewiſe of medicine. I have often known dyſenteries cured by it, after pompous medicines had proved ineffectual *.

* The manner of making this broth is, to take a ſheep's head and feet with the ſkin upon them, and to burn the wool off with a hot iron, in the manner they do in Scotland. Afterwards to boil them till the broth is quite a jelly. A little cinnamon or mace may be added to give the broth an agreeable flavour, and the patient may take a little of it warm with toaſted bread, three or four times a-day. A clyſter of it may likewiſe be given twice a day. Such as cannot uſe the broth made in this way, may have the head and feet ſkinned; but we have reaſon to believe that this hurts the medicine. It is not our buſineſs here to reaſon upon the nature and qualities of medicines, otherwiſe this might be ſhewn to poſſeſs virtues

ANOTHER kind of food very proper in the dyſentery, which may be uſed by ſuch as cannot take the broth mentioned above, is made by boiling a few handfuls of fine flower, tied in a cloth, for ſix or ſeven hours, till it becomes as hard as ſtarch. Two or three table ſpoonfuls of this may be grated down, and boiled in ſuch a quantity of new milk and water as to be of the thickneſs of pap. This may be ſweetened to the patient's taſte, and taken for his ordinary food *.

THE patient may likewiſe be allowed to eat freely of moſt kinds of good ripe fruit; as apples, grapes, currant-berries, ſtrawberries, &c. Theſe

virtues every way ſuited to the cure of a dyſentery which does not proceed from a putrid ſtate of the humours. One thing we know, which is preferable to all reaſoning, that whole families have often been cured by it. after they had uſed many other medicines in vain. It will however be proper that the patient take a vomit, and a doſe or two of rhubarb, before he begins to uſe the broth. It will likewiſe be neceſſary to continue the uſe of it for a conſiderable time, and to make it the principal food.

* The learned Dr Rutherford, late profeſſor of medicine in the univerſity of Edinburgh, uſed to mention this medicine in his public lectures with great encomiums. He directed it to be made by tying three or four handfuls of the fineſt flower, as tight as poſſible, in a linnen rag, afterwards to dip it frequently in water, and to dridge the outſide with flower till a cake or cruſt be formed around it, which prevents the water from ſoaking into it while boiling. It is then to be boiled till it becomes a hard dry maſs, as directed above. This will not only anſwer the purpoſe of food, but may likewiſe be given in clyſters.

These may either be eat raw or boiled, with or without milk, as the patient chuses. The prejudice against fruit in this disease is so great, that many believe it to be the common cause of dysenteries. This however is an egregious mistake. Both reason and experience shew, that good fruit is one of the best medicines, both for the prevention and cure of the most dangerous kind of dysentery. In a dysentery arising from a putrid state of the humours, fruit is in every respect calculated to counteract that tendency to putrefaction, from whence all the danger proceeds. The patient in such a case ought therefore to be allowed to eat as much fruit as he pleases, provided it be good *.

The most proper drink in this disorder is whey. The dysentery has often been cured by the

* I lately attended a young gentleman who had been seized with a dysenetry in North America. All means had been tried for his relief, but to no purpose. At length, tired out with disappointments from medicine, and reduced to skin and bone, he came over to Britain, rather with a view to die among his relations than with any hopes of a cure. After trying sundry medicines here with no better success than abroad, I advised him to leave off the use of drugs, and to trust entirely to a diet of milk and fruits, with gentle exercise. Strawberries was the only fruit he could procure at that season. These he eat with milk twice, and sometimes thrice a-day. The consequence was, that in a short time his stools were reduced from upwards of twenty in a day, to three or four, and sometimes not so many. He used the other fruits as they came in, and was, in a few weeks, so well as to leave the part of the country where I was with a view to return to America.

the uſe of clear whey alone. It may be taken both for drink, and in form of clyſter. When whey cannot be had, barley water ſharpened with cream of tartar may be drank, or a decoction of barley and tamarinds; two ounces of the former and one of the latter may be boiled in two Engliſh quarts of water to one. Warm water, water-gruel, or water wherein hot iron has been frequently quenched, are all very proper, and may be drank in turns. Camomile-tea, if the ſtomach will bear it, is an exceeding proper drink. It both ſtrengthens the ſtomach, and by its antiſeptic quality tends to prevent a mortification of the bowels.

MEDICINE.—— At the beginning of this diſeaſe it is always neceſſary to cleanſe the firſt paſſages. For this purpoſe a vomit of ipecacoanha muſt be given, and wrought off with weak camomile tea. Strong vomits are ſeldom neceſſary here. A ſcruple, or at moſt half a dram of ipecacoanha, is generally ſufficient for an adult, and ſometimes a very few grains will ſuffice. The day after the vomit, half a dram, or two ſcruples of rhubarb, muſt be taken. This doſe may be repeated every other day for two or three times. Afterwards ſmall doſes of ipecacoanha may be taken for ſome time. Two or three grains of the powder may be mixed in a table ſpoonful of the ſyrup of poppies, and taken three times a-day.

THESE evacuations, and the regimen preſcribed above, will ſeldom fail to perform the cure,

cure. Should it however happen otherwise, the following astringent medicines must be used.

A clyster of starch or fat mutton broth, with twenty or thirty drops of liquid laudanum in it, may be administered twice a-day. At the same time an ounce of gum arabic, and half an ounce of gum tragacanth, may be dissolved in an English pint of barley water, over a slow fire, and a table-spoonful of it taken every hour.

If these have not the desired effect, the patient may take, four times a-day, about the bulk of a nutmeg of the *Japonic confection*, drinking after it a tea cupful of the decoction of logwood; which may be thus made:

Boil three or four ounces of the shavings of logwood in two English quarts of water to one; towards the end add two drams of cinnamon-bark. This decoction gives the stools a reddish colour, which is sometimes mistaken for blood. We mention this circumstance to prevent the patient from being alarmed at their appearance.

Some have treated dysenteries very successfully, by giving the patient white wax dissolved in milk. Others extol the virtues of the *Connessi* root, the *Simaruba* bark, &c. for the cure of this disease. When other medicines fail, these strong astringents may be tried; but we hope they will seldom be found necessary. At any rate, astringent, or binding medicines, never are to be used till proper evacuations have been premised,

ſed, otherwiſe they will fix the diſeaſe inſtead of removing it.

PERSONS who have been cured of this diſeaſe are very liable to relapſe; to prevent which, great circumſpection with reſpect to diet is neceſſary. The patient muſt abſtain from all fermented liquors, except now and then a glaſs of good wine; but he muſt drink no kind of malt-liquor. He muſt likewiſe abſtain from animal food, as fiſh and fleſh, and muſt live principally upon milk and vegetables.

GENTLE exerciſe and wholeſome air are likewiſe of importance. The patient ſhould go to the country as ſoon as his ſtrength will permit, and ſhould take exerciſe daily on horſeback, or in a machine. He may likewiſe uſe bitters infuſed in wine or brandy, and may drink twice a-day a gill of lime-water mixed with an equal quantity of new milk.

WHEN dyſenteries prevail, we would recommend a ſtrict attention to cleanlineſs, a ſpare uſe of animal food, and the free uſe of ſound ripe fruits, and other vegetables. The night-air is to be carefully avoided, and all communication with the ſick. Bad ſmells are likewiſe to be ſhunned, eſpecially thoſe which ariſe from putrid animal ſubſtances. The office-houſes where the ſick go are very dangerous. Nothing is more apt to occaſion the diſeaſe than being greatly afraid of it.

WHEN the firſt ſymptoms of the dyſentery appear,

appear, the patient ought immediately to take a vomit, to go to bed, and drink plentifully of weak warm liquor, to promote a ſweat. This, with a doſe or two of rhubarb, would often carry off the diſeaſe at the beginning. In countries where dyſenteries prevail, we would adviſe ſuch as are liable to them, to take either a vomit or a doſe of phyſic every ſpring and autumn, as a preventive.

THERE are ſundry other fluxes of the belly, as the LIENTERY and COELIAC PASSION, which, tho' leſs dangerous than the dyſentery, yet merit conſideration. Theſe diſeaſes generally proceed from a relaxed ſtate of the ſtomach and inteſtines, which is ſometimes ſo great, that the food paſſes through them without almoſt any ſenſible alteration; and the patient dies merely from the want of nouriſhment.

WHEN the lientery or cœliac paſſion ſucceed a dyſentery, they often prove fatal. They are always dangerous in old age, eſpecially when the conſtitution has been broken by exceſs or acute diſeaſes. If the ſtools be very frequent, and quite crude, the thirſt great, with little urine, the mouth ulcerated, and the face marked with ſpots of different colours, the danger is very great.

THE treatment of the patient is in general the ſame as in the dyſentery. In all obſtinate fluxes of the belly, from whatever cauſe, the cure muſt be attempted, by firſt cleaning the ſtomach and bowels with gentle vomits and purges,

ges. Afterwards ſuch a diet as has a tendency to brace and ſtrengthen the bowels, with opiates and aſtringent medicines, will generally perfect the cure.

THIS obſervation likewiſe holds with reſpect to a TENESMUS, or frequent deſire of going to ſtool. It reſembles the dyſentery ſo much, both in its ſymptoms and method of cure, that we think it needleſs to inſiſt upon it.

OF A DIABETES, OR EXCESSIVE DISCHARGE OF URINE.

THE diabetes may be called a flux of the kidneys. It is ſeldom to be met with among young people; but I have often known it happen to labourers in the decline of life, eſpecially thoſe who followed the more violent employments, and who had been hard drinkers in their youth.

CAUSES.—— A diabetes is often the conſequence of acute diſeaſes, as fevers, fluxes, &c. where the patient has ſuffered exceſſive evacuations; it may alſo be occaſioned by exceſſive fatigue, as riding long journeys upon a hard-trotting horſe, carrying heavy burdens, running, &c. It may be brought on by the uſe of ſtrong ſtimulating diuretic medicines, as tincture of cantharides, ſpirits of turpentine, and ſuch like. It is often the effect of drinking large quantities of mineral waters. Many imagine that theſe will do them no ſervice unleſs they be drank in large

large quantities, by which miſtake it happens that they often occaſion worſe diſcaſes than thoſe they were taken to cure. In a word, this diſeaſe may either proceed from too great a laxity of the organs which ſecrete the urine, from ſomething that ſtimulates the kidneys too much, or from a thin diſſolved ſtate of the blood, which makes too great a quantity of it run off by the urinary paſſages.

SYMPTOMS.—— In a diabetes the urine generally exceeds in quantity all the liquid food and drink which the patient takes. It is thin and pale, of a ſweetiſh taſte, and an agreeable ſmell. The patient has a continual thriſt, with ſome degree of fever; his mouth is dry, and he ſpits frequently a frothy ſpittle The ſtrength fails, the appetite decays, and the fleſh waſtes away till the patient is reduced to ſkin and bone. There is a heat of the bowels; and frequently the loins, teſticles, and feet are ſwelled.

THIS diſeaſe may be cured at the beginning; but, after it has continued long, the cure becomes very difficult. In drunkards, and very old people, a cure is not to be expected.

REGIMEN.—— Every thing that ſtimulates the urinary paſſages, or tends to relax the habit, muſt be avoided. The patient ſhould live chiefly on ſolid food. His thirſt may be quenched with acids, as ſorrel, juice of lemon, or vinegar. The mucilaginous vegetables, as rice, ſago, and ſalop, with milk, are the moſt proper food.

Of animal ſubſtances, ſhell-fiſh are to be preferred, as oyſters, crabs, &c.

THE drink may be Briſtol-water. When that cannot be obtained, lime-water with milk may be drank. This will be better if an ounce of gum arabic be diſſolved in every pound of it. The white decoction, with iſinglaſs diſſolved in it, is likewiſe a very proper drink. It is made by boiling two ounces of calcined hartſhorn, and half an ounce of gum-arabic, in three Engliſh pints of water, to two, and afterwards ſtraining it.

THE patient ought daily to take exerciſe, but it ſhould be ſo gentle as not to fatigue him. He ſhould lie upon a hard bed or mattreſs. Nothing hurts the kidneys more than lying too ſoft. A warm dry air, the uſe of the fleſh bruſh, and every thing that promotes perſpiration, is of ſervice. For this reaſon the patient ought to wear flannel next his ſkin. A large ſtrengthening plaſter may be applied to the back; or, what will anſwer the ſame end, a broad girdle may be worn about the loins.

MEDICINE.—— Gentle purges, if the patient be not too much weakened by the diſeaſe, have a good effect. They tend to promote a flux of the humours towards the inteſtines, and of courſe to leſſen the diſcharge by the kidneys. They may conſiſt of rhubarb, with cardamum ſeeds, or any other ſpiceries, infuſed in wine, and may be taken in ſuch quantities as to keep the belly gently open.

THE patient muſt next have recourſe to aſtringents

ſtringents and corroborants. Half a dram of powder made of equal parts of allum and the gum called *dragon's blood,* may be taken four times a-day, or oftner if the ſtomach will bear it. The allum muſt firſt be melted in a crucible; afterwards they may both be pounded together. Along with every doſe of this powder the patient may take a tea cupful of the tincture of roſes. It is made by infuſing in a ſtone-ware veſſel, for four hours, an ounce of the dried leaves of red roſes, with one dram of ſpirit of vitriol, in two Engliſh pints of boiling water. Afterwards the tincture may be filtred, and four or five ounces of white ſugar added to it.

If the patient's ſtomach cannot bear the allum in ſubſtance, whey may be made of it, and taken in the doſe of three or four ounces three times a-day. The allum-whey is prepared by boiling two Engliſh quarts of milk over a ſlow fire, with three drams of allum, till it be turned into whey.

Opiates are of ſervice in this diſeaſe, even though the patient reſts well. They take off ſpaſm and irritation, and at the ſame time leſſen the force of the circulation. Ten or twelve drops of liquid laudanum may be taken in a cup of the patient's drink two or three times a-day.

The beſt corroborants which we know, are the jeſuits bark and wine. A dram of bark may be taken in a glaſs of red port or claret three times a-day. The medicine will be more efficacious and leſs diſagreeable, if fifteen or twenty ty drops of the acid elixir of vitriol be added to every doſe. Such as cannot take the bark in ſubſtance may uſe the decoction, mixed with an equal quantity of red wine, and ſharpened as above.

THERE is a diſeaſe pretty incident to labouring people in the decline of life, called *an INCONTINENCY of urine.* This differs intirely from a diabetes, as the water paſſes off involuntarily by drops, and does not exceed the uſual quantity. This diſeaſe is rather troubleſome than dangerous. It is owing to a relaxation of the ſphincter of the bladder, and is often the effect of a palſy. Sometimes it proceeds from hurts, or injuries occaſioned by blows, bruiſes, preternatural labours, &c. Sometimes it is the effect of a fever. It may likewiſe be occaſioned by a long uſe of ſtrong diuretics, or of ſtimulating medicines injected into the bladder.

THIS diſeaſe may be mitigated by the uſe of aſtringent and corroborating medicines, ſuch as have been mentioned above; but we do not remember ever to have ſeen it cured.

OF A SUPPRESSION OF URINE.

IT has already been obſerved, that a ſuppreſſion of urine may proceed from various cauſes; as an inflammation of the kidneys, or bladder; ſmall ſtones or gravel lodged in the urinary paſſages, hard *fæces* lying in the *rectum,* a ſpaſm or or contraction of the neck of the bladder, clotted blood in the bladder, a swelling of the hæmorrhoidal veins, &c.

SOME of these cases require the cathater, both to remove the obstructing matter, and to draw off the urine; but as this instrument can only be managed with safety by persons skilled in surgery, we shall say nothing further of its use.

WE would chiefly recommend, in all obstructions of urine, fomentations and evacuations. If the patient be young, of a full habit, and if his pulse be hard, frequent bleeding will be necessary, especially where there are symptoms of a topical inflammation. Bleeding in this case not only abates the fever, by lessening the force of the circulation, but, by relaxing the solids, takes off the spasm or stricture upon the vessels, which occasioned the obstruction.

AFTER bleeding, fomentations must be used. These may either consist of warm water alone, or of decoctions of mild vegetables; as mallows, camomile-flowers, &c. Cloths dipped in these may either be applied to the part affected, or a large bladder filled with the decoction may be kept continually upon it. Some put the herbs themselves into a flannel-bag, and apply them to the part, which is far from being a bad method. These continue longer warm than cloths dipped in the decoction, and at the same time keep the part equally moist.

IN all obstructions of urine the belly ought

to

to be kept open. This is not however to be attempted by brisk purgatives, but by emollient clysters, or gentle infusions of senna and manna. Clysters in this case not only open the belly, but answer the purpose of an internal fomentation, and greatly assist in removing spasms of the bladder, &c.

THE food must be light, and taken in small quantities. The drink may be weak broth, or decoctions and infusions of mucilaginous vegetables, as marsh mallow roots, lime-tree buds, &c. A tea spoonful of the sweet spirits of nitre, or a dram of Castile soap, may be frequently put into the patient's drink; and if there be no inflammation, he may drink small gin punch without acid.

IN a suppression of urine, nature often attempts to relieve the patient by a sweat, looseness, spitting, gulping up of clear water from the stomach, &c. These discharges ought not to be suppressed, but encouraged, as the patient's life often depends on them.

PERSONS subject to a suppression of urine ought to live very temperate. Their diet should be light, and their liquor diluting. They ought to avoid all acids, and wines that abound with tartar; they should likewise take plenty of exercise, lie hard, and avoid study and sedentary occupations.

OF

OF COSTIVENESS.

No perſon can long enjoy good health who does not go regularly to ſtool. There is however a very great difference of perſons in this reſpect, ſome being able to bear coſtiveneſs much longer than others. We do not here mean to treat of thoſe aſtrictions of the bowels which are the ſymptoms of diſeaſes, as in the colic, the iliac paſſion, &c. but only to take notice of that infrequency of ſtools which ſometimes happens, and which in ſome particular conſtitutions may occaſion diſeaſes.

COSTIVENESS may proceed from an exceſſive heat of the liver; drinking rough red wines, or other aſtringent liquors; too much exerciſe, eſpecially on horſeback: It may likewiſe proceed from a long uſe of cold inſipid food, which does not ſufficiently ſtimulate the inteſtines. Sometimes it is owing to the bile not deſcending to the inteſtines, as in the jaundice; and at other times it proceeds from diſeaſes of the inteſtines themſelves, as a palſy, ſpaſms, tumors, a cold dry ſtate of the inteſtines, &c.

WHEN coſtiveneſs is conſtitutional, it may be born a long time without any bad effects; but when it proceeds from an inflammation or tumor in the inteſtines, it is dangerous. Coſtiveneſs, when long continued, is apt to occaſion pains of the head, vomiting, colics, &c. It is peculiarly hurtful to hypochondriac and hyſteric perſons, as it generates wind and other grievous ſymptoms.

PERSONS who are liable to be coſtive ſhould live upon a moiſtening and laxative diet, as roaſted or boiled apples, pears, ſtewed prunes, raiſins, gruels with currants, butter, honey, and ſugar, &c. Green broths with ſpinage, leeks, and other ſoft pot-herbs, are likewiſe proper. Rye-bread, or that which is made of a mixture of wheat and rye together, ought to be eat. No perſon troubled with coſtiveneſs ſhould eat wheat-bread alone, eſpecially that which is made of fine flower. The beſt bread for keeping the belly ſoluble is what the Engliſh call *meſlin.* It is made of equal parts of wheat and rye; or more commonly of two parts of the former to one of the latter.

COSTIVENESS is increaſed by keeping the body too warm, and by every thing that promotes the perſpiration; as wearing flannel, lying too long a-bed, &c. Intenſe thought, and a ſedentary life, are likewiſe hurtful. All the ſecretions and excretions are promoted by moderate exerciſe without doors, and by a gay, cheerful, ſprightly temper of mind.

THE drink ſhould be of an opening quality. All ardent ſpirits, auſtere and aſtringent wines, as port, claret, &c. ought to be avoided. Malt-liquor that is fine, and of a moderate ſtrength, is very proper. Butter-milk, whey, and other watery liquors, are likewiſe proper, and may

be

be drank in turns, as the patient's inclination directs.

* THOSE who are troubled with coſtiveneſs ought, if poſſible, to remedy it by diet, as the conſtant uſe of medicines for that purpoſe is attended with many inconveniencies, and often with bad conſequences. I never knew any one get into a habit of taking medicine for keeping the belly open, who could leave it off. In time the cuſtom becomes neceſſary, and generally ends in a total relaxation of the bowels, indigeſtion,

* THE learned Dr Arbuthnot adviſes thoſe who are troubled with coſtiveneſs to uſe animal oils, as freſh butter, cream, marrow, fat broths, eſpecially thoſe made of the internal parts of animals, as the liver, heart, midriff, &c He likewiſe recommends the expreſſed oils of mild vegetables, as olives, almonds, paſtaches, and the fruits themſelves; all oily and mild fruits, as figs; decoctions of mealy vegetables; theſe lubricate the inteſtines; ſome ſaponaceous ſubſtances which ſtimulate gently, as honey, hydromel, or boiled honey and water, unrefined ſugar, &c.

THE doctor obſerves, that ſuch lenitive ſubſtances are proper for perſons of dry atrabilarian conſtitutions, who are ſubject to aſtriction of the belly, and the piles, and will operate when ſtronger medicinal ſubſtances are ſometimes ineffectual; but that ſuch lenitive diet hurts thoſe whoſe bowels are weak and lax. He likewiſe obſerves that all watery ſubſtances are lenitive, and that even common water whey, ſour milk and butter-milk have that effect;——That new milk, eſpecially aſſes milk, ſtimulates ſtill more when it ſours on the ſtomach; and that whey turned ſour will purge ſtrongly — That moſt garden fruits are likewiſe laxative; and that ſome of them, as grapes, will throw ſuch as take them immoderately, into a cholera morbus, or incurable diarrhœa.

geſtion, loſs of appetite, waſting of the ſtrength, and death.

When the belly cannot be kept open without medicine, we would recommend gentle doſes of rhubarb to be taken twice or thrice a-week. This is not near ſo injurious to the ſtomach as aloes, jalap, or the other draſtic purgatives ſo much in uſe. Infuſions of ſenna and manna may likewiſe be taken, or half an ounce of ſoluble tartar diſſolved in water-gruel. About the ſize of a nutmeg of lenitive electuary taken twice or thrice a-day, generally anſwers the purpoſe very well.

Of INVOLUNTARY DISCHARGES OF BLOOD.

Spontaneous, or involuntary diſcharges of blood, often happen from various parts of the body. They are ſeldom however attended with great danger, and prove often ſalutary. When ſuch diſcharges are critical, which is frequently the caſe in fevers, they ought not to be ſtopped. Nor indeed is it proper at any time to ſtop them, unleſs they be ſo great as to endanger the patient's life. Moſt people, afraid of the ſmalleſt appearance of blood from any part of the body, flie immediately to the uſe of ſtiptic and aſtringent medicines, by which means an an inflammation of the brain, or ſome other fatal diſeaſe, is occaſioned, which, had the diſcharge been allowed to go on, might have been prevented.

PERIODICAL diſcharges of blood, from whatever part of the body they proceed, muſt not be ſtopped. Theſe are always the efforts of nature to relieve herſelf, and fatal diſeaſes have often been the conſequence of obſtructing them. It may indeed be ſometimes neceſſary to check the violence of ſuch diſcharges; but even this requires the greateſt caution. Inſtances may be given where the ſtopping of a ſmall periodical flux of blood, from one of the fingers, has proved fatal to the perſon's health.

IN the early period of life, bleeding at the noſe is moſt common. Thoſe who are farther advanced in life are more liable to a hæmoptoe, or diſcharge of blood from the lungs. After the middle period of life, hæmorrhoidal fluxes are moſt common, and in the decline of life, diſcharges of blood from the urinary paſſages.

INVOLUNTARY fluxes of blood may proceed from very different, and often from quite oppoſite cauſes. Sometimes they are hereditary, or owing to a particular conſtruction of the body, as a ſanguine temperament, a lax or plethoric habit, &c. Sometimes they proceed from a determination of the blood towards one particular part, as the head, the hæmorrhoidal veins, &c. They may likewiſe proceed from an an inflammatory diſpoſition of the blood, in which caſe there is generally ſome degree of fever: this likewiſe happens when the flux is occaſioned by an obſtructed perſpiration, or a ſtricture upon the ſkin, the bowels, or any particular part of the ſyſtem.

But a diſſolved ſtate of the blood will likewiſe occaſion hæmorrhages. Thus, in putrid fevers, the ſcurvy, the malignant ſmall pox, &c. there are often very great diſcharges of blood from different parts of the body. They may likewiſe be brought on by the uſe of any medicines which tend to diſſolve the blood, as mercury, cantharides, and the volatile alcaline ſalts, &c. Food of an acrid or irritating quality may likewiſe occaſion hæmorrhages; as alſo ſtrong purges and vomits, or any thing that greatly ſtimulates the bowels.

Violent paſſions or agitations of the mind will alſo occaſion hæmorrhages. Theſe often cauſe bleeding at the noſe, and I have known them ſometimes occaſion an hæmorrhage in the brain. Violent efforts of the body, by overſtraining or hurting the veſſels, may likewiſe bring on hæmorrhages, eſpecially when the body is long kept in an unnatural poſture, as hanging the head very low, &c.

The cure of an hæmorrhage muſt be adapted to its cauſe. When it proceeds from too much blood, or a tendency to inflammation, bleeding, with gentle purges and other evacuations, will be neceſſary. It will likewiſe be proper for the patient

patient in that caſe to live chiefly upon a vegetable diet, to avoid all ſtrong liquors, and food that is of an acrid, hot, or ſtimulating quality. The body ſhould be kept cool, and the mind eaſy.

WHEN an hæmorrhage is owing to a putrid or diſſolved ſtate of the blood, the patient ought to live chiefly upon acid fruits with milk, and vegetables of a nouriſhing nature, as ſago, ſalop, &c. His drink may be wine diluted with water, and ſharpened with the juice of lemon, vinegar, or ſpirits of vitriol. The beſt medicine in this caſe is the jeſuits bark. It may be taken as directed pages 387. and 388.

WHEN a flux of blood is the effect of acrid food, or of ſtrong ſtimulating medicines, the cure is to be effected by ſuch ſoft and mucilaginous diet as is recommended in the dyſentery or bloody flux. The patient may likewiſe take frequently about the bulk of a nutmeg of Locatelli's balſam, or the ſame quantity of ſperma ceti.

WHEN an obſtructed perſpiration, or a ſtricture upon any part of the ſyſtem, is the cauſe of an hæmorrhage, it may be removed by drinking warm diluting liquors, lying a-bed, bathing the extremities in warm water, &c.

OF BLEEDING AT THE NOSE.

A bleeding at the noſe is commonly preceded by ſome degree of quickneſs of the pulſe, a fluſhing in the face, pulſation of the temporal arteries, heavineſs in the head, dimneſs of the ſight heat and itching of the noſtrils &c.

To perſons who abound with blood this diſcharge is very ſalutary. It often cures a vertigo, the headach, a phrenzy, and even an epilepſy. In fevers where there is a great determination of blood towards the head, it is of the utmoſt ſervice. It is likewiſe beneficial in inflammations of the liver and ſpleen, and often in the gout and rheumatiſm. In all diſeaſes where evacuations are neceſſary, a ſpontaneous diſcharge of blood from the noſe, is of much more ſervice than the ſame quantity let with a lancet.

In a diſcharge of blood from the noſe, the great point is to determine whether it ought to be ſtopped or not. It is a common practice to ſtop the bleeding without conſidering whether it be a diſeaſe, or the cure of a diſeaſe. This conduct proceeds from fear; but it has many bad and ſometimes even fatal conſequences.

When a diſcharge of blood from the noſe happens in an inflammatory diſeaſe, there is always reaſon to believe that it may prove ſalutary; and therefore it ſhould be ſuffered to go on, at leaſt

leaſt as long as the patient ſeems to bear it well.

When it happens to perſons in perfect health, who are full of blood, it ought not to be ſtopped; eſpecially if the ſymptoms of plethora, mentioned above, have preceded it. In this caſe it cannot be ſtopped without riſking the patient's life.

In fine, whenever bleeding at the noſe relieves any bad ſymptom, and does not proceed ſo far as to endanger the patient's life, it ought not to be ſtopped. But when it returns frequently, or continues till the pulſe becomes very low, the extremities begin to grow cold, the lips pale, or the patient complains of being ſick, or like to faint, it muſt immediately be ſtopped.

The patient ſhould be ſet nearly upright, with his head inclining a little backwards, and his legs immerſed in water about the warmth of new milk. His hands ought likewiſe to be put in lukewarm water, and his garters may be tied a little tighter than uſual, about three inches above the knee. Ligatures may likewiſe be applied to the arms, about the place where they are uſually made for bleeding, and with nearly the ſame degree of tightneſs. Theſe muſt be gradually ſlackened as the blood begins to ſtop, and removed intirely as ſoon as it gives over.

Sometimes dry lint put up the noſtrils will ſtop the bleeding. When this does not ſucceed, doſſils of lint dipped in ſtrong ſpirits of wine, may be put up the noſtrils, or, if that cannot

cannot be had, they may be dipped in brandy. Roman vitriol diſſolved in water may likewiſe be uſed for this purpoſe, or a tent dipped in the white of an egg well beat up, may be rolled in a powder made of equal parts of white ſugar, burnt allum, and white vitriol, and put up the noſtril from whence the blood iſſues.

INTERNAL medicines can hardly take place here, as they have ſeldom time to operate. It may not however be amiſs to give the patient half an ounce of Glauber's ſalt, and the ſame quantity of manna, diſſolved in four or five ounces of barley-water. This may be taken at a draught, and repeated if it does not operate in a few hours. Ten or twelve grains of nitre may be taken in a glaſs of cold water and vinegar every hour, or oftener, if the ſtomach will bear it. If a ſtronger medicine be neceſſary, a tea-cupful of the tincture of roſes, made as directed page 387. with twenty or thirty drops of the ſmall ſpirit of vitriol, may be taken every hour. When theſe things cannot be had, the patient may drink water, with a little common ſalt in it, or equal parts of water and vinegar.

IF the genitals be immerſed in cold water, it will generally ſtop a bleeding at the noſe.—I have never known this fail.

SOMETIMES when the blood is ſtopped outwardly, it continues to bleed inwardly. This is very dangerous, and requires particular attention, as the patient is apt to be ſuffocated with the blood, eſpecially if he falls aſleep, which

which he is very ready to do after loſing a great quantity of blood.

After the bleeding is ſtopped, the patient ought to be kept as eaſy and quiet as poſſible. He ought not to pick his noſe, nor to take away the tents or clotted blood, till they fall off of their own accord, and ſhould not lie with his head too low.

Those who are affected with frequent bleeding at the noſe ought to bathe their feet often in warm water, and keep them warm and dry. They ought to wear nothing tight about their necks, to keep their body as much in an erect poſture as poſſible, and never to view any object obliquely. If they have too much blood, a vegetable diet, with now and then a doſe of phyſic, is the ſafeſt way to leſſen it.

But when the diſeaſe proceeds from a thin diſſolved ſtate of the blood, the diet ſhould be rich and nouriſhing; as ſtrong broths with bread, ſago-gruel with wine and ſugar, &c. Infuſions of the jeſuits bark in wine ought likewiſe to be taken and perſiſted in for a conſiderable time.

OF THE BLEEDING AND BLIND PILES.

A diſcharge of blood from the hæmorrhoidal veſſels is called the *bleeding piles*. When the veſſels only ſwell, and diſcharge no blood, but are exceeding painful, the diſeaſe is called the *blind piles*.

PERSONS of a looſe ſpungy texture, of a bulky ſize, who live high, and lead a ſedentary inactive life, are moſt ſubject to this diſeaſe. It is often owing to a hereditary diſpoſition. Where this is the caſe, it attacks perſons more early in life than when it is accidental. Men are more liable to it than women, eſpecially thoſe of a ſanguine plethoric habit, or of a melancholly diſpoſition.

THE piles may be occaſioned by an exceſs of blood, by ſtrong aloetic purges, high ſeaſoned food, drinking great quantities of ſweet wines, the neglect of bleeding, or other cuſtomary evacuations, much riding, great coſtiveneſs, or any thing that occaſions hard or difficult ſtools. Anger, grief, and other violent paſſions, will likewiſe occaſion the piles. I have often known them brought on by cold, eſpecially about the *anus*. A pair of thin breeches will occaſion the diſorder in a perſon who is ſubject to it, and and ſometimes even in thoſe who never had it before. Pregnant women are often afflicted with the piles.

A flux of blood from the *anus* is not always to be reckoned a diſeaſe. It is even more ſalutary than bleeding at the noſe, and often prevents or carries off diſeaſes. It is peculiarly beneficial in the gout, rheumatiſm, aſthmas, and hypochondriacal complaints, and often proves critical in colics, and inflammatory fevers.

IN

In the treatment of this diſeaſe regard muſt be had to the patient's habit of body, his age, ſtrength, and manner of living. A diſcharge which might be exceſſive and prove hurtful to one, may be very moderate, and even ſalutary to another. That only is to be eſteemed dangerous which continues ſo long, and in ſuch quantity, as to waſte the patient's ſtrength, hurt the digeſtion, nutrition, and other functions neceſſary to life.

When that is the caſe, the diſcharge muſt be checked by a proper regimen, and aſtringent medicines. The DIET muſt be cool but nouriſhing, conſiſting chiefly of bread, milk, cooling vegetables and broths. The DRINK may be chalybeate water, orange whey, decoctions or infuſions of the aſtringent and mucilaginous plants, as the tormentil root, the marſh mallow roots, &c.

Old conſerve of red roſes is a very good medicine in this caſe. It may be mixed with new milk, and taken in the quantity of an ounce three or four times a-day. This medicine is in no great repute, owing to its being ſeldom taken in ſuch quantity as to produce any effects; but when taken as here directed, and duly perſiſted in, I have known it perform very extraordinary cures in violent hæmorrhages, eſpecially when aſſiſted by the tincture of roſes; a teacupful of which may be taken about an hour after every doſe of the conſerve. The method

of

of preparing this tincture is mentioned page 387.

The jesuits bark is likewise proper in this case, both as a strengthener and astringent. It may be taken in red wine, sharpened with the spirit of vitriol.

The bleeding piles are sometimes periodical, and return regularly once a month, or once in three weeks. In this case they are always to be considered as a salutary discharge, and by no means to be stopped. Some have intirely ruined their health by stopping a periodical discharge of blood from the hæmorrhoidal veins.

In the *blind piles* bleeding is generally of use. The diet must be light and thin, and the drink cool and diluting. It is likewise necessary that the belly be kept gently open. This may be done by small doses of flower of brimstone and cream of tartar. These may be mixed in equal quantities, and a tea spoonful taken two or three times a-day, or as often as is necessary to keep the belly easy. Or an ounce of flower of brimstone and half an ounce of purified nitre may be mixed with three or four ounces of the lenitive electuary, and a tea-spoonful of it taken three or four times a-day.

Emollient clysters are likewise beneficial; but there is sometimes such an astriction of the *anus*, that they cannot be thrown up. In this case I have known a vomit have an exceeding good effect.

When

When the piles are exceeding painful and ſwelled, but diſcharge nothing, the patient muſt ſit over the ſteams of warm water. He may likewiſe apply a linen-cloth dipped in warm ſpirits of wine to the part, or poultices made of bread and milk, or of leeks fried with butter. If theſe do not produce a diſcharge, and the piles appear large, leeches muſt be applied as near the piles as poſſible, or if they will fix upon the piles themſelves ſo much the better. When leeches will not fix, the piles may be opened with a lancet. The operation is very eaſy, and is attended with no danger.

Various ointments, and other external applications, are recommended in the piles; but I do not remember ever to have ſeen any effects from theſe worth mentioning. Their principal uſe is to keep the part ſoft, which may be done equally well by a ſoft poultice or an emollient cataplaſm.

SPITTING OF BLOOD.

We only mean here to treat of that diſcharge of blood from the lungs, which commonly goes by the name of an *hæmoptoe*, or *ſpitting of blood.* Perſons of a ſlender make, and a lax fibre, who have long necks and ſtrait breaſts, are moſt liable to this diſeaſe. It is moſt common

common in the ſpring, and generally attacks people before they arrive at the prime or middle period of life. It is a common obſervation, that thoſe who have been ſubject to bleeding at the noſe when young, are afterwards moſt liable to an hæmoptoe.

CAUSES.——An hæmoptoe may proceed from exceſs of blood, from a peculiar weakneſs of the lungs, or a bad conformation of the breaſt. It is often occaſioned by exceſſive drinking, running, wreſtling, ſinging, or ſpeaking aloud. Such as have weak lungs ought to avoid all violent exertions of that organ, as they value life. They ſhould likewiſe guard againſt violent paſſions, and every thing that occaſions a rapid circulation of the blood.

THIS diſeaſe may likewiſe proceed from wounds of the lungs. Theſe may either be received from without, or they may be occaſioned by hard bodies getting into the wind pipe, and ſo falling down upon the lungs, and hurting their tender veſſels. The obſtruction of any cuſtomary evacuation may occaſion a ſpitting of blood; as the neglect of bleeding or purging at the uſual ſeaſons, the ſtoppage of the bleeding piles in men, or the menſes in women, &c. It may likewiſe proceed from a polypus, ſchirrous concretions, or any thing that obſtructs the circulation of the blood in the lungs. It is often the effect of a long and violent cough; in which caſe it is generally the forerunner of a conſumption. A violent degree of cold ſuddenly applied

plied to the external parts of the body will occasion an hæmoptoe. It may likewiſe be occaſioned by breathing in air which is too much rarified to be able properly to expand the lungs. This is often the caſe with thoſe who work in hot places, as furnaces, glaſs-houſes, &c. It may likewiſe happen to ſuch as aſcend to the top of very high mountains, as the peak of Teneriff, &c.

SPITTING of blood is not always to be conſidered as a primary diſeaſe. It is often only a ſymptom, and in ſome caſes not an unfavourable one. This is the caſe in pleuriſies, peripneumonies, and ſundry other fevers. In a dropſy, ſcurvy, or conſumption, it is a bad ſymptom, and ſhews that the lungs are ulcerated.

SYMPTOMS.—— Spitting of blood is generally preceded by a ſenſe of weight, and oppreſſion of the breaſt, a dry tickling cough, hoarſeneſs, and a difficulty of breathing. Sometimes it is uſhered in with ſhivering, coldneſs of the extremities, coſtiveneſs, great laſſitude, flatulence, pains of the back and loins, &c. As theſe ſhew a general ſtricture upon the veſſels, and a tendency of the blood to inflammation, they are commonly the forerunners of a very copious diſcharge. Theſe ſymptoms do not attend a diſcharge of blood from the gums or fauces, by which means they may always be diſtinguiſhed from an hæmoptoe. Sometimes the blood that is ſpit up is thin, and of a florid red colour; and at other times it is thick, and of a dark or blackiſh colour; nothing however can be inferred from this circumſtance, but that the blood has lain a longer or ſhorter time in the breaſt before it was diſcharged.

SPITTING of blood, in a ſtrong healthy perſon, of a ſound conſtitution, is ſeldom dangerous; but when it attacks the tender and delicate, or perſons of a weak lax fibre, it is not eaſily removed. When it proceeds from a ſchirrus or polypus of the lungs, it is bad. The danger is greater when the diſcharge proceeds from the rupture of a large veſſel than of a ſmall one. When the extravaſated blood is not ſpit up, but lodges in the breaſt, it corrupts, and greatly increaſes the danger. When the blood proceeds from an ulcer in the lungs, it is generally fatal.

REGIMEN.—— The patient ought to be kept cool, and perfectly at reſt. Every thing that heats the blood, or quickens the circulation, increaſes the danger. The mind ought likewiſe to be ſoothed, and every occaſion of exciting the paſſions avoided. The diet ſhould be ſoft, cooling, and ſlender; as rice boiled with milk, ſmall broths, barley gruels, panada, &c. The diet, in this caſe can ſcarce be too low. Even water-gruel is ſufficient to ſupport the patient for ſome days. All ſtrong liquors muſt be avoided. The patient may drink milk and water, barley-water, whey, butter-milk, and ſuch like. Every thing ſhould be drank cold, and in ſmall quantities at a time. The patient muſt

muſt obſerve the ſtricteſt ſilence, or at leaſt ſpeak with a very low voice.

MEDICINE.—— This, like the other involuntary diſcharges of blood, ought not to be ſuddenly ſtopped by aſtringent medicines. More miſchief is often done by theſe than if it were ſuffered to go on. It may however proceed ſo far as to weaken the patient, and even endanger his life, in which caſe proper means muſt be uſed for reſtraining it.

THE belly ſhould be kept gently open by laxative diet; as roaſted apples, ſtewed prunes, &c. If theſe ſhould not have the effect, a tea-ſpoonful of the lenitive electuary may be taken twice or thrice a-day, as is found neceſſary. If the bleeding proves violent, ligatures may be applied to the extremities, as directed for the bleeding at the noſe.

IF the patient be hot or feveriſh, bleeding and ſmall doſes of nitre will be of uſe; a ſcruple or half a dram may be taken in a cup of his ordinary drink twice or thrice a-day. His drink may likewiſe be ſharpened with acids, as juice of lemon, or a few drops of the ſpirit of vitriol; or he may take frequently a cup of the tincture of roſes, as directed page 387.

BATHING the feet and legs in lukewarm water, by taking off ſpaſm, has a very good effect in this diſeaſe. Opiates too are ſometimes beneficial for that purpoſe; but theſe muſt be given with the greateſt caution. Ten or twelve drops of laudanum may be given in a cup of barley-water twice a-day, and continued for ſome time, provided they be found beneficial.

THE conſerve of roſes is likewiſe a very good medicine in this caſe, provided it be taken in ſufficient quantity, and long enough perſiſted in. It may be taken to the extent of three or four ounces a day; and, if the patient be troubled with a cough, it ſhould be made into an electuary with balſamic ſyrup, and a little of the ſyrup of poppies.

IF ſtronger aſtringents be found neceſſary, fifteen or twenty drops of the acid elixir of vitriol may be taken in a glaſs of water, three or four times a day.

THOSE who are ſubject to frequent returns of this diſeaſe, ſhould be careful to avoid all exceſs. Their diet ſhould be light and cool, conſiſting chiefly of milk and vegetables. Above all, let them beware of vigorous efforts of the body, and violent agitations of the mind.

VOMITING OF BLOOD.

THIS is not ſo common as the other diſcharges of blood which have already been mentioned; but it is more dangerous, and requires the greateſt attention.

VOMITING of blood is generally preceded by pains in the ſtomach, ſickneſs and nauſea, and

and is accompanied with great anxiety, and frequent fainting fits.

VOMITING of blood is ſometimes periodical; in which caſe it is leſs dangerous. It often proceeds from an obſtruction of the menſes in women; and ſometimes from the ſtopping of the hæmorrhoidal flux in men. It may be occaſioned by any thing that greatly ſtimulates or wounds the ſtomach, as ſtrong vomits or purges, acrid poiſons, ſharp or hard ſubſtances taken into the ſtomach, &c. It is often the effect of obſtructions in the liver, the ſpleen, or ſome of the other viſcera. It may likewiſe proceed from external violence, as blows or bruiſes, or from any of the cauſes which produce inflammation.

A great part of the danger in this diſeaſe ariſes from the extravaſated blood lodging in the bowels, and becoming putrid, by which means a dyſentery or putrid fever may be occaſioned. The beſt way of preventing this, is to keep the belly gently open, by frequently exhibiting emollient clyſters. Purges muſt not be given till the diſcharge is ſtopt, otherwiſe they will irritate the ſtomach, and increaſe the diſorder. All the food and drink muſt be of a mild cooling nature, and taken in ſmall quantities. Even drinking cold water has ſometimes proved a remedy. When there are ſigns of an inflammation, bleeding may be neceſſary; but the patient's weakneſs will ſeldom permit it. Aſtringents can ſeldom be uſed, as they ſtimulate

ſtimulate the ſtomach, and of courſe increaſe the diſeaſe. Opiates may be of uſe; but they muſt be given in very ſmall doſes, as four or five drops of liquid laudanum twice or thrice a-day. After the diſcharge is over, as the patient is generally troubled with gripes, occaſioned by the acrimony of the blood lodged in the inteſtines, gentle purges will be neceſſary.

OF BLOODY URINE.

THIS diſorder is commonly called *piſſing of blood.* It is a diſcharge of blood, with or without urine, from the veſſels of the kidneys or bladder, which may be either enlarged, broken, or eroded. It is more or leſs dangerous according to the different circumſtances which attend it.

WHEN pure blood is voided ſuddenly without interruption and without pain, it proceeds from the kidneys; but if the blood be in ſmall quantity, of a dark colour, and emitted with heat and pain about the bottom of the belly, it proceeds from the bladder. When bloody urine is occaſioned by a large rough ſtone deſcending from the kidneys to the bladder, which wounds the *ureters*, it is attended with a ſharp pain in the back and difficulty of making water. If the coats of the bladder are hurt by a ſtone, and bloody urine follows, it is attended-ed with the moſt acute pain, and a previous ſtoppage of urine.

BLOODY urine may likewiſe be occaſioned by falls, blows, the lifting or carrying of heavy burdens, hard riding, or any violent motion. It may alſo proceed from ulcers or eroſions of the bladder, from a ſtone lodged in the kidneys, or from violent purges, or ſharp diuretic medicines, eſpecially cantharides.

BLOODY urine is always attended with ſome degree of danger; but it is peculiarly ſo when mixed with purulent matter, as this ſhews an ulcer ſomewhere in the urinary paſſages. Sometimes this diſcharge proceeds from exceſs of blood, in which caſe it is rather to be conſidered as a ſalutary evacuation than a diſeaſe. If the diſcharge however be very great, it may waſte the patient's ſtrength, and occaſion an ill habit of body, a dropſy, or a conſumption, &c.

THE treatment of this diſorder muſt be varied according to the different cauſes from which it proceeds.

WHEN it is owing to a ſtone in the bladder, the cure depends upon an operation, which it is not our buſineſs to deſcribe.

IF it be attended with a plethora, and ſymptoms of an inflammation, bleeding will be neceſſary. The belly muſt likewiſe be kept open by emollient clyſters, or cooling purgative medicines; as cryſtals of tartar, rhubarb, manna, or ſmall doſes of lenitive electuary.

WHEN bloody urine proceeds from a diſſolved

ved ſtate of the blood, it is commonly the ſymptom of ſome malignant diſeaſe; as the ſmall pox, a putrid fever, or the like. In this caſe the patient's life depends on the liberal uſe of the jeſuits bark and acids, as has already been ſhewn.

WHEN there is reaſon to ſuſpect an ulcer in the kidneys or bladder, the patient's diet muſt be cool, and his drink of a ſoft, healing, balſamic quality, as decoctions of marſhmallow roots with liquorice, ſolutions of gum arabic, &c. Three ounces of marſhmallow roots, and half an ounce of liquorice, may be boiled in two Engliſh quarts of water to one; two ounces of gum-arabic, and half an ounce of purified nitre, may be diſſolved in the ſtrained liquor, and a tea-cupful of it taken four or five times a-day.

THE early uſe of aſtringents in this diſeaſe has often bad conſequences. When the flux is ſtopped too ſoon, the grumous blood, by being confined in the veſſels, may produce inflammations, abſceſs, and ulcers. If however the caſe be urgent, or the patient ſeem to ſuffer from the loſs of blood, gentle aſtringents may be neceſſary. In this caſe the patient may take three or four ounces of * lime-water, with half an ounce

* LIME-WATER is prepared by pouring two Engliſh gallons of water gradually upon a pound of quicklime; when the ebullition is over, let the whole ſtand to ſettle for two days, then filter the liquor through paper. It ſhould be kept in veſſels cloſely ſtopped.

ounce of the tincture of jesuits bark three times a-day. Or he may take an ounce or two of the conserve of roses three or four times a day, drinking a tea cupful of the tincture of roses after it. If stronger styptics be necessary, a dram of Armenian bole may be taken in a cup of whey three or four times a day.

OF VOMITING.

VOMITING may proceed from various causes; as excess in eating or drinking; a foul stomach; the acrimony of the aliments; the translation of the morbific matter of ulcers, the gout, the erysipelas, and other diseases, to the stomach. It may likewise proceed from a looseness, or flux of blood being too suddenly stopped, or from the stoppage of any customary evacuation, as the bleeding piles, the *menses*, &c. Vomiting may proceed from the weakness of the stomach, the colic, the iliac passion, a rupture, a fit of the gravel, worms, or from any kind of poison taken into the stomach. It is an usual symptom of hurts of the brain; as contusions, compressions, &c. It is likewise a symptom of wounds, or inflammations of the diaphragm, intestines, spleen, liver, kidneys, &c.

VOMITING may be occasioned by unusual motions; as riding backwards in a cart or coach, sailing, &c. It may likewise be excited by violent passions, or by the idea of nauseous objects,

jects, especially of such things as have formerly produced vomiting. Sometimes it proceeds from a regurgitation of the bile into the stomach; in this case what the patient vomits is generally of a yellow or greenish colour, and has a bitter taste. Persons who are subject to nervous affections are often suddenly seized with violent fits of vomiting. Lastly, Vomiting is a common symptom of pregnancy. In this case it generally comes on about two weeks after the stopping of the *menses*, and continues during the first three or four months.

WHEN vomiting proceeds from a foul stomach or indigestion, it is not to be considered as a disease, but as the cure of a disease. It ought therefore to be promoted by drinking lukewarm water, or thin gruel. If this does not put a stop to the vomiting, a dose of ipecacuanha may be taken, and wrought off with weak camomile-tea.

WHEN the retrocession of gouty matter, or the obstruction of customary evacuations occasion vomiting, all means must be used to restore these discharges; or, if that cannot be effected, their place must be supplied by others, as bleeding, purging, bathing the extremities in warm water, opening issues, setons, perpetual blisters, &c.

WHEN vomiting proceeds from pregnancy, it may generally be relieved by bleeding, and keeping the belly gently open. The bleeding however ought to be in small quantities at a time,

time, and the purgatives ſhould be of the mildeſt kind, as figs, ſtewed prunes, manna or ſenna. Pregnant women are moſt apt to vomit in the morning, immediately after geting out of bed, which is owing partly to the change of poſture, but more to the emptineſs of the ſtomach. It may generally be prevented by taking a diſh of tea, or ſome light breakfaſt in bed. Pregnant women who are afflicted with vomiting ought to be kept eaſy both in body and mind. They ſhould neither allow their ſtomachs to be quite empty, nor ſhould they eat much at once. Cold water is a very good drink in this caſe; if the ſtomach be weak, a little brandy may be added to it. If the ſpirits be low, and the perſon apt to faint, a ſpoonful of cinnamon-water, with a little marmalade of quinces or oranges, may be taken.

If vomiting proceeds from weakneſs of the ſtomach, bitters will be of ſervice, as the Gentian root, camomile and ſnake-root, infuſed in brandy or wine. To theſe may be added as much rhubarb as will keep the belly gently open. The jeſuits bark is likewiſe an excellent medicine for bracing and ſtrengthening the ſtomach. It may be drank in form of tea, or infuſed in wine or brandy, &c. The elixir of vitriol is alſo a good medicine in this caſe. It may be taken in the doſe of fifteen or twenty drops, twice or thrice a-day, in a glaſs of wine or water.

A vomiting which proceeds from acidities

 in

in the ſtomach is relieved by alkaline purges. The beſt medicine of this kind is the magneſia alba, a tea ſpoonful of which may be taken in a diſh of tea or a little milk, twice or thrice a-day, or oftener if neceſſary, to keep the belly open.

WHEN vomiting proceeds from violent paſſions, or affections of the mind, all kind of evacuations muſt be avoided, eſpecially vomits. Theſe are exceeding dangerous. The patient in this caſe ought to be kept perfectly eaſy and quiet, to have the mind ſoothed, and to take ſome gentle cordial, as negas, or a little brandy and water. A few drops of liquid laudanum may likewiſe be taken, to calm the ſpirits, and take off the irritation upon the nerves.

WHEN vomiting proceeds from ſpaſmodic affections of the ſtomach, muſk, caſtor, and other antiſpaſmodic medicines, are of uſe. Aromatic plaſters have likewiſe a good effect. The ſtomach plaſter of the London or Edinburgh diſpenſatory may be applied to the pit of the ſtomach, or rather a little towards the left ſide, ſo as to cover a part of the falſe ribs. Aromatic medicines may likewiſe be taken inwardly, as cinnamon-tea, mint-tea, wine with ſpiceries boiled in it, &c. The region of the ſtomach may be rubbed with æther, or, if that cannot be had, with ſtrong brandy, or other ſpirits. The belly ſhould be fomented with warm water, or the patient immerſed up to the breaſt in a warm bath.

I have always found the ſaline draughts moſt effectual in ſtopping a vomiting, from whatever cauſe it proceeded. Theſe may be made by diſſolving a dram of the ſalt of tartar in an ounce and half of freſh lemon juice, adding to it an ounce of peppermint water, and half an ounce of ſpirituous cinnamon-water. This draught may be ſweetened with a little white ſugar, and taken in the act of efferveſcence. It muſt be repeated every two hours, or every hour, if the vomiting be very violent. I do not remember to have ſeen this medicine, when duly perſiſted in, fail to ſtop a vomiting.

As the leaſt motion will often bring on the vomiting again, even after it has been ſtopped, the patient muſt avoid all manner of action. His diet muſt be ſo regulated as to ſit eaſy upon the ſtomach, and he ſhould take nothing that is hard of digeſtion. We do not however mean that the patient is to live upon ſlops. Solid food, in this caſe, often ſits eaſier on the ſtomach than liquids.

OF THE HEAD ACH.

THE head-ach is produced by various cauſes, and attended with different ſymptoms, according to its different degrees, and the part where it is ſituated. When it is ſlight, and affects a particular part of the head, it is called *cephalalgia*;

lalgia; when the whole head is affected *cephalæa*; and when one fide only, *hemicrania*. A fixed pain in the forehead, which may be covered with the end of the thumb, is called *clavis hystericus*.

THERE are alfo other diftinctions. Sometimes the pain is internal, fometimes external; fometimes it is an original difeafe, and at other times only fymptomatic. When the head ach proceeds from a hot bilious habit, the pain is very acute and throbbing, with a confiderable heat of the part affected. When from a cold phlegmatic habit, the patient complains of a dull heavy pain and has a fenfe of coldnefs in the part. This kind of head ach is fometimes attended with a degree of ftupidity or folly.

WHATEVER obftructs the free circulation of the blood through the veffels of the head, may occafion a head-ach. In perfons of a full habit, who abound with blood, or other humours, the head-ach often proceeds from the fuppreffion of cuftomary evacuations; as bleeding at the nofe, fweating of the feet, &c. It may likewife proceed from any caufe that determines a greater flux of blood towards the head; as coldnefs of the extremities, hanging of the head, &c. Whatever prevents the return of the blood from the head will likewife occafion a head-ach; as looking long at any object obliquely, wearing any thing tight about the neck, &c.

WHEN a head ach proceeds from the ftoppage of a running of the nofe, there is a heavy, obtufe, preffing preſſing pain in the forepart of the head, in which there ſeems to be ſuch a weight, that the patient can ſcarce hold it up. When it is occaſioned by the cauſtic matter of the venereal diſeaſe, it generally affects the ſkull, and often produces a *caries* of the bones.

SOMETIMES the head-ach proceeds from the repulſion, or retroceſſion of the morbific matter of the gout, the eryſipelas, the ſmall pox, meaſles, itch, or other eruptive diſeaſes. A *hemicrania* generally proceeds from crudities or indigeſtion.

THERE is likewiſe a moſt violent, fixed, conſtant, and almoſt intolerable head-ach, which occaſions great debility both of body and mind, prevents ſleep, diſturbs digeſtion, deſtroys the appetite, cauſes a *vertigo*, dimneſs of ſight, a noiſe in the ears, convulſions, epileptic fits, and ſometimes vomiting, coſtiveneſs, coldneſs of the extremities, &c.

THE head ach is often ſymptomatic in continual and intermitting fevers, eſpecially quartans. It is likewiſe a very common ſymptom of hyſteric and hypochondriac complaints.

AN external pain of the head is ſeldom dangerous. When it attends an acute fever, with pale urine, it is an unfavourable ſymptom. In exceſſive head achs, coldneſs of the extremities is a bad ſign. When the diſeaſe continues long, and is very violent, it often terminates in blindneſs, an apoplexy, deafneſs, a *vertigo*, the palſy, epilepſy, &c.

THE

THE cool regimen in general is to be obferved in this difeafe. The diet ought to confift of fuch emollient fubftances as will correct the acrimony of the humours, and keep the belly open; as apples boiled in milk, fpinage, turnips, and fuch like. The drink ought to be diluting; as barley-water, infufions of mild mucilaginous vegetables, decoctions of the fudorific woods, * &c. The feet and legs ought to be kept warm, and frequently bathed in lukewarm water; the head fhould be fhaved, and bathed with water and vinegar. The patient ought, as much as poffible, to keep an erect pofture, and not to lie with his head too low.

WHEN the head-ach is owing to excefs of blood, and in hot bilious conftitutions, bleeding is neceffary. The patient may be bled in the jugular vein, and the operation repeated if there be occafion. Cupping alfo, or the application of leeches to the temples, and behind the ears, may be of fervice. Afterwards a bliftering plafter may be applied to the neck, or behind the ears, or to any part of the head that is

* THE decoction of woods is thus made. Take fhavings of guaiacum wood, three ounces; raifins of the fun, ftoned, two ounces; faffafras wood, fhaved, one ounce; liquorice fliced. half an ounce. Boil the guaiacum and raifins in an Englifh gallon of water, over a gentle fire, to the confumption of one half; adding towards the end the faffafras and liquorice Strain the liquor, and having fuffered it to fettle for fome time, pour off the clear liquor from the fœces. This may be taken at pleafure for ordinary drink.

is moſt affected. In ſome caſes it will be proper to bliſter the whole head. In perſons of a groſs habit, iſſues or perpetual bliſters will be of ſervice. The belly ought likewiſe to be kept open by gentle laxatives.

BUT when the head-ach proceeds from a copious vitiated *ſerum* ſtagnating in the membranes, either within or without the ſkull, with a dull, heavy, continual pain, which will neither yield to bleeding nor gentle laxatives, then more powerful purgatives are neceſſary, as pills made of aloes, reſin of jalap, or the like. It will alſo be neceſſary in this caſe to bliſter the whole head, and to keep the back part of the neck open for a conſiderable time by a perpetual bliſter.

WHEN the head-ach is occaſioned by a ſtoppage of the running of the noſe, the patient ſhould frequently ſmell to a bottle of volatile ſalts; he may likewiſe take ſnuff, or any thing that will irritate the noſe, ſo as to promote a diſcharge from it; as the herb maſtich, ground-ivy, &c.

A *hemicrania*, eſpecially a periodical one, is generally owing to a foulneſs in the ſtomach, for which gentle vomits will be beneficial, as alſo purges of rhubarb. After the bowels have been ſufficiently cleared, chalybeate waters, and ſuch bitters as ſtrengthen the ſtomach, will be neceſſary.

WHEN the head-ach ariſes from a vitiated ſtate of the humours, as in the ſcurvy and venereal

nereal diſeaſe, the patient, after proper evacuations, muſt drink freely of the decoction of woods, recommended above, or the decoction of ſarſaparilla with raiſins and liquorice *. Theſe promote perſpiration, ſweeten the humours, and, if duly perſiſted in, will produce very happy effects. When a collection of matter is felt under the ſkin, it muſt be diſcharged by an inciſion, otherwiſe it will render the bone carious.

WHEN the head-ach is ſo intolerable as to endanger the patient's life, or is attended with continual watching, delirium, &c. recourſe muſt be had to opiates. Theſe, after proper evacuation by clyſters, or mild purgatives, may be applied both externally and internally. The affected part may be rubbed with Bate's anodyne balſam, or a cloth dipped in it may be applied to the part. The patient may, at the ſame time, take twenty drops of laudanum, in a cup of valerian or pennyroyal tea, twice or thrice a-day. This is only to be done in caſe of extreme pain. Proper evacuations ought always to accompany and follow the uſe of opiates.

WHEN the patient cannot bear the loſs of blood, his feet ought frequently to be bathed in lukewarm water, and well rubbed with a coarſe cloth. Cataplaſms with muſtard or horſe-radiſh

* This is made by boiling three ounces of freſh ſarſaparilla, an ounce of raiſins, and half an ounce of liquorice, in three Engliſh quarts of water to one. The liquor muſt be ſtrained, and an Engliſh pint of it drank daily.

radiſh ought likewiſe to be applied to them. This courſe is peculiarly neceſſary when the pain proceeds from a gouty humour affecting the head.

When the head ach is occaſioned by great heat, hard labour, or violent exerciſe of any kind, it may be allayed by cooling medicines; as the ſaline draughts with nitre, &c.

OF THE TOOTH-ACH.

This diſeaſe is ſo well known, that it needs no deſcription. It has great affinity with the rheumatiſm, and often ſucceeds pains of the ſhoulders and other joints.

It may proceed from various cauſes; as obſtructed perſpiration or catching cold; or from any of the common cauſes of inflammation. I have often known the tooth ach occaſioned by neglecting ſome part of the uſual coverings of the head, by ſitting with the head bare near an open window, or its being any how expoſed to a draught of cold air. Food or drink taken either too hot or too cold, is very hurtful to the teeth. Great quantities of ſugar, or other ſweet-meats, are likewiſe hurtful. Nothing is more deſtructive to the teeth than cracking nuts, or chewing any kind of hard ſubſtances. Picking the teeth with pins, needles, or with any thing that may hurt the enamel with which they are covered, does great miſchief; as the tooth is ſure to be ſpoilt whenever the air gets into it. Pregnant women are very ſubject to the tooth ach, eſpecially during the firſt three or four months of pregnancy. The tooth ach often proceeds from ſcorbutic humours affecting the gums. In this caſe the teeth are ſometimes waſted, and fall out without any conſiderable degree of pain. The proximate or immediate cauſe of the tooth ach is a rotten or *carious* tooth.

In order to relieve the tooth ach, we muſt endeavour to draw off or divert the humours from the part affected. This may be done by mild purgatives, bleeding, and bathing the feet frequently in warm water. The perſpiration ought likewiſe to be promoted, by drinking freely of weak wine whey, or other diluting liquors, with ſmall doſes of nitre. Vomits too have often an exceeding good effect in the tooth ach. It is ſeldom ſafe to adminiſter opiates, or any kind of heating medicines, or even to draw a tooth till proper evacuations have been premiſed, and theſe alone will often effect the cure.

Next to evacuations we recommend fomenting the part with warm water, or decoctions of emollient vegetables. Bags filled with boiled camomile flowers, flowers of elder, or the like, may be applied to the part affected, with as great a degree of warmth as the patient can bear, and renewed as they grow cool. The patient may likewiſe receive the ſteams of warm water in-

to

to his mouth, through an inverted funnel, or by holding his head over the mouth of a porringer filled with warm water, &c.

GARGLES are likewise of use to make a discharge from the part. Rob of elder dissolved in small beer makes a very proper gargle, or an infusion of sage or mulberry leaves.

SUCH things as promote the discharge of saliva, or cause the patient to spit, are always proper. For this purpose bitter, hot, or pungent vegetables may be chewed; as gentian, calamus aromaticus, or pellatory of Spain. Allen recommends the root of *yellow water flower de luce* in this case. This root may either be rubbed upon the tooth or chewed. Brookes says, he hardly ever knew it fail to ease the tooth-ach.

MANY other herbs, roots, and seeds, &c. are recommended for curing the tooth-ach; as the leaves or roots of millefoil or yarrow chewed, tobacco smoaked or chewed, or the ashes put into the hollow tooth, staves acre, or the seeds of mustard chewed, &c. These bitter, hot, and pungent things, by occasioning a great flow of *saliva*, frequently give ease in the tooth-ach.

OPIATES often relieve the tooth-ach. For this purpose a little cotton wet with laudanum may be held between the teeth; or a piece of sticking plaster, about the bigness of a sixpence, with a bit of opium in the middle of it, of a size not to prevent the sticking of the other, may be be laid on the temporal artery, where the pulſation is moſt ſenſible. *De la Motte* affirms, that there are few caſes wherein this will not give relief. If there be a hollow tooth, a ſmall pill made of equal quantities of camphire and opium, put into the hollow, is often beneficial. When this cannot be had, the hollow tooth may be filled with gum maſtich, wax, lead, or any ſubſtance that will ſtick in it, and keep the external air out.

FEW applications give more relief in the tooth-ach than bliſtering plaſters. Theſe may be applied betwixt the ſhoulders, but they have the beſt effect when put behind the ears, and made ſo large as to cover a part of the lower jaw. Burning the nerve within the affected tooth with a hot iron, has frequently given eaſe; but this operation ought to be done with care. Applying a hot iron to the *antetragus*, or what is called *the inner bar of the ear*, is likewiſe a noted cure for the tooth-ach. Bliſtering however is more ſafe than either of theſe, and is not leſs efficacious.

HOFFMAN ſays, When every thing elſe failed, that he had often great ſucceſs from the following pills.

TAKE of aromatic pill one dram, ſtorax pill half a dram, extract of ſaffron ſix grains. Make them into nine pills; of which ſix or eight are to be taken at bed time for a doſe.

AFTER all, when a tooth is carious, it is often impoſſible to remove the pain, without draw-

drawing the tooth; and, as a ſpoilt tooth never becomes ſound again, it is prudent to draw it ſoon, leſt it ſhould affect the reſt. Tooth-drawing, like bleeding, is very much practiced by mechanics as well as perſons of the medical profeſſion. The operation however is not without danger, and ought always to be done with care. A perſon unacquainted with the ſtructure of the parts will be in danger of breaking the jaw-bone, or of drawing a ſound tooth inſtead of a rotten one, &c.

WHEN a ſound tooth has been drawn, if it be replaced immediately, it will grow in again. It is now a common practice to draw a rotten tooth, and put a ſound one, taken from the mouth of ſome other perſon, in its place. It is likewiſe an eaſy matter to fix artificial teeth ſo neatly, as to anſwer moſt of the purpoſes of the natural; but theſe are matters which do not properly fall under our conſideration.

WHEN the tooth-ach returns periodically, and the pain chiefly affects the gums, it may be cured by the bark.

SOME pretend to have found great benefit in the tooth-ach, from the application of an artificial magnet to the affected tooth. We ſhall not attempt to account for its mode of operation, but, if it be found to anſwer, though only in particular caſes, it certainly deſerves a trial, as it is attended with no expence, and cannot do any harm.

PERSONS who have returns of the tooth-ach

at

at certain ſeaſons, as ſpring and autumn, might often prevent it by taking a doſe of phyſic at theſe times.

Keeping the teeth clean has no doubt a tendency to prevent the tooth ach. The beſt method of doing this is to waſh them daily with ſalt and water, or with cold water alone. All bruſhing and ſcraping of the teeth is dangerous, and, unleſs it be performed with great care, muſt do miſchief.

OF THE EAR-ACH.

This diſorder chiefly affects the membrane which lines the inner cavity of the ear called the *meatus auditorius*. It is often ſo violent as to occaſion great reſtleſſneſs and anxiety, and even delirium. Sometimes epileptic fits, and other convulſive diſorders, have been brought on by extreme pain in the ear.

The ear-ach may proceed from any of the cauſes which produce inflammation. It often proceeds from a ſudden ſuppreſſion of perſpiration, or from the head being expoſed to cold when covered with ſweat. It may alſo be occaſioned by worms, or other inſects getting into the ear, or being bred there; or from any hard body ſticking in the ear. Sometimes it proceeds from the tranſlation of morbific matter to the ear. This often happens in the decline of malignant fevers,

fevers, and occasions deafness, which is generally reckoned a favourable symptom.

WHEN the ear ach proceeds from insects, or any hard body sticking in the ear, every method must be taken to remove them as soon as possible. The membranes may be relaxed by dropping into the ear oil of sweat almonds, or olive oil. Afterwards the patient should be made to sneeze, by taking snuff, or some strong sternutatory. If this should not force out the body, it must be extracted by art. I have seen insects, which had got into the ear, come out of their own accord upon pouring in oil upon them, which is a thing they cannot bear.

WHEN the pain of the ear proceeds from inflammation, it must be treated like other topical inflammations, by a cooling regimen and opening medicines. Bleeding at the beginning, either in the arm or jugular vein, or cupping in the neck, will be proper. The ear may likewise be fomented with steams of warm water, or flannel-bags filled with boiled mallows and camomile flowers may be applied to it warm; or bladders filled with warm milk and water. An exceeding good method of fomenting the ear is to apply it close to the mouth of a jug filled with a strong decoction of camomile flowers.

THE patient's feet should be frequently bathed in lukewarm water, and he ought to take small doses of nitre and rhubarb, viz. a scruple of the former, and ten grains of the latter three times a-day. His drink may be whey, or decoctions of barley and liquorice with figs or raisins, &c. The parts behind the ear ought frequently to be rubbed with camphorated oil, or the volatile liniment; and a few drops of the camphorated spirit of wine may be put into the ear with wool or cotton.

When the inflammation cannot be resolved, a poultice of bread and milk, or roasted onions, may be applied to the ear, and frequently renewed, till it breaks, or the abscess can be opened. Afterwards the humours may be diverted from the part by gentle laxatives, blisters, or issues; but the discharge must not be suddenly dried up by any external application.—I have often known the sudden drying of a running of the ear produce fatal consequences.

OF THE HEART-BURN.

What is called the *heart burn* is not a disease of that organ, but an uneasy sensation of heat or acrimony about the pit of the stomach, which is sometimes attended with anxiety, nausea, and vomiting.

It may proceed from indigestion; from the acidity of the fluids, or contents of the stomach; or from bilious humours. Stale liquors, vinegar, greasy aliment, wind, &c. will cause the heart-burn. In some constitutions it is occasioned

oned by the uſe of acids, and in others by aromatics. Pregnant women are very ſubject to it.

WHEN the heart burn proceeds from indigeſtion, or a foul ſtomach, the patient ought to take a vomit, and afterwards a purge. After the ſtomach has been cleanſed, he may drink twice or thrice a day a cup of camomile tea, with fifteen or twenty drops of elixir of vitriol in it, in order to ſtrengthen the ſtomach and promote digeſtion.

WHEN acidity or ſourneſs of the ſtomach occaſions the heart-burn, abſorbents are the proper medicines. In this caſe chalk and water, or what is called the chalk julep, often anſwers very well. It is made by mixing an ounce of powdered chalk, half an ounce of fine ſugar, and a quarter of an ounce of gum arabic, in two Engliſh pints of water. A tea cupful of this may be taken at pleaſure. When the gum arabic cannot be had, the chalk may be mixed with milk, or taken in water alone. The teſtacious powders are very proper here. A tea-ſpoonful of prepared oyſter-ſhells, or the powder called crab's eyes, may be taken in a glaſs of peppermint-water, or ſimple cinnamon-water, as often as there is occaſion.

BUT the ſafeſt abſorbent which we know is the *magneſia alba*. This not only acts as an abſorbent, but by its purging quality cleanſes the bowels; whereas the chalk, and other abſorbents of that ſort, are apt to lie in the inteſtines, and occaſion obſtructions. This pow-

 der,

der is no way disagreeable, and may be taken in a cup of tea, a little milk, or a glass of peppermint water. A large tea-spoonful is the usual dose, but there is no danger in taking a much greater quantity, and it may be repeated as often as is found necessary.

When the heart burn proceeds from bilious humours, a tea spoonful of the sweat spirits of nitre in a glass of water, or a cup of tea or coffee, will generally give ease. If it be caused by fat or greasy aliments, a dram of brandy, or rum may be taken.

If wind be the cause of this complaint, the medicines called carminatives are proper; as aniseeds, juniper-berries, cardamom-seeds, &c. These may either be chewed, or a glass of their distilled waters taken at pleasure. These, and other warm aromatics, as ginger, cannella alba, &c. give ease, but they ought never to be used unless when necessary. They are only drams in a dry form, and very pernicious to the stomach. One of the safest medicines of this kind is the tincture made by infusing an ounce of rhubarb, and a quarter of an ounce of the lesser cardamoms, in an English pint of brandy. This must digest for two days; afterwards it should be strained, and four ounces of white sugar candy in powder added to it. It must stand to digest again till the sugar be dissolved. A table spoonful may be taken for a dose.

I have frequently known the heart-burn cured by the patient chewing green tea.

PAIN

PAIN of the STOMACH.

THIS may proceed from various cauſes; as indigeſtion; wind; the acrimony of the bile; or from ſharp, acrid, or poiſonous ſubſtances taken into the ſtomach. It may likewiſe proceed from worms; the ſtoppage of cuſtomary evacuations; or from a tranſlation of gouty matter to the ſtomach, &c.

WOMEN in the decline of life are very liable to this diſeaſe eſpecially ſuch as are afflicted with hyſteric complaints. It is likewiſe very common to hypochondriac men of a ſedentary and luxurious life. In ſuch perſons it often proves ſo extremely obſtinate, as to baffle all attempts of medicine.

WHEN the pain of the ſtomach is moſt violent after eating, there is reaſon to ſuſpect that it proceeds from ſome fault either in the digeſtion or the food. In this caſe the patient ought to change his diet, till he finds what kind of food agrees beſt with his ſtomach, and ſhould continue chiefly to uſe that. If a change of diet does not remove the complaint, the patient may take a gentle vomit, and afterwards a doſe or two of rhubarb. He ought likewiſe to take an infuſion of camomile-flowers, or ſome other ſtomachic bitter either in wine or water. I have often known exerciſe remove this complaint, eſpecially ſailing, or a long journey on horſeback, or in a machine.

WHEN a pain of the ſtomach proceeds from flatulencies, the patient is conſtantly belching up wind, and feels an uneaſy diſtenſion of the ſtomach after meals. This is a moſt deplorable diſeaſe and is ſeldom cured. In general, the patient ought to avoid all windy diet, and every thing that ſours on the ſtomach, as greens, roots, &c. This rule however admits of ſome exceptions. I have known ſeveral inſtances of perſons very much troubled with wind, who received great benefit from eating parched peas *, though that grain is well known to be of a windy nature. This complaint may likewiſe be greatly relieved by exerciſe, eſpecially digging, walking, or riding, &c. I have found the elixir of vitriol anſwer very well in flatulencies. It may be taken as directed page 433.

WHEN a pain of the ſtomach is occaſioned by the ſwallowing of acrid or poiſonous ſubſtances, they muſt be diſcharged by vomit; this may be excited by butter, oils, or other ſoft things, which ſheath and defend the ſtomach from the acrimony of its contents.

WHEN pain of the ſtomach proceeds from a tranſlation of gouty matter, warm cordials are neceſſary. Some have drank a whole bottle of brandy or rum, in this caſe, in a few hours, without being in the leaſt intoxicated, or even feeling the ſtomach warmed by it. Generous wines however

* THESE are prepared by ſteeping or ſoaking peas in water, and afterwards drying them in a pot or kiln till they be quite hard. They may be uſed at pleaſure.

ever are more ſafe, as genuine Madeira, &c. It is impoſſible to aſcertain the quantities neceſſary upon theſe occaſions. This muſt be left to the feelings and diſcretion of the patient. It is however the ſafer way not to go too far. When there is an inclination to vomit, it may be promoted by drinking an infuſion of camomile-flowers or *carduus benedictus*.

If a pain of the ſtomach proceeds from the ſtoppage of cuſtomary evacuations, bleeding will, in ſome caſes, be neceſſary, eſpecially in ſanguine and very full habits. It will likewiſe be of uſe to keep the belly gently open by mild purgatives; as rhubarb or ſenna, &c. When this diſeaſe affects women in the decline of life, after the ſtoppage of the *menſes*, making an iſſue in the leg or arm will be of peculiar ſervice.

When the diſeaſe is occaſioned by worms, they muſt be deſtroyed, or expelled by ſuch means as are recommended in the following ſection.

OF WORMS.

These are chiefly of three kinds, viz. the *tænia*, or tape worm; the *teres*, or round and long worm, and the *aſcarides*, or round and ſhort worm. There are many other kinds of worms found in the human body; but as they proceed, in a great meaſure, from ſimilar cauſes, have nearly the ſame ſymptoms, and require

quire almoſt the ſame method of cure, we ſhall not ſpend time in enumerating them.

THE tape-worm is white, very long, and all over jointed. It is generally bred either in the ſtomach or ſmall inteſtines. The round and long worm is likewiſe bred in the ſmall guts, and ſometimes in the ſtomach. The round and ſhort worms commonly lodge in the *rectum*, or what is called the end-gut, and occaſion a diſagreeable itching about the *anus*.

THE long round worms occaſion ſqueamiſhneſs, vomiting, an ill breath, gripes, looſeneſs, ſwelling of the belly, ſwoonings, loathing of food, and at other times a voracious appetite, a dry cough, convulſions, epilectic fits, and ſometimes a privation of ſpeech. Theſe worms have been known to perforate the inteſtines, and get into the cavity of the belly. The effects of the tape-worm are nearly the ſame with thoſe of the long and round, but rather more violent.

ANDRY ſays, the following ſymptoms particularly attend the *ſolium*, which is a ſpecies of the tape-worm, viz. ſwoonings, privation of ſpeech, and a voracious appetite. The round worms called *aſcarides*, beſides an itching of the *anus*, cauſe ſwoonings, and teneſmus, or an inclination to go to ſtool.

CAUSES.—— Worms may proceed from various cauſes; but they are ſeldom found except in weak and relaxed ſtomachs, where the digeſtion is bad. Sedentary perſons are more liable to them than the active and laborious. Thoſe who

who eat great quantities of unripe fruit, or who live much on raw herbs and roots, are generally ſubject to worms. Worms are often a ſymptom of fevers, and other acute diſeaſes. There ſeems to be a hereditary diſpoſition in ſome perſons to this diſeaſe. I have often ſeen all the children of a family ſubject to worms of a particular kind. They ſeem likewiſe frequently to be owing to the nurſe. Children of the ſame family, nurſed by one woman, have often worms, when thoſe nurſed by another have none.

CHILDREN are more liable to this diſeaſe than adults, eſpecially after two years of age. Infants while on the breaſt are ſeldom troubled with worms. To this however there are ſeveral exceptions. I lately ſaw an inſtance of a child who paſſed worms before it was three months old. They were indeed of a very particular kind, being real caterpillars. Some of them were above an inch long; they had red heads, and were ſo briſk as to jump about; they lived ſeveral days after the child had paſſed them. Another child ſuckled by the ſame woman paſſed the ſame kind of worms when upon the breaſt, and both children ſuffered extremely before the worms came away.

SYMPTOMS.—— The common ſymptoms of worms are, paleneſs of the countenance, and, at other times, an univerſal fluſhing of the face; itching of the noſe, this however is doubtful,

doubtful, as children pick their noſes in all diſeaſes; ſtarting, and grinding of the teeth in ſleep; the appetite ſometimes bad, at other times quite voracious; looſeneſs; a ſour or ſtinking breath; a hard ſwelled belly; great thirſt; the urine frothy, and ſometimes of a whitiſh colour; gripping, or colic pains; an involuntary diſcharge of *ſaliva*, eſpecially when aſleep; frequent pains of the ſide, with a dry cough, and unequal pulſe; palpitations of the heart; ſwoonings; drowſineſs; cold ſweats; palſy; epilectic fits, with many other unaccountable nervous ſymptoms, which were formerly attributed to witchcraft, or the influence of evil ſpirits. Small bodies in the excrements reſembling melon or cucumber ſeeds are ſymptoms of the tape worm.

THO' this is a very common diſeaſe, yet it is leſs ſo than is generally imagined. Nurſes impute moſt of the diſeaſes of children to worms, and often give medicine to kill theſe vermine where they do not exiſt. Even phyſicians are often deceived with reſpect to worms. I have frequently opened children who were thought to have been killed by them, and found none. In ſhort, there is no certain proof of worms exiſting in the inteſtines, but their being paſſed; and that will ſometimes happen where no previous ſymptoms appeared.

MEDICINES.—— Though numberleſs medicines are extolled for killing and expelling

ing worms *, yet no disease more frequently baffles the physician's skill. In general, the most proper medicines for their expulsion are strong purgatives; and to prevent their breeding, stomachic-bitters, with now and then a glass of good wine.

The best purge for an adult is jalap and calomel. Five and twenty or thirty grains of the former, with six or seven of the latter, mixed in syrup, may be taken for a dose. This should be taken early in the morning. It will be proper that the patient keep the house all day, and drink nothing cold. The dose may be repeated once or twice a week, for a fortnight or three weeks. On the intermediate days the patient may take a dram of the powder of tin, twice or thrice a-day, mixed with syrup, honey, or treacle.

Those who do not chuse to take calomel may make use of the bitter purgatives; as aloes, hiera picra, tincture of senna and rhubarb, &c.

Oily medicines are likewise of use for expelling worms. An ounce of salad oil and a table-spoonful of common salt, may be taken in a glass of red port wine thrice a-day, or oftener if the stomach will bear it. But the more common form of using oil is in clysters. Oily

* A medical writer of the present age has enumerated upwards of fifty British plants, all famous for killing and expelling worms out of the body.

clysters sweetned with sugar or honey, are very efficacious in bringing away the short round worms called *ascarides*.

The Harrowgate water is an excellent medicine for expelling worms, especially the *ascarides*. As this water evidently abounds with sulphur, we may hence infer, that sulphur alone must be a good medicine in this case; this is found to be true in fact. Many practitioners give flower of sulphur in very large doses, and with great success. It may be made into an electuary with honey or treacle, and taken in such quantity as to purge the patient.

Where Harrowgate-water cannot be obtained, sea-water may be used, which is far from being a contemptible medicine in this case. If sea-water cannot be had, common salt may be dissolved in water and drank. I have often seen this used by country nurses, when they suspected their children were troubled with worms, with very good effect.

But worms, tho' expelled, will soon breed again, if the stomach remains weak and relaxed; to prevent this, we would recommend the jesuits bark. Half a dram of bark in powder may be taken in a glass of red port-wine, three or four times a-day, after the above medicines have been used. Lime water is likewise good for this purpose, or a table spoonful of the chalybeate

wine

wine * taken twice or thrice a-day. Infusions or decoctions of bitter herbs may likewise be drank; as the infusion of tansy, water-trefoil, camomile flowers, tops of wormwood, the lesser centaury, &c.

The above directions are calculated for adults; but for children the medicines must be more agreeable, and given in smaller doses.

For a child of four or five years old, ten grains of rhubarb, five of jalap, and two of calomel, may be mixed in a spoonful of syrup or honey, and given in the morning. The child should keep the house all day, and have nothing cold. This dose may be repeated twice a-week for three or four weeks. On the intermediate days the child may take a scruple of powdered tin and ten grains of æthiops mineral in a spoonful of treacle twice a day. These doses must be increased or diminished according to the age of the patient.

I have frequently known those big bellies, which in children are commonly reckoned a sign of worms, quite removed by giving them white soap in their pottage, or other food. Tansy, garlic, and rue, are all good against worms, and may be used various ways. We might here mention many plants, both for external and

* The chalybeate wine is made by digesting three ounces of filings of iron, and half a dram of cochineal, in two English pints of Rhenish wine for three weeks, frequently shaking the vessel. Afterwards the liquor must be filtered.

and internal uſe, but think the powder of tin with æthiops mineral, and the purges of rhubarb and calomel are much more to be depended on. It will not however be amiſs to give a child who is troubled with worms a glaſs of red wine now and then, as every thing that braces and ſtrengthens the ſtomach is good both for preventing and expelling theſe vermine.

Parents who would preſerve their children from worms ought to allow them plenty of exerciſe in the open air, to ſee that their food be wholeſome and ſufficiently ſolid, and, as far as poſſible, to prevent their eating raw herbs, roots, or green traſhy fruits *.

OF THE JAUNDICE.

This diſeaſe is firſt obſervable in the white of the eye, which appears of a yellowiſh colour. Afterwards the whole ſkin puts on a yellow, and ſometimes a blackiſh appearance. The urine

* We think it neceſſary here to warn people of their danger who buy worm-cakes and powders at random from quacks, and give them to their children without proper care. The principal ingredient in moſt of theſe medicines is mercury, which is never to be trifled with. I lately ſaw a ſhocking inſtance of the danger of this conduct. A girl who had taken a doſe of worm-powder, bought of a travelling quack, went out, and I believe might be ſo imprudent as to drink cold water during its operation. She immediately ſwelled, and died that very day, with all the ſymptoms of having been poiſoned.

urine too is of a ſaffron hue, and dyes a white cloth, if put into it, of the ſame colour.

CAUSES.——The immediate cauſe of the jaundice is an obſtruction of the bile. The remote or occaſional cauſes are, the bites of poiſonous animals, as the viper, mad dog, &c. the bilious or hyſteric colic; violent paſſions, as grief, anger, &c. Strong purges or vomits will likewiſe occaſion the jaundice. Sometimes it proceeds from obſtinate agues, or from that diſeaſe being prematurely ſtopped by aſtringent medicines. In infants it is often occaſioned by the *meconium* not being ſufficiently purged off. Pregnant women are very ſubject to it. It is likewiſe a ſymptom in ſeveral kinds of fevers. Catching cold, or the ſtopping of cuſtomary evacuations, as the *menſes*, the bleeding piles, iſſues, &c. will occaſion the jaundice.

SYMPTOMS.—— The patient at firſt complains of exceſſive wearineſs, and has great averſion to any kind of motion. His ſkin is dry, and he generally feels a kind of itching or pricking pain over the whole body. The ſtools are of a whitiſh or clay colour, and the urine, as was obſerved above, is yellow. The breathing is difficult, and the patient complains of an unuſual load or oppreſſion on his breaſt. There is a heat in the noſtrils, a bitter taſte in the mouth, loathing of food, ſickneſs at the ſtomach, vomiting, flatulency, and frequently all objects appear to the eye of a yellow colour.

If the patient be young, and the diſeaſe complicated

plicated with no other malady, it is ſeldom dangerous; but in old people, where it continues long, returns frequently, or is complicated with the dropſy or hypochondriac ſymptoms, it generally proves fatal. The black jaundice is more dangerous than the yellow.

REGIMEN.—— The diet ſhould be cool, light, and diluting, conſiſting chiefly of ripe fruits and mild vegetables; as apples boiled or roaſted, ſtewed prunes, preſerved plumbs, boiled ſpinage, &c. Veal or chicken-broth, with light bread, are likewiſe very proper. The drink ſhould be butter milk, whey ſweetened with honey, or decoctions of cool opening vegetables; as marſh mallow roots, with liquorice, &c.

THE patient ſhould take as much exerciſe as he can bear, either on horſe-back or in a machine; walking, running, and even jumping, are likewiſe proper, provided he can bear them without pain, and there be no ſymptoms of inflammation. Patients have been often cured of this diſeaſe by a long journey, after medicines had proved ineffectual.

AMUSEMENTS are likewiſe of great uſe in the jaundice. The diſeaſe is often occaſioned by a ſedentary life, joined to a dull melancholy diſpoſition. Whatever therefore tends to promote muſcular motion, and to cheer the ſpirits, muſt have a good effect; as dancing, laughing, ſinging, &c.

MEDICINE.—— If the patient be young, of a full ſanguine habit, and complains of pain in in the right ſide, about the region of the liver, bleeding will be neceſſary. After this a vomit muſt be adminiſtered, and if the diſeaſe proves obſtinate, it may be repeated once or twice. No medicines are more beneficial in the jaundice than vomits, eſpecially where it is not attended with inflammation. Half a dram of ipecacuanha in powder will be a ſufficient doſe for an adult. It may be wrought off with weak camomile-tea, or lukewarm water.

THE belly muſt likewiſe be kept open by mild purgatives. Caſtile ſoap, if taken in ſufficient quantities, anſwers this purpoſe extremely well. It may be taken from half an ounce to an ounce daily, for a conſiderable time. As few people have reſolution to ſwallow ſuch large quantities of ſoap, I generally give pills made of ſoap, aloes, and rhubarb, which anſwer the ſame intention in a ſmaller doſe. They may be prepared in the following manner:

TAKE ſocotrine aloes and Turkey rhubarb in powder, of each a dram, Caſtle ſoap an ounce. Beat them all together, with a little ſyrup, into a proper conſiſtence for pills. Let them be formed into pills of an ordinary ſize, and five or ſix of them taken three times a-day. They muſt be continued for ſome time, and the quantity regulated by the patient's ſtools, of which he ought at leaſt to have one or two every day.

FOMENTING the parts about the region of the ſtomach and liver, and rubbing them with a warm hand or fleſh-bruſh, are likewiſe beneficial;

cial; but it is ſtill more ſo for the patient to ſit in a veſſel of warm water up to the breaſt. He ought to do this frequently, and ſhould continue in it as long as his ſtrength will permit.

MANY dirty things are recommended for the cure of the jaundice; as lice, the millepedes, &c. But theſe do more harm than good, as people truſt to them, and neglect more valuable medicines; beſides, they are ſeldom taken in ſufficient quantity to produce any effects. People always expect that theſe *out of the way things* ſhould act as charms, and conſequently ſeldom perſiſt in the uſe of them. Vomits, purges, fomentations, and exerciſe, will ſeldom fail to cure the jaundice when it is a ſimple diſeaſe; and when complicated with the dropſy, or other chronic complaints, it is hardly to be cured by any means.

NUMBERLESS Brittiſh herbs are extolled for the cure of this diſeaſe. Dr Short, in his *medicina Britannica*, mentions near a hundred, all famous for curing the jaundice. The fact is, this diſeaſe often goes off of its own accord; in which caſe the laſt medicine is always ſaid to have performed the cure. I have however ſeen conſiderable benefit, in a very obſtinate jaundice, from a decoction of hemp-ſeed. Four ounces of the ſeed may be boiled in two Engliſh quarts of ale, and ſweetened with coarſe ſugar. The doſe is half an Engliſh pint every morning. It may be continued for eight or nine days.

I have known Harrowgate water cure a very obſtinate

obſtinate jaundice. I have known patients, after taking many medicines without effect, go thither in the middle of winter, and in a few weeks return quite well. They both drank the ſulphur water, and bathed.

OF THE DROPSY.

THE dropſy is a preternatural ſwelling of the whole body, or ſome part of it, occaſioned by a collection of watery humour. It is diſtinguiſhed by different names, according to the part affected, as the *anaſarca*, or a collection of water under the ſkin; the *aſcites*, or a collection of water in the belly; the *hydrops pectoris*, or dropſy of the breaſt; the *hydrocephalus*, or dropſy of the brain, &c. There is likewiſe a ſpecies of dropſy called *tympany*, which is occaſioned by rarified air pent up in the cavities or cells of the body.

CAUSES.—— A very common cauſe of the dropſy is a hereditary diſpoſition. It may likewiſe proceed from drinking ardent ſpirits, or other ſtrong liquors. It is true, almoſt to a proverb, that great drinkers die of a dropſy. The want of exerciſe is alſo a very common cauſe of the dropſy. Hence it is juſtly reckoned among the diſeaſes of the ſedentary. It often proceeds from exceſſive evacuations, as frequent and copious bleedings, ſtrong purges

 often

often repeated, frequent salivations, &c. The sudden stoppage of customary or necessary evacuations, as the *menses*, the hæmorrhoids, or fluxes of the belly. may likewise cause a dropsy.

I have often known the dropsy occasioned by drinking large quantities of cold, weak, watery liquor after violent exercise, while the body was hot. A low, damp, or marshy situation is likewise a frequent cause of it. Hence it is a common disease in moist, flat, fenny countries. It may also be brought on by a long course of poor watery diet, or the use of viscous aliment that is hard of digestion. It is often the effect of other diseases, as the jaundice, a schirrus of the liver, a violent ague of long continuance, a diarrhœa, a dysentery, an empyema, or a consumption of the lungs. In short, whatever obstructs the circulation of the blood, or prevents its being duly prepared, may occasion a dropsy.

SYMPTOMS.—— This disease generally begins with a swelling of the feet and ancles towards night, which, for some time, disappears in the morning. In the evening the parts, if pressed with the finger, will pit. The swelling gradually ascends towards the belly, which at length grows big. When it is struck with the hand, a fluctuation may be felt, and sometimes heard. Afterwards the breathing becomes difficult, the urine is in small quantity, and the thirst great, the belly is bound, and the perspiration is greatly obstructed. To these succeed torpor, heaviness, a slow wasting fever, and

and a troublesome cough. This last is generally a fatal symptom, as it shews the lungs so be affected. In a tympany the belly when struck sounds like a drum.

WHEN the disease comes suddenly on, and the patient is young and strong, there is reason to hope for a cure, especially if medicine be given early. But if the patient be old, has led an irregular or a sedentary life, or if there be reason to suspect that the liver, lungs, or any of the viscera are unsound, there is great ground to fear that the consequences will prove fatal.

REGIMEN.——The patient must abstain, as much as possible, from all drink, especially weak and watery liquors, and must quench his thirst with acids, as juice of lemons, oranges, sorrel, &c. His aliment ought to be dry of a heating and diuretic quality, as toasted bread, the flesh of birds, or other wild animals, roasted; pungent and aromatic vegetables, as garlic, mustard, onions, cresses, horse-radish, rocambole, shalot, &c. They may also eat sea-biscuit dipt in wine or a little brandy. This is not only nourishing, but tends to quench thirst. Some have been actually cured of a dropsy by a total abstinence from all liquids, and living entirely upon such things as are mentioned above. If the patient must have drink, the spaw-water, or Rhenish wine, with diuretic medicines infused in it, are the best.

EXERCISE is of the greatest importance in a dropsy. If the patient be able to walk, run, dance,

dance, or jump about, he ought to continue theſe exerciſes as long as he can. If he be not able to walk, &c. he muſt ride on horſe-back, or in a machine, and the more violent the motion ſo much the better, provided he can bear it. His bed ought to be hard, and the air of his apartments warm and dry. If he lives in a damp country, he ought to be removed into a dry one, and, if poſſible, into a warmer climate. In a word, every method muſt be taken to promote the perſpiration and to brace the ſolids. For this purpoſe it will likewiſe be proper to rub the patient's body, two or three times a day, with a hard cloth or the fleſh-bruſh, and he ought conſtantly to wear flannel next his ſkin.

MEDICINE. ---If the patient be young, his conſtitution good, and the diſeaſe has come on ſuddenly, it may generally be removed by ſtrong vomits, briſk purges, and ſuch medicines as promote a diſcharge of ſweat and urine. For an adult half a dram of ipecacuanha in powder, and half an ounce of oxymel of ſquills, will be a proper vomit. This may be repeated three or four times, if neceſſary, three or four days intervening betwixt each doſe. The patient muſt not drink much after the vomit, otherwiſe he deſtroys its effect. A cup or two of camomile tea will be ſufficient to work it off.

BETWIXT each vomit, on one of the intermediate days, the patient may take the following purge. Take jalap in powder half a dram, cream of tartar two drams, calomel ſix grains. Theſe

Theſe may be made into a bolus with a little ſyrup of pale roſes, and taken early in the morning. The leſs the patient drinks after it the better. If he be much griped, he may take now and then a cup of chicken-broth.

THE patient may likewiſe take every night at bedtime the following bolus: Take four or five grains of camphor, one grain of opium, and as much ſyrup of orange-peel as is ſufficient to make them into a bolus. This will generally promote a gentle ſweat, which ſhould be encouraged by drinking now and then a ſmall cup of wine whey, with a tea-ſpoonful of the ſpirits of hartſhorn in it.

THE patient may take, three or four times a day, a tea cupful of the following infuſion: Take juniper berries, muſtard-ſeed, and horſe-radiſh, of each half an ounce, aſhes of broom half a pound; infuſe them in a quart of Rheniſh wine or ſtrong ale for a few days, and afterwards ſtrain off the liquor. Such as cannot take this infuſion, may uſe the decoction of ſeneka-root, which is both diuretic and ſudorific. It may be prepared and taken as directed page 199.

As this diſeaſe is very apt to return; after the water has been drained off, to prevent its collecting again, the patient muſt continue to take exerciſe, to uſe a dry diet, and ſuch medicines as ſtrengthen and brace the ſolids, as wine with ſteel or bark infuſed in it; warm and aromatic bitters are likewiſe proper, as the Virginian ſnake-root, *canella alba*, orange peel, &c. infuſed in in wine or brandy: The patient muſt avoid all great evacuations, and ought, if he can, to make choice of a dry warm ſituation.

The above courſe will often cure an incidental dropſy, if the conſtitution be good; but when the diſeaſe proceeds from a bad habit, or an unſound ſtate of the viſcera, ſtrong purges and vomits are not to be ventured upon. In this caſe, the ſafer courſe is to palliate the ſymptoms by the uſe of ſuch medicines as promote the ſecretions, and to ſupport the patient's ſtrength by warm and nouriſhing cordials.

The diſcharge of urine may be greatly promoted by nitre. Brookes ſays he knew a young woman who was cured of a dropſy by taking a dram of nitre every morning in a draught of ale, after ſhe had been given over as incurable. The powder of ſquills is likewiſe a good diuretic. Six or eight grains of it, with a ſcruple of nitre, may be given twice a day in a glaſs of ſtrong cinnamon water. Ball ſays a large ſpoonful of unbruiſed muſtard ſeed taken every night and morning, and drinking half an Engliſh pint of the decoction of the tops of green broom after it, has produced a cure, after other powerful methods had proved ineffectual.

To promote perſpiration, the patient may uſe the decoction of ſeneka-root, as directed above; or he may take two ſpoonfuls of * Mindererus's

* This ſpirit is prepared by gradually pouring diſtilled vinegar upon any quantity of the volatile ſalt ammoniac till the effervеſcence ceaſes; occaſionally ſhaking the veſſel to promote the action of the vinegar on the ſalt.

ſpirit,

ſpirit, in a cup of wine-whey, three or four times a day. The ſaline draughts recommended page 177. are likewiſe very proper in this caſe. Theſe medicines, with the regimen mentioned above, if they do not cure will at leaſt alleviate the diſeaſe, which, in worn-out conſtitutions, is a ſafer courſe than attempting to extirpate it. When other means fail, recourſe muſt be had to tapping, which is a very ſafe and eaſy operation, tho' it ſeldom produces a radical cure.

OF THE GOUT.

THERE is no diſeaſe which ſhews the imperfection of the medical art more than the gout. Nor does any malady ſhew the advantages of temperance and exerciſe in a ſtronger light. Few who pay a proper regard to theſe are troubled with the gout, unleſs when it is hereditary. This points out the true ſource from whence that peſt originally ſprung,. viz. *exceſs* and *idleneſs*. Few perſons are affected with the gout till the decline of life, except thoſe who inherit it from their parents. Men are more liable to it than women, eſpecially thoſe of a full, groſs habit.

CAUSES.——One very common cauſe of the gout is a hereditary diſpoſition. Perſons who know themſelves to be tainted this way, ought therefore to guard againſt its attack, by ſteadily purſuing a courſe directly oppoſite to that

that which occaſions the diſeaſe. Full living, but eſpecially indulging in rich, pungent, or ſtimulating ſauces and generous wines, has a great tendency to bring on the gout. Intenſe thought or application of the mind to obſtruſe ſubjects, particularly night-ſtudies, has likewiſe this effect. The plentiful uſe of acids, as ſour punch, prickt wines, &c. are alſo hurtful; but nothing more certainly induces this diſeaſe than exceſs of venery, eſpecially in the early period of life.

SOMETIMES the gout has been known to prove infectious; but this is rarely the caſe. It may proceed from an obſtruction or defect of any of the uſual diſcharges, as the perſpiration, ſweating of the feet, the menſes, &c. A ſudden chilling of the feet after ſweat, or drying them at the fire after being wet and cold, are likewiſe bad. The modern cuſtom of eating a hot fleſh-ſupper, drinking warm ſtrong liquors after it, and ſitting up the greater part of the night, is one very great cauſe of the gout, and indeed of many other diſeaſes.

SYMPTOMS.——A fit of the gout is generally preceded by indigeſtion, drowſineſs, wind, a ſlight head ach, ſickneſs, and ſometimes vomiting. The patient complains of wearineſs and dejection of ſpirits, and has often a pain in the limbs, with a ſenſation as if wind or cold water were paſſing down the thigh. The appetite is often remarkably keen a day or two before the fit, and there is a ſlight pain in paſſing urine, and ſometimes an involuntary ſhedding

ding of tears: Sometimes theſe ſymptoms are much more violent, eſpecially upon the near approach of the fit; and ſome obſerve, that as the fever which uſhers in the gout is, ſo will the fit be; if the fever be ſhort and ſharp, the fit will be ſo likewiſe; if it be feeble, long, and lingering, the ſit will be ſuch alſo. But this obſervation can only hold with reſpect to very regular fits of the gout.

THE regular gout generally makes its attack in the ſpring, or beginning of winter, in the following manner: About two or three in the morning the patient is ſeized with a pain in his great toe, ſometimes in the heel, and at other times in the ancle or calf of the leg. This pain is accompanied with a ſenſation, as if cold water were poured upon the part, which is ſucceeded by a ſhivering, with ſome degree of fever. Afterwards the pain increaſes, and fixing among the ſmall bones of the foot, the patient feels all the different kinds of torture, as if the part were ſtretched, burnt, ſqueezed, gnawed, or torn in pieces, &c. The part at length becomes ſo exquiſitely ſenſible, that the patient cannot bear to have it touched, nor even ſuffer any perſon to walk acroſs the room.

THE patient is generally in exquiſite torture for twenty four hours, from the time of the coming on of the fit: He then becomes eaſier, the part begins to ſwell, appears red, and is covered with a little moiſture. Towards morning he drops aſleep, and generally falls into a gentle breathing ſweat. This terminates the firſt paroxyſm, a number of which conſtitutes a fit of the gout; which is longer or ſhorter according to the patient's age, ſtrength, the ſeaſon of the year, and the diſpoſition of the body to this diſeaſe.

THE patient is always worſe towards night, and eaſier in the morning. The paroxyſms however generally grow milder every day, till at length the matter is diſcharged by perſpiration, urine, and the other evacuations. In ſome patients this happens in a few days; in others it requires weeks, and in ſome months, to finiſh the fit. Thoſe whom age and frequent fits of the gout have greatly debilitated, ſeldom get free of it before the approach of ſummer, and ſometimes not till it be pretty far advanced.

REGIMEN.—— As there are no medicines, yet known, that will cure the gout, we ſhall confine our obſervations moſtly to regimen, both in and out of the fit.

IN THE FIT, if the patient be young and ſtrong, his diet ought to be thin and cooling, and his drink of a diluting nature; but where the conſtitution is weak, and the patient has been accuſtomed to live high, this is not a proper time to retrench. In this caſe he muſt keep nearly to his uſual diet, and ſhould take frequently a cup of ſtrong negas, or a glaſs of generous wine. Wine whey is a very proper drink in this caſe, as it promotes the perſpiration

tion without heating the patient. It will anſwer this purpoſe better if a tea ſpoonful of *ſal volatile oleoſum*, or ſpirits of hartſhorn, be put into a cup of it twice or thrice a day. It will likewiſe be proper for the patient to take at bed-time a tea ſpoonful of the volatile tincture of *guaiacum* in a large draught of warm wine-whey. This will greatly promote perſpiration thro' the night.

As we know no ſafe way of diſcharging the gouty matter but by perſpiration, this ought to be kept up by all means, eſpecially in the part affected. For this purpoſe the leg and foot affected ſhould be wrapt in ſoft flannel, fur, or wool. The laſt is moſt readily obtained, and ſeems to anſwer the purpoſe as well, if not better, than any thing elſe. The people of Lancaſhire look upon wool as a kind of ſpecific in the gout. They wrap a great quantity of it combed about the leg and foot affected, and cover it with a ſkin of ſhamoy leather. This they ſuffer to continue for eight or ten days, and ſometimes for a fortnight or three weeks, or longer if the pain does not ceaſe. I never knew any external application anſwer ſo well in the gout. I have often ſeen it applied when the ſwelling and inflammation were very great, with violent pain; and have found all theſe ſymptoms relieved by it in a few days. The wool which they uſe is generally greaſed. and carded or combed. They chuſe the ſofteſt which

which can be had, and ſeldom or never remove it till the fit be entirely gone off.

THE patient ought likewiſe to be kept quiet and eaſy during the fit. Every thing that affects the mind diſturbs the paroxyſm, and tends to throw the gout upon the nobler parts. For the ſame reaſon all external applications that repel the matter are to be avoided as death. They do not cure the diſeaſe, but remove it from a ſafe to a more dangerous part of the body, where it often proves fatal. A fit of the gout is rather to be conſidered as Nature's method of curing a diſeaſe than a diſeaſe itſelf, and all that we can do, with ſafety, is to promote her intentions, and to aſſiſt her in expelling the enemy in her own way. Evacuations by bleeding, ſtool, &c. are likewiſe hurtful. They do not remove the cauſe of the diſeaſe, and, by weakening the patient, they generally prolong the fit.

MANY things will indeed ſhorten a fit of the gout, and ſome will drive it off altogether; but nothing has yet been found which will do this with ſafety to the patient. In pain we eagerly graſp at any thing that promiſes immediate eaſe, and even hazard life itſelf for a momentary relief. This is the true reaſon why ſo many infallible remedies have been propoſed for the gout, and why ſuch numbers have loſt their lives by them. It would be as prudent to ſtop the ſmall pox from riſing, and to drive them into the blood, as to attempt to repel the

the gout. The latter is as much an effort of Nature to free herſelf from an offending cauſe as the former, and ought equally to be promoted. In fine, there is no diſeaſe which Nature makes a greater effort to cure than the gout; nor is it difficult to ſee which way her endeavours tend. She always attempts to throw the diſeaſe upon the extremities, and when that is accompliſhed, her work is half done. It may ſafely lodge theie till it be gradually expelled by the vital powers, and it cannot lodge ſafely any where elſe, nor be expelled in any other way.

AFTER the fit is over, the patient ought to take a doſe or two of the bitter tincture of rhubarb, or ſome other warm ſtomachic purge. He ſhould alſo drink a weak infuſion of ſtomachic bitters in ſmall wine or ale, as Gentian, with cinnamon or Virginian ſnake root, and orange peel. The diet at this time ſhould be light, but nouriſhing, and gentle exerciſe ſhould be taken on horſe-back or in a machine, &c.

OUT OF THE FIT, it is in the patient's power to do many things towards preventing a return of the diſorder, or rendering the fit, if it ſhould return, leſs ſevere. This however is not to be attempted by medicine. I have frequently known the gout kept off for ſeveral years by the jeſuits bark and other medicines; but in all the caſes where I had occaſion to ſee this tried the perſons died ſuddenly, and, to all appearance, for want of a regular fit of the gout.

One

One would be apt, from hence, to conclude, that a ſit of the gout, to ſome conſtitutions, in the decline of life, is rather ſalutary than hurtful.

Tho' it may be dangerous to ſtop a fit of the gout by medicine, yet if the conſtitution can be ſo changed by diet and exerciſe, as to leſſen or totally prevent its return, there certainly can be no danger in following ſuch a courſe. It is well known that the whole humours may be ſo altered by a proper courſe of diet, as quite to eradicate this diſeaſe; and thoſe only who have reſolution enough to perſiſt in ſuch a courſe have reaſon to expect a cure.

The courſe which we would recommend for preventing the gout, is as follows: In the firſt place, *univerſal temperance*. In the next place, plenty of *exerciſe*. By this we do not mean ſauntering about in an indolent manner, but labour, ſweat, and toil. Theſe only can render the humours wholeſome, and keep them ſo. Going early to bed, and riſing by times, are of great importance. It is likewiſe proper to avoid night ſtudies, and all intenſe thought. The ſupper ſhould be light, and taken early. All ſtrong liquors, eſpecially generous wines and ſour punch, are to be avoided. Above all, we would recommend a milk diet. The uſe of milk is not to be gone into all at once, but increaſed gradually, till it becomes the principal part of the diet.

We would likewiſe recommend ſome doſes of *magneſia alba* and rhubarb to be taken every ry ſpring and autumn; and afterwards a courſe of ſtomachic bitters, as tanſy or water trefoil tea, an infuſion of gentian and camomile flowers, or a decoction of burdock-root, &c. Any of theſe, or an infuſion of any wholeſome bitter that is more agreeable to the patient, may be drank for two or three weeks twice a-day. An iſſue or perpetual bliſter has a great tendency to prevent the gout. If theſe were more generally uſed, in the decline of life, they would not only often prevent the gout, but alſo many other maladies. Such as can afford to go to Bath will find great benefit from bathing and drinking the water. It both promotes digeſtion and invigorates the habit.

When the gout attacks the head or lungs, every method muſt be taken to draw it towards the feet. They muſt be frequently bathed in warm water, and acrid cataplaſms applied to the ſoles. Bliſtering plaſters ought likewiſe to be applied to the ancles or calves of the legs. Bleeding in the feet or ancles is alſo neceſſary, and warm ſtomachic purges. The patient ought to keep in bed for the moſt part, if there be any ſigns of inflammation, and ſhould be very careful not to catch cold.

If it attacks the ſtomach with a ſenſe of cold, the moſt warm cordials are neceſſary; as ſtrong wine, cinnamon water, peppermint water, and even brandy or rum. The patient ſhould keep in bed, and endeavour to promote a ſweat by drinking warm liquors; and if he ſhould be troubled

troubled with a nauſea, or inclination to vomit, he may drink camomile tea or ſmall poſſet.

WHEN the gout attacks the kidneys, and imitates gravel pains, the patient ought to drink freely of a decoction of marſh-mallows, and to have the parts fomented with warm water. An emollient clyſter ought likewiſe to be given, and afterwards an opiate. If the pain be very violent, twenty or thirty drops of laudanum may be taken in a cup of the decoction.

PERSONS who have had the gout ſhould be very attentive to any complaints that may happen to them about the time when they have reaſon to expect a return of the fit. The gout imitates many other diſorders, and by being miſtaken for them, and treated accordingly, is often diverted from its proper courſe, to the great danger of the patient's life.

THOSE who never had the gout, but who, from their conſtitution or manner of living, have reaſon to expect it, ought likewiſe to be very circumſpect with regard to its firſt approach. If the diſeaſe, by wrong conduct or improper medicines, be diverted from its proper courſe, the miſerable patient has a chance to be ever after tormented with head-achs, coughs, pains of the ſtomach and inteſtines; and generally falls, at laſt, a victim to its attack upon ſome of the more noble parts.

OF

OF THE RHEUMATISM.

THIS diſeaſe has great affinity with the gout. It generally attacks the joints with exquiſite pain, and is ſometimes attended with inflammation and ſwelling. It is moſt common in the ſpring and towards the end of autumn. It is uſually diſtinguiſhed into acute and chronic; or the rheumatiſm attended with a fever, and that which is not.

CAUSES.—— The cauſes of a rheumatiſm are frequently the ſame as thoſe of an inflammatory fever; viz. an obſtructed perſpiration, the immoderate uſe of ſtrong liquors, &c. Sudden changes of the weather, and all quick tranſitions from heat to cold, are very apt to occaſion the rheumatiſm. The moſt extraordinary caſe of a rheumatiſm that I ever ſaw, where almoſt every joint of the body was diſtorted, was in a man who uſed to work one part of the day by the fire, and the other part of it in the water. Very obſtinate rheumatiſms have likewiſe been brought on by perſons, not accuſtomed to it, allowing their feet to continue long wet. The ſame effects are often produced by wet cloaths, damp beds, or lying upon the ground, eſpecially in the night,

THE rheumatiſm may either be occaſioned by exceſſive evacuations, or the ſtoppage of uſual diſcharges. It is often the effect of chronic diſeaſes, which vitiate the humours; as the ſcurvy, the *lues venerea*, obſtinate autumnal agues, &c.

THE rheumatiſm prevails moſt in low, damp, marſhy countries. It is likewiſe very common amongſt the poorer ſort of peaſants, who are ill clothed, live in low, cold houſes, and eat coarſe unwholeſome food, which contains but little nouriſhment, and is not eaſy aſſimilated.

SYMPTOMS.—— The *acute* rheumatiſm commonly begins with wearineſs, ſhivering, a quick pulſe, reſtleſſneſs, thirſt, and other ſymptoms of fever. Afterwards the patient complains of flying pains, which are increaſed by the leaſt motion. Theſe at length fix in the joints, which are often affected with ſwelling and inflammation If blood be let in this diſeaſe, it has generally the ſame appearance as in the pleuriſy.

IN this kind of rheumatiſm the treatment of the patient is nearly the ſame as in an acute or inflammatory fever. If he be young and ſtrong, bleeding is neceſſary, which may be repeated according to the exigencies of the caſe. The belly ought likewiſe to be kept open by emollient clyſters, or cool opening liquors; as decoctions of tamarinds and liquorice, cream tartar whey, &c. The diet ſhould be light, and in ſmall quantity, conſiſting chiefly of roaſted apples, groat gruel, or very weak chicken broth. After the feveriſh ſymptoms have abated, if the pain ſtill continues, the patient muſt keep his bed,

bed, and take ſuch things as promote perſpiration; as wine whey with *ſpiritus Mindereri*, in the manner directed pages 454. and 455. The patient may likewiſe take, for a few nights, at bed time, in a cup of wine whey, a dram of cream of tartar, and half a dram of gum guaiacum in powder.

WARM bathing, after proper evacuations, has often an exceeding good effect. The patient may either be put into a bath of warm water, or have cloths wrung out of it applied to the parts affected. Great care muſt be taken that he do not catch cold after bathing.

THE *chronic* rheumatiſm is ſeldom attended with any conſiderable degree of fever, and is generally confined to ſome particular part of the body, as the ſhoulders, the back, or the loins. There is ſeldom any inflammation or ſwelling in this caſe. Perſons in the decline of life are moſt ſubject to the chronic rheumatiſm. In ſuch patients it often proves extremely obſtinate, and ſometimes incurable.

IN this kind of rheumatiſm the regimen ſhould be nearly the ſame as in the acute. Cool and diluting diet, conſiſting chiefly of vegetable ſubſtances, as ſtewed prunes, coddled apples, currants or gooſeberries boiled in milk, is moſt proper. Arbuthnot ſays "If there be a ſpecific in aliment for the rheumatiſm, it is certainly whey," and adds, That he knew a perſon ſubject to this diſeaſe, who could never be cured by any other me-

method but a diet of whey and bread.' He likewiſe ſays, 'That cream of tartar in water-gruel, taken for ſeveral days, will eaſe rheumatic pains conſiderably.' This I have often experienced, but found it always more efficacious when joined with gum guaiacum, as directed above. In this caſe the patient may take the doſe mentioned above twice a day, and likewiſe a tea-ſpoonful of the volatile tincture of gum guaiacum at bed time in wine whey.

This courſe may be continued for a week, or longer, if the caſe proves obſtinate, and the patient's ſtrength will permit. It ought then to be omitted for a few days, and repeated again. At the ſame time leeches or a bliſtering plaſter may be applied to the part affected. What I have generally found anſwer better than either of theſe, in obſtinate fixed rheumatic pains, is the *warm plaſter*. It is made by melting over a gentle fire, an ounce of gum plaſter with two drams of bliſtering plaſter. This may be ſpread upon ſoft leather, and applied to the part affected. It ſhould be taken off and wiped every three or four days, and may be renewed once a fortnight. Cupping upon the part affected is likewiſe often very beneficial, and is greatly preferable to the application of leeches.

Tho' this diſeaſe may not ſeem in the leaſt to yield to medicines for a long time, yet they ought ſtill to be perſiſted in. Perſons who are ſubject to frequent returns of the rheumatiſm, will

will often find their account in uſing medicines, whether they be immediately affected with it or not. The chronic rheumatiſm is ſimilar to the gout in this reſpect, that the moſt proper time for uſing medicines to extirpate it, is when the patient is moſt free from it.

To thoſe who can afford to go thither, we would recommend the warm baths of Buxton or Matlock in Derbyſhire. Theſe have often cured very obſtinate rheumatiſms, and are always ſafe either in or out of the fit. When the rheumatiſm is complicated with ſcorbutic complaints, which is not ſeldom the caſe, the Harrowgate waters and thoſe of Moffat are proper. They ſhould both be drank and uſed as a warm bath.

There are ſeveral of our own domeſtic plants which may be uſed with advantage in the rheumatiſm. One of the beſt of them is the white *muſtard ſeed.* A table ſpoonful of this may be taken twice or thrice a-day, in a glaſs of water or ſmall wine. The water-trefoil is likewiſe of great uſe in this complaint. It may be infuſed in wine or ale, or drank in form of tea. The ground-ivy, camomile, and ſeveral other bitters, are alſo beneficial, and may be uſed in the ſame manner. No benefit however is to be expected from theſe unleſs they be uſed for a conſiderable time. Excellent medicines are often deſpiſed in this caſe becauſe they do not perform a cure inſtantaneouſly; whereas nothing would be more certain than their effect, were

were they duly perſiſted in. The want of perſeverance in the uſe of medicines is one great cauſe why chronic diſeaſes are ſo ſeldom cured.

COLD bathing, eſpecially in ſalt water, often cures the rheumatiſm. We would alſo recommend riding on horſe-back, and wearing flannel next the ſkin. A flannel ſhirt, in an obſtinate rheumatiſm, eſpecially if the patient be old, is one of the beſt medicines we know. Iſſues are likewiſe very proper; they have often been known to cure a chronic rheumatiſm. If the pain affects the ſhoulders, an iſſue may be made in the arm; but if it affects the loins, it ſhould be put in the leg or thigh. Rheumatic perſons ought to make choice of a dry warm air, to avoid wet cloaths as much as poſſible, and make frequent uſe of the fleſh-bruſh.

OF THE SCURVY.

THIS diſeaſe prevails chiefly in cold northern countries, eſpecially in low damp ſituations, near large marſhes, or great quantities of ſtagnating water. Sedentary people of a dull melancholy diſpoſition are moſt ſubject to it. It proves often fatal to ſailors in long voyages, particularly in ſhips that are not properly ventilated, and have many people on board.

CAUSES.—— The ſcurvy is occaſioned by cold moiſt air; by the long uſe of ſalted or ſmoke-

ſmoke-dried proviſions, or of any kind of food that is hard of digeſtion, and affords little nouriſhment. It may alſo proceed from exceſſive evacuations, or the ſuppreſſion of cuſtomary diſcharges; as the *menſes* hæmorrhoidal flux, &c. It is ſometimes owing to a hereditary taint, in which caſe a very ſmall cauſe will excite the latent diſorder. Grief, fear, and other depreſſing paſſions, have a great tendency to produce this diſeaſe. It may likewiſe proceed from neglect of cleanlineſs; bad cloathing; the want of proper exerciſe; confined air; exceſs in eating or drinking; or from any diſeaſe which greatly weakens the body or vitiates the humours.

SYMPTOMS.—— This diſeaſe may be known by unuſual wearineſs, heavineſs of the body, and difficulty of breathing, eſpecially after bodily motion; rottenneſs of the gums, which are apt to bleed on the ſlighteſt touch; a ſtinking breath; frequent bleeding of the noſe; difficulty of walking; ſometimes a ſwelling and ſometimes a falling away of the legs, on which there are livid yellow or violet coloured ſpots; the face is generally of a pale or leaden colour. As the diſeaſe advances, other ſymptoms come on; as rottenneſs of the teeth, hæmorrhages, or diſcharges of blood from various parts of the body, foul obſtinate ulcers, which no applications will cure; the patient complains of pains in various parts of the body, eſpecially about the breaſt, and his body is covered

covered with dry ſcaly eruptions. At laſt a waſting or hectic fever comes on, and the miſerable patient is often carried off by a dyſentery, a diarrhœa, a dropſy, the palſy, fainting fits, or a mortification of ſome of the bowels.

CURE —— We know no method of curing this diſeaſe but by purſuing a courſe directly oppoſite to that which brought it on. It proceeds from a vitiated ſtate of the humours, occaſioned by errors in diet, air, or exerciſe; and this can be removed no other way than by a proper attention to theſe important articles.

If the patient has been obliged to breathe a cold, damp, or confined air, he ſhould be removed, as ſoon as poſſible, to a dry, open, and moderately warm one. If the diſeaſe proceeds from a ſedentary life, or depreſſing paſſions, as grief, fear, &c. the patient muſt take daily as much exerciſe in the open air as he can bear, and his mind ſhould be diverted by cheerful company and other amuſements. Nothing has a greater tendency either to prevent, or remove this diſeaſe, than conſtant cheerfulneſs and good humour. But this, alas, is ſeldom the lot of perſons afflicted with the ſcurvy; they are generally ſurly, peeviſh, ſour, moroſe, and dull.

When the ſcurvy has been brought on by a long uſe of ſalted proviſions, the proper medicine is a diet conſiſting chiefly of freſh vegetables; as oranges, lemons, apples, tamarinds, water-creſſes, ſcurvy-graſs, brook lime, &c. The uſe of

theſe,

these, with milk, pot herbs, new bread, and fresh beer or cyder, will seldom fail to remove a scurvy of this kind, if taken before it be too far advanced; but to have this effect they must be persisted in for a considerable time. When fresh vegetables cannot be had, pickled or preserved ones may be used; and if these cannot be obtained, the chymical acids may be taken in their stead. All the patient's food and drink must be sharpened with cream of tartar, elixir of vitriol, vinegar, or the spirit of sea salt, &c.

THESE things however will more certainly prevent than cure the scurvy; for which reason seafaring people, especially on long voyages, ought to lay in plenty of them. Cabbage, onions, gooseberries, and many other vegetables, may be kept a long time by *pickling*, *preserving*, &c. When these fail, the chymical acids, mentioned above, which will keep for any length of time, may be used. We have reason to believe, if ships were well ventilated, good store of fruits, greens, and portable soup, &c. laid in, and a proper regard paid to cleanliness and warmth, that sailors would be the most healthy people in the world, and would seldom suffer either from the scurvy or putrid fevers, which are so fatal to that useful set of men; but it is too much the temper of such people to despise all precaution; they will not think of any calamity till they find it, when it is too late to ward off the blow.

It muſt indeed be owned, that many of them have it not in their power to make the proviſion we are ſpeaking of; but in this caſe it is the buſineſs of their employers to make it for them; and no man ought to engage in a long voyage without having this article ſecured.

I have often ſeen very extraordinary effects in the ſcurvy from a milk-diet. This preparation of nature is a mixture of animal and vegetable properties, which of all others is the moſt fit for reſtoring a decayed conſtitution, and removing that particular acrimony of the humours, which ſeems to conſtitute the very eſſence of the ſcurvy and many other diſeaſes. But men deſpiſe this wholeſome and nouriſhing food, becauſe it is cheap, and guzzle down fleſh, and fermented liquors, while milk is only deemed fit for their hogs.

The moſt proper drink in the ſcurvy is whey or butter-milk. When theſe cannot be had, ſound cyder or perry may be uſed. Wort has been found to be a proper drink in the ſcurvy, and may be uſed at ſea, as malt will keep during the longeſt voyage. A decoction of the tops of the ſpruce fir is alſo good. It may be drank in the quantity of an Engliſh pint twice a day. Tar water may likewiſe be uſed for this purpoſe, or decoctions of any of the mild mucilaginous vegetables; as ſarſaparilla, marſhmallow roots, &c. Infuſions of the bitter plants, as ground-ivy, the leſſer centaury, marſh trefoil,

foil, &c. are likewife beneficial. I have feen the peafants in fome parts of Britain exprefs the juice of the laft mentioned plant, and drink it with good effects in thofe foul fcorbutic eruptions with which they are often troubled in the fpring feafon.

THE Harrowgate-water is certainly an excellent medicine in the fcurvy. I have often feen patients in the moft deplorable condition from that difeafe, greatly relieved by drinking the fulphur-water, and bathing in it. The chalybeate-water may alfo be ufed with advantage, efpecially with a view to brace the ftomach after drinking the fulphur-water, which, though it fharpens the appetite, never fails to weaken the powers of digeftion.

A flight degree of fcurvy may be carried off by frequently fucking a little of the juice of a bitter orange, or lemon. When the difeafe affects the gums only, this practice, if continued for fome time, will generally carry it off. We would however recommend the bitter orange as greatly preferable to lemon. It feems to be as good an acid, and is not near fo hurtful to the ftomach. Perhaps our own forrel may be little inferior to either of them. All kinds of falad are good in the fcurvy, and ought to be eat in great plenty, as fpinage, lettice, parfley, celery, endive, radifh, dandelion, &c. It is amazing to fee how foon frefh vegetables in the fpring cure the brute animals

animals of any ſcab or foulneſs which is upon th ir ſkins. Is it not natural to ſuppoſe that their effects ſhould be as great upon the human ſpecies?

THE LEPROSY, which was ſo common in this country long ago, ſeems to have been near akin to the ſcurvy. Perhaps its appearing ſo ſeldom now may be owing to the inhabitants of Britain eating more vegetable food than formerly, living more upon tea and other diluting diet, uſing far leſs ſalted meat, and being greatly more cleanly, and better cloathed, &c. ——Where this diſeaſe happens, we would recommend the ſame courſe of diet and medicine as in the ſcurvy.

Of the SCROPHULA or KING's EVIL.

THIS diſeaſe chiefly affects the glands, eſpecially thoſe of the neck. Children and young perſons of a ſedentary life are moſt ſubject to it. It is one of thoſe diſeaſes that may be removed by proper regimen, but ſeldom yields to medicine. The inhabitants of cold, damp, marſhy countries are moſt liable to the ſcrophula.

CAUSES.——This diſeaſe may proceed from a hereditary taint, infection, a ſcrophulous nurſe, &c. Children who have the misfortune to be born of ſickly parents, whoſe conſtitutions

tions have been worn out by the French-pox, or other chronic diſeaſes, are apt to be affected with the ſcrophula. It may likewiſe proceed from ſuch diſeaſes as weaken the habit or vitiate the humours, as the ſmall pox, meaſles, &c. External injuries as blows, bruiſes, compreſſions, &c. ſometimes produce ſcrophulous ulcers; but there is reaſon to believe, when this happens, that it is owing either to a prediſpoſition in the habit to this diſeaſe, or to the confinement of the patient. In ſhort, whatever tends to vitiate the humours or relax the ſolids prediſpoſes to this diſeaſe, as the want of exerciſe, too much heat or cold, confined air, unwholeſome food, bad water, the long uſe of poor, weak, watery aliments, the neglect of cleanlineſs, or ſuffering children to continue long wet, &c.

SYMPTOMS.—— At firſt ſmall knots appear under the chin or behind the ears, which gradually increaſe in number and ſize, till they form one large hard tumour. This often continues for a long time without breaking, and when it does break, it only diſcharges a thin *ſanies* or watery humour. Other parts of the body are likewiſe liable to its attack, as the armpits, groins, feet, hands, eyes, breaſts, &c. Nor are the internal parts exempt from it. It often affects the lungs, liver or ſpleen; and I have frequently ſeen the glands of the meſentery greatly enlarged by it.

THESE

THESE obſtinate ulcers which break out upon the feet and hands with ſwelling, and little or no redneſs, commonly called the *ſpina ventoſa*, are of the ſcrophulous kind. They ſeldom diſcharge good matter, and are exceeding difficult to cure. The *white ſwellings* of the joints ſeem likewiſe to be of this kind. They can ſeldom be brought to a ſuppuration, and when opened they only diſcharge a thin ichor. There is not a more general ſymptom of the ſcrophula than a ſwelling of the upper lip and noſe. It likewiſe frequently begins in a ſingle toe or finger, which continues long ſwelled, with no great degree of pain, till at length the bone becomes carious.

REGIMEN.——As this diſeaſe proceeds, in a great meaſure, from relaxation, the diet ought to be generous and nouriſhing, but at the ſame time light and of eaſy digeſtion, as good light bread, the fleſh and broth of young animals, with now and then a glaſs of generous wine, or good ale. The air ought to be open, dry, and not too cold, and the patient ſhould take as much exerciſe as he can bear. Exerciſe is here of the utmoſt importance. Children will ſeldom be troubled with the ſcrophula who have enough of exerciſe, and if they be, it alone has the greateſt chance to cure them.

MEDICINE——The vulgar are remarkably credulous with regard to the cure of the ſcrophula, many of them believing in the virtue of the royal touch, that of the ſeventh ſon,

&c.

&c. The truth is, we know but little either of the nature or cure of this diſeaſe, and where reaſon or medicines fail, ſuperſtition always comes in their place. Hence it is, that in diſeaſes which are the moſt difficult to underſtand, we always hear of the greateſt number of miraculous cures being performed. Here however, the deception is eaſily accounted for. The ſcrophula at a certain period of life, often cures of itſelf; and, if the patient happens to be touched about this time, the cure is imputed to the touch, and not to nature, who is really the phyſician. In the ſame way the inſignificant noſtrums of quacks and old women often gain applauſe when they deſerve none.

There is nothing more pernicious, than the cuſtom of doſing children with ſtrong purgative medicines in the ſcrophula. People imagine, that it proceeds from humours which muſt be purged off, without conſidering, that theſe purgatives increaſe the relaxation and aggravate the diſeaſe. It has indeed been found that keeping the belly gently open, eſpecially with ſea-water, has a good effect; but this ſhould only be given in ſuch quantity as to procure one, or at moſt two ſtools every day. Bathing in the ſalt water has likewiſe a very good effect, eſpecially in the warm ſeaſon. I have often known a courſe of bathing in ſalt water, and drinking it in ſuch quantities as to keep the belly gently open, cure a ſcrophula, after many medicines had been tried in vain. When

ſalt water

ſalt-water cannot be had, the patient may be bathed in freſh-water, and his belly kept open by ſmall quantities of ſalt and water, or ſome other mild purgative.

NEXT to cold bathing and drinking the ſalt-water, we would recommend the jeſuits bark. The cold bath may be uſed in ſummer, and the bark in winter. It may either be taken in ſubſtance mixed with wine, or if the patient cannot be brought to uſe it in that form, a decoction of it may be drank. An ounce of the jeſuits bark, and a dram of Winter's bark groſsly powdered, may be boiled in an Engliſh quart of water to a pint; towards the end, half an once of ſliced liquorice-root, and a handful of raiſins may be added, which will both render the medicine leſs diſagreeable and make it take up more of the bark. The liquor muſt be ſtrained, and two, three, or four ſpoonfuls, according to the age of the patient, taken three times a day. The patient ought at the ſame time to take, twice or thrice a day, a glaſs of good wine, with ten, twenty, or thirty drops of volatile tincture of guaiacum in it. I have often given the bark in obſtinate ſcrophulous caſes with very good effect. An adult may take at leaſt two drams of it daily, and muſt continue to uſe it for ſeveral months.

THE Moffat and Harrowgate waters are likewiſe very proper medicines in the ſcrophula, eſpecially the latter. They ought not howe-

ver

ver to be drank in large quantities, but ſhould be taken ſo as to keep the belly gently open, and muſt be uſed for a conſiderable time.

As to external applications, they are of little avail. Before the tumour breaks, nothing ought to be applied to it, unleſs a piece of flannel, or ſomething to keep it warm. After it breaks, the ſore may be dreſſed with ſome digeſtive ointment. What I have always found to anſwer beſt, was the yellow baſilicon mixed with about a ſixth or eight part of its weight of red precipitate. The ſore may be dreſſed with this twice a day; and if it be very fungous, and does not digeſt well, a larger proportion of the precipitate may be added.

MEDICINES which mitigate this diſeaſe, tho' they do not cure it, are not to be deſpiſed. If the patient can be kept alive by any means till he arrives at the age of puberty, he has a great chance to get well; but, if he does not recover at this time, in all probability he never will. Perſons afflicted with this diſeaſe ought not to marry. There is no malady which parents are ſo apt to communicate to their offspring as the ſcrophula, and ſurely it is a cruel thing to entail miſery on poſterity.

FOR the means of preventing this diſeaſe, we muſt refer the reader to the obſervations on nurſing, at the beginning of the book.

Of the RICKETS.

THIS diſeaſe generally attacks children betwixt the age of nine months and two years. It appeared firſt in England, about the time when manufactures began to be introduced, and ſtill prevails moſt in towns where the inhabitants follow ſedentary employments, and by that means neglect either to take proper exerciſe themſelves, or to give it to their children. It has a great reſemblance to the foregoing diſeaſe both in its cauſes and method of cure.

CAUSES.—— One cauſe of the rickets in children is diſeaſed parents. Mothers of a weak relaxed habit, who neglect exerciſe, and live upon weak watery diet, can neither be expected to bring forth ſtrong and healthy children, nor to be able to nurſe them, after they are brought forth. Accordingly we find, that the children of ſuch women generally die of the rickets, the ſcrophula, conſumptions, &c. Children begotten by men in the decline of life, who are afflicted with the gout, the gravel, or other chronic diſeaſes, or who have been often affected with the venereal diſeaſe in their youth, are likewiſe very liable to the rickets.

ANY diſorder that weakens the conſtitution, or relaxes the habit of children, as the ſmall-pox, meaſles, teething, the hooping-cough, &c. prediſpoſes them to this diſeaſe. It may likewiſe be occaſioned by improper diet, as food that is either too weak and watery, or ſo viſcid that the ſtomach cannot digeſt it. Too great

a

a quantity of rich and nouriſhing diet may likewiſe vitiate the humours and occaſion the rickets. Bad nurſing is often the cauſe of this diſeaſe. When the nurſe is either diſeaſed, or has not enough of milk to nouriſh the child, it muſt ſuffer. But children ſuffer oftener by want of care in nurſes than want of food. Allowing an infant to continue long wet, or not keeping it thoroughly clean in its cloaths, &c. has the moſt pernicious effects. Wet ſhoes, ſtockings, and other cloaths, relax the bodies of children, and greatly obſtruct their growth. The want of free air, is likewiſe very hurtſul to children in this reſpect. A nurſe who lives in a cloſe, ſmall houſe, where the air is damp and confined, and who is too indolent to carry her child abroad into the open air, will hardly fail to give it the rickets. But want of exerciſe is the chief cauſe of this diſeaſe. A healthy child ſhould always be in motion, unleſs when aſleep; but if it be ſuffered to lie, or ſit, inſtead of being toſſed and dandled about, it can hardly eſcape this baneful malady.

SYMPTOMS.——At the beginning of this diſeaſe the child's fleſh grows ſoft and flabby; its ſtrength is diminiſhed; it loſes its wonted cheerfulneſs, looks more grave and compoſed than is natural for its age, and does not care to be moved. The head and belly become too large in proportion to the other parts; the face appears full, and the complexion florid. Afterwards the bones begin to be affected, eſpecially

ſpecially in the more ſoft and ſpungy parts, or towards the ends. Hence the wriſts and ancles become thicker than uſual; the ſpine or back-bone puts on an unnatural ſhape; the breaſt is likewiſe often deformed; and the bones of the arms and legs grow crooked. All thoſe ſymptoms vary according to the violence of the diſeaſe. The pulſe is generally quick, but feeble; the appetite and digeſtion, for the moſt part, bad; the teeth come ſlowly and with difficulty, and they often rot and fall out afterwards. Ricketty children generally have great acuteneſs of mind, and an underſtanding above their years. Whether this be owing to their being more in the company of adults than other children, or the enlargement of the brain, we ſhall not pretend to determine.

REGIMEN.—As this diſeaſe is always attended with evident ſigns of weakneſs and relaxation, our chief aim in the cure muſt be to brace and ſtrengthen the ſolids, and to promote the digeſtion and due preparation of the fluids. Theſe important ends will be beſt promoted by wholeſome nouriſhing diet, ſuited to the age and ſtrength of the patient, and often repeated; by open dry air, and plenty of exerciſe. If the child has a bad nurſe, who either neglects her duty, or has not enough of milk, ſhe ſhould be changed. If the ſeaſon be cold, the child ought to be kept warm; and when the weather is hot it ought to be kept cool; as ſweating is very

very apt to weaken it; and too great a degree of cold has the ſame effect. The limbs ſhould be rubbed frequently with a warm hand, and the child ſhould be kept as cheerful as poſſible.

The diet ought to be light and dry, as good bread, roaſted fleſh, &c. Biſcuit is generally reckoned the beſt bread; and pigeons, pullets, veal, rabbets, or mutton roaſted or minced, are the moſt proper fleſh. If the child be too young for fleſh meats, he may have rice, millet, or pearl barley boiled with raiſns, to which may be added a little wine and ſpice. His drink may be good claret, of which he may take half a glaſs three or four times a day. Thoſe who cannot afford claret, may give the child now and then a wine glaſs of fine mild ale.

MEDICINE.——Medicines are here of little avail. The diſeaſe may often be cured by the nurſe, but ſeldom by the phyſician. In children of a groſs habit, gentle purges or vomits may ſometimes be of uſe; but they will never carry off the malady. That muſt depend upon bracing alone: For which purpoſe, beſides the regimen mentioned above, we would recommend the cold bath, eſpecially in the warm ſeaſon. It muſt however be adminiſtred with prudence, as ſome ricketty children cannot bear it. The beſt time for uſing the cold bath is in the morning, and the child ſhould be well rubbed with a dry cloth immediately after. If the

child

child ſhould be weakened by the uſe of the cold bath, it muſt be diſcontinued.

SOMETIMES iſſues have been found beneficial both in this and the foregoing diſeaſe. They are peculiarly neceſſary for children who abound with groſs humours. An infuſion of the jeſuits bark in wine or ale, is likewiſe of uſe; but it is ſcarce poſſible to bring children to take it. We might here mention many other medicines which have been recommended for the rickets; but, as there is far more danger in truſting to theſe than in neglecting them altogether, we chuſe rather to paſs them over, and to depend entirely on regimen.

OF THE ITCH.

THE ITCH is a diſeaſe of the ſkin, and is generally communicated by infection. It ſeems originally to proceed from the want of cleanlineſs, bad air, or unwholeſome diet; as the inmates of jails, hoſpitals, and ſuch as live upon ſalted and ſmoked dried proviſions are ſeldom free from it.

IT generally appears in form of ſmall watery puſtules, firſt about the wriſts, or betwixt the fingers, and afterwards it affects the arms, legs, and thighs, &c. Theſe puſtules are attended with an intolerable itching, eſpecially when the patient is warm in bed, or ſits near the fire.

Sometimes

Sometimes the ſkin is covered with large blotches or ſcabs, and at other times with a white ſcurf, or ſcaly eruption. This laſt is called the dry itch, and is the moſt difficult to cure.

The itch is ſeldom a dangerous diſeaſe, unleſs when it is rendered ſo by neglect or improper treatment. If it be ſuffered to continue too long, it may vitiate the whole maſs of humours; and, if it be ſuddenly drove in, without proper evacuations, it may occaſion fevers, inflammations of the viſcera, or other internal diſorders.

The ſafeſt medicine for the itch is ſulphur, which ought to be applied both externally and internally. The parts moſt affected may be rubbed with an ointment made of common ſulphur and flower of brimſtone, each an ounce; crude ſal ammoniac, finely powdered, two drams; hog's lard, or butter, four ounces. A ſcruple, or half a dram of the eſſence of lemon may be added, to take away the diſagreeable ſmell. About the bulk of a nutmeg of this may be rubbed upon the extremities; at bed-time, twice or thrice a week. It is ſeldom neceſſary to rub any part but the extremities, and even theſe ought not to be all rubbed at the ſame time, but by turns, as it is dangerous to ſtop too many pores at once.

Before the patient begins to uſe the ointment, he ought, if he be of a full habit, to bleed and take a purge or two. It will likewiſe be proper, during the uſe of it, to take every

very night and morning as much of the flower of brimſtone, in a little treacle or new-milk, as will lie upon a ſhilling. He ſhould beware of catching cold, ſhould wear more cloaths than uſual, and take every thing warm. The ſame cloaths, the linen excepted, ought to be kept on all the time of uſing the ointment; and ſuch cloaths as have been worn while the patient was under the diſeaſe, are not to be uſed again, unleſs they have been fumigated with brimſtone, and thoroughly cleaned, otherwiſe they will communicate the infection anew.

I never knew brimſtone, if uſed as directed above, fail to cure the itch; and I have reaſon to believe, that, if duly perſiſted in, it never will fail; but if it be only uſed once or twice, and cleanlineſs be neglected, it is no wonder if the diſorder returns. The great ſecret both for preventing and curing the itch is CLEANLINESS. Where it prevails, the itch will ſeldom approach, and if it ſhould, it will ſoon be baniſhed. The quantity of ointment mentioned above will generally be ſufficient for the cure of one perſon; but, if any ſymptoms of the diſeaſe ſhould appear again, the medicine may be repeated. It is both more ſafe and efficacious when perſiſted in for a conſiderable time, than when a large quantity is applied at once It will likewiſe be proper that the patient, while he is uſing the ointment, ſhould take a purge once a week.

PEOPLE ought to be extremely cautious not to miſtake other eruptions for the itch; as the

ſtoppage

ſtoppage of theſe may be attended with fatal conſequences. Many of the eruptive diſeaſes to which children are liable, have a near reſemblance to the itch; and I have often known infants killed by being rubbed with greaſy ointments that made theſe eruptions ſtrike ſuddenly in, which nature had thrown out to preſerve the patient's life, or prevent ſome other diſeaſe.

MUCH miſchief is likewiſe done by the uſe of mercury in this diſeaſe. I have known ſome perſons mad enough to waſh the parts affected with a ſtrong ſolution of the corroſive ſublimate, which had almoſt proved fatal. Others uſe the mercurial ointment without taking the leaſt care either to avoid cold or obſerve a proper regimen. The conſequences of ſuch conduct may be eaſily gueſſed. I have known even the mercurial girdles produce tragical effects, and would adviſe every perſon, as he values his health, to beware how he uſes them. Mercury ought never to be uſed as a medicine without the greateſt care. Ignorant people look upon theſe girdles as a kind of charm, without conſidering that the mercury enters the blood.

As ſulphur is both the moſt ſafe and efficacious medicine for the itch, we ſhall not recommend any other. Other medicines may be uſed by perſons of ſkill, but are not to be ventured upon by the ignorant. Thoſe who would avoid this deteſtable diſeaſe ought to beware of infected perſons, to uſe wholeſome food, and to ſtudy univerſal cleanlineſs.

OF THE ASTHMA.

THE aſthma is a diſeaſe of the lungs, which ſeldom admits of a cure. Perſons in the decline of life are moſt liable to this diſeaſe. It is divided into the moiſt and dry, or humoural and nervous. The former is attended with expectoration or ſpitting; but in the latter the patient ſeldom ſpits, unleſs ſometimes a little tough phlegm by the mere force of coughing.

CAUSES.—— The aſthma is ſometimes hereditary. It may likewiſe proceed from a bad formation of the breaſt; the fumes of metals or minerals taken into the lungs *; violent exerciſe, eſpecially running; the obſtruction of cuſtomary evacuations, as the menſes, hæmorrhoids, &c.; the ſudden retroceſſion of the gout, or ſtriking in of eruptions, as the ſmall-pox, meaſles, &c.; violent paſſions of the mind, as ſudden fear, or ſurpriſe. In a word, the diſeaſe may proceed from any cauſe that either impedes the circu-

* I knew a perſon whoſe lungs were ſet in a manner ſtock-ſtill, by the fumes of antimony. It happened in the night, after he had been preparing a great quantity of the regulus of antimony through the day. He was relieved by clyſters, fomentations and oily emulſions.

circulation of the blood through the lungs, or prevents their being duly expanded by the air.

SYMPTOMS.—— An aſthma is known by a quick laborious reſpiration, which is generally performed with a kind of wheezing noiſe. Sometimes the difficulty of breathing is ſo great that the patient is obliged to keep an erect poſture, otherwiſe he is in danger of being ſuffocated. A fit or paroxyſm of the aſthma is very apt to happen after a perſon has been expoſed to cold eaſterly winds, or has been abroad in thick foggy weather, or has got wet, or continued long in a damp place under ground, or the like.

A fit of the aſthma is generally uſhered in with great liſtleſſneſs, want of ſleep, hoarſeneſs, cough, belching of wind, a ſenſe of heavineſs about the breaſt, and difficulty of breathing. To theſe ſucceed heat, fever, pain of the head, ſickneſs and nauſea, great oppreſſion of the breaſt, palpitation of the heart, a weak and ſometimes intermitting pulſe, an involuntary flow of tears, bilious vomitings, &c. All the ſymptoms grow worſe towards night; the patient is eaſier when up than in bed, and is very deſirous of cool air.

REGIMEN.—— The food ought to be light, and of eaſy digeſtion. Boiled meats are generally preferred to roaſted, and the fleſh of young animals to that of old. All windy food, and whatever is apt to ſwell upon the ſtomach, is to be avoided. Light puddings, white broths, and ripe fruits baked, boiled or roaſted, are proper.

per. Strong liquor of all kinds, eſpecially malt-liquor, is hurtful. The patient ſhould eat a very light ſupper, or rather none at all. His cloathing ſhould be warm, eſpecially in the winter-ſeaſon. A flannel ſhirt or waſtecoat, and thick ſhoes, are of great ſervice; as all diſorders of the breaſt are much relieved by keeping the feet warm, and promoting the perſpiration.

But nothing is of ſo great importance in the aſthma as pure and moderately warm air. Aſthmatic people can ſeldom bear either the cloſe heavy air of a large town, or the ſharp, keen atmoſphere of a bleak hilly country; a medium between theſe is therefore to be choſen. The air near a large town is often better than at a diſtance, provided the patient be removed ſo far as not to be affected by the ſmoke. Some aſthmatic patients indeed breathe eaſier in town than in the country; but this is ſeldom the caſe, eſpecially in towns where much coal is burnt. Aſthmatic perſons who are obliged to be in town all day, ought, at leaſt, to ſleep out of it. Even this will often prove of great ſervice. Thoſe who can afford it ought to travel into a warmer climate. Many aſthmatic perſons who cannot live in Britain enjoy very good health in the ſouth of France, or in Spain or Italy.

Exercise is likewiſe of very great importance in the aſthma, as it promotes the digeſtion, and greatly aſſiſts in the preparation of the

the blood. The blood of aſthmatic perſons is ſeldom duly prepared, owing to the proper action of the lungs being impeded. For this reaſon ſuch people ought daily to take as much exerciſe, either on foot, horſeback, or in a machine, as they can bear.

MEDICINE.—— Almoſt all that can be done by medicine in this diſeaſe, is to relieve the patient when ſeized with a violent fit. This indeed requires the greateſt expedition, as the diſeaſe often proves ſuddenly fatal. In the paroxyſm or fit, the body is generally bound, a clyſter ought therefore to be adminiſtered, and if there be occaſion, it may be repeated two or three times. The patient's feet ought to be put into warm water, and afterwards rubbed with a warm hand, or dry cloth. If there be a violent ſpaſm about the breaſt or ſtomach, warm fomentations, or bladders filled with warm milk and water, may be applied to the part affected, and warm cataplaſms to the ſoles of the feet. The patient muſt drink freely of diluting liquors, and may take a tea-ſpoonful of the tincture of caſtor and ſaffron, mixed together in a cup of valerian-tea, twice or thrice a-day. Sometimes a vomit has a very good effect, and ſnatches the patient, as it were, from the jaws of death. This will be more ſafe after other evacuations have been premiſed.

OUT OF THE FIT. In the moiſt aſthma, ſuch things as promote expectoration or ſpitting, ought to be uſed; as the ſyrup of ſquills, gum-ammo-

ammoniac, and ſuch like. A common ſpoonful of the ſyrup or oxymell of ſquills, mixed with an equal quantity of cinnamon-water, may be taken three or four times a-day. Any quantity of gum-ammonaic, with an equal quantity of aſafœtida, may be made into pills, and four or five of them taken every night at bed-time.

In the convulſive or nervous aſthma, anti-ſpaſmodics and bracers are the moſt proper medicines. The patient may take a tea ſpoonful of the paregoric elixir twice a-day. The jeſuits bark is likewiſe proper in this caſe. It may be taken in ſubſtance, or infuſed in wine. In ſhort, every thing that braces the nerves, or takes off ſpaſm, may be of uſe in a nervous aſthma. It is often relieved by the uſe of aſſes milk; I have likewiſe known cows milk drank warm of a morning, have a very good effect in this caſe.

In every ſpecies of aſthma iſſues have a good effect; they may either be made in the back or ſide, and ſhould never be allowed to dry up. We ſhall here, once for all, obſerve, that in moſt chronic diſeaſes, iſſues are extremely proper. They are both a ſafe and efficacious remedy; and tho' they do not always cure the diſeaſe, yet they will often prolong the patient's life.

OF

OF THE APOPLEXY.

THE apoplexy is a ſudden loſs of ſenſe and motion, wherein the patient is to all appearance dead, only the heart and lungs ſtill continue to move. This diſeaſe, by a little care, might often be prevented, but can ſeldom be cured. It chiefly attacks ſedentary perſons of a groſs habit, who uſe a rich and plentiful diet, and indulge in ſtrong liquors. People in the decline of life are moſt ſubject to the apoplexy. It prevails moſt in winter, eſpecially in long rainy ſeaſons, and very low ſtates of the barometer.

CAUSES.——The immediate cauſe of an apoplexy is a compreſſion of the brain, occaſioned by an effuſion of blood, or of watery humours on that part. The former is called a *ſanguine*, and the latter a *ſerous apoplexy*. It may be produced by any cauſe that increaſes the circulation towards the brain, or prevents the return of the blood from the head; as intenſe ſtudy; violent paſſions *; viewing objects for a long time obliquely;

* I knew a woman who in a violent fit of anger was ſeized with a ſanguine apoplexy. She at firſt complained of extreme pain, *as if daggers had been thruſt thro' her head, as ſhe expreſſed it*. Afterwards ſhe became comatoſe and dull, her pulſe ſunk very low, and was exceeding ſlow. By the help of bleeding, bliſtering, and other evacuations, ſhe was kept alive for about a forthnight. When her head was opened, a large quantity of extravaſated blood was found in the left ventricle of the brain.

liquely; wearing any thing too tight about the neck; a rich and luxurious diet; ſuppreſſion of urine; ſuffering the body to cool ſuddenly after having been very hot; continuing long in a warm bath; the exceſſive uſe of ſpiceries, or high-ſeaſoned food; exceſs of venery; the ſudden ſtriking in of any eruption; ſuffering iſſues, ſeatons, &c. ſuddenly to dry up, or the ſtoppage of any cuſtomary evacuation; a mercurial ſalivation ſuddenly checked by cold; wounds or bruiſes on the head, long expoſure to exceſſive cold; poiſonous exhalations: &c.

SYMPTOMS, and method of cure.—— The uſual forerunners of an apoplexy are giddineſs, pain, and ſwimming of the head; loſs of memory; drowſineſs; noiſe in the ears; the night-mare; a ſpontaneous flux of tears, and laborious reſpiration. When perſons of an apoplectic make obſerve theſe ſymptoms, they have reaſon to fear the approach of a fit, and ſhould endeavour to prevent it by plentiful bleeding, low diet, and opening medicines.

In the ſanguine apoplexy, if the patient does not die ſuddenly, the countenance appears florid, the face is ſwelled or puffed up, and the blood-veſſels, eſpecially about the neck and temples, are turged; the pulſe beats ſtrong; the eyes are prominent and fixed, and the breathing is difficult, and performed with a ſnorting noiſe. The excrements and urine are often voided ſpontaneouſly, and the patient is ſometimes ſiezed with a vomiting.

In

In this caſe every method muſt be taken to leſſen the force of the blood towards the head. The patient ſhould be kept perfectly eaſy and cool. His head ſhould be raiſed pretty high, and his feet ſuffered to hang down. His cloaths ought to be looſened, eſpecially about the neck, and freſh air admitted into his chamber. His garters ſhould be tied pretty tight, by which means the motion of the blood from the lower extremities will be retarded. As ſoon as the patient is placed in a proper poſture, he ſhould be bled pretty freely in the neck or arm, and, if there be occaſion, the operation may be repeated in two or three hours. A laxative clyſter with plenty of ſweet oil, or freſh butter and a large ſpoonful of common ſalt in it, may be adminiſtred every two hours; and bliſtering plaſters applied betwixt the ſhoulders, and to the calves of the legs.

As ſoon as the ſymptoms are a little abated, and the patient is able to ſwallow, he ought to drink freely of ſome diluting opening liquor, as a decoction of tamarinds and liquorice, cream-tartar-whey, or common whey with cream of tartar diſſolved in it. Or he may take any cooling purge, as Glauber's ſalts, or manna diſſolved in an infuſion of ſenna, or the like. All ſpirits and other ſtrong liquors are to be avoided. Even volatile ſalts held to the noſe do miſchief. Vomits, for the ſame reaſon, ought not to be given, nor any thing that may increaſe the motion of the blood towards the head.

In the ſerous apoplexy, the ſymptoms are nearly ſimilar, only the pulſe is not ſo ſtrong, the countenance is leſs florid, and the breathing leſs difficult. Bleeding is not ſo neceſſary here, as in the former caſe. It may however generally be performed once with ſafety and advantage; but ſhould not be repeated. The patient ſhould be placed in the ſame poſture as directed above, and ſhould have bliſtering plaſters applied, and receive opening clyſters in the ſame manner. Purges are here likewiſe neceſſary, and the patient may drink ſtrong balm tea. If he be inclined to ſweat, it ought to be promoted by drinking ſmall wine whey, or an infuſion of carduus benedictus. A plentiful ſweat kept up for a conſiderable time, has often carried off a ſerous apoplexy.

When apoplectic ſymptoms proceed from opium, or other narcotic ſubſtances taken into the ſtomach, vomits are neceſſary. The patient is generally relieved, as ſoon as he has diſcharged the poiſon in this way.

Persons of an apoplectic make, or thoſe who have been attacked by it, ought to uſe a very ſpare and ſlender diet, avoiding all ſtrong liquors, ſpiceries, and high ſeaſoned food. They ought likewiſe to guard againſt all violent paſſions, and to avoid the extremes of heat and cold. The head ſhould be ſhaved, and daily waſhed with cold water. The feet ought to be kept warm, and never ſuffered to continue long wet. The belly muſt, by all means, be kept open,

pen, either by food or medicine, and blood ought to be let every ſpring and fall. Moderate exerciſe ſhould likewiſe be taken; but it ought never to be continued too long. Nothing has a greater effect in preventing an apoplexy than iſſues or perpetual bliſters; but great care muſt be taken never to ſuffer them to dry up, without opening others in their ſtead. Apoplectic perſons ought never to go to ſleep with a full ſtomach, nor to ly with their heads too low, or wear any thing tight about their necks.

Of the PALSY.

THE palſy is a loſs or diminution of ſenſe, or motion, or of both, in one or more parts of the body. It is more or leſs dangerous, according to the importance of the part affected. A palſy of the heart, lungs, or any part neceſſary for life, is mortal. When it affects the ſtomach, the inteſtines, or the bladder, it is highly dangerous. If the face be affected, the caſe is bad, as this ſhews, that the diſeaſe proceeds from the brain. If the part affected feels cold, is inſenſible, or waſtes away, there is ſmall hopes of a cure, eſpecially, if the judgement and memory begin to fail.

CAUSES. THE immediate cauſe of palſy is whatever prevents the regular exertion of the

the nervous power upon any particular muſcle or part of the body. The occaſional and predisposing cauſes are various, as drunkenneſs; wounds of the brain, or ſpinal marrow; preſſure upon the brain or nerves; very cold or damp air; the ſuppreſſion of cuſtomary evacuations; ſudden fear; want of exerciſe; or whatever greatly relaxes the ſyſtem, as drinking much tea, * or coffee, &c. Wounds of the nerves themſelves, or any thing that obſtructs the regular action of that vital power contained in them, will occaſion a palſy. It may likewiſe proceed from the poiſonous fumes of metals or minerals, as mercury, lead, arſenick, &c.

In young perſons of a full habit, where there are ſymptoms of inflammation, the palſy muſt be treated in the ſame manner as the ſanguine apoplexy. The patient muſt be bled, bliſtered; and have his belly kept open by ſharp clyſters or purgative medicines. But, in old age, or when the diſeaſe proceeds from relaxation or debility, which is generally the caſe, a quite contrary courſe muſt be purſued. The diet muſt be warm and attenuating, conſiſting chiefly of ſpicy and aromatic

* Many people imagine, that tea has no tendency to hurt the nerves, and that drinking the ſame quantity of warm water would be equally pernicious. This however ſeems to be a miſtake. I know many perſons who daily drink three or four cups of warm milk and water without feeling any bad conſequences; yet the ſame quantity of tea will make their hands ſhake for twenty four hours.

aromatic vegetables, as muſtard, horſe-radiſh, &c. The drink may be generous wine, muſtard-whey, or brandy and water. Friction with the fleſh bruſh, or a warm hand, is extremely proper, eſpecially on the parts affected. Bliſtering-plaſters may likewiſe be applied to the affected parts with advantage. When this cannot be done, they may be rubbed with the volatile liniment, or the nerve-ointment of the Edinburgh diſpenſatory. But the beſt external application is electricity. The ſhocks ſhould be received on the part affected; and they ought daily to be repeated for ſeveral weeks. This is not only proper for curing, but alſo for preventing a palſy.

VOMITS are very beneficial in this kind of palſy, and ought to be frequently adminiſtred. Cæphalic ſnuff, or any thing that makes the patient ſneeze, is likewiſe uſeful. Some pretend to have found great benefit from rubbing the parts affected with nettles; but this does not ſeem to be any ways preferable to bliſtering. If the tongue be affected, the patient may gargle his mouth frequently with brandy and muſtard; or he may hold a bit of ſugar in his mouth wet with the palſy-drops or compound ſpirits of lavender. The wild valerian root is a very proper medicine in this caſe. It may either be taken in an infuſion with ſage leaves, or half a dram of it in powder may be given in a glaſs of wine three times a day. If the patient cannot uſe the valerian, he may take of *ſal volatile oleoſum*, compound ſpirits of lavender, and tincture of caſtor,

caſtor, each half an ounce; mix theſe together, and take forty or fifty drops in a glaſs of wine, three our four times a day. A table ſpoonful of muſtard-ſeed taken frequently is a very good medicine. The patient ought likewiſe to chew cinnamon bark, ginger, or other warm ſpiceries.

EXERCISE is of the utmoſt importance in the palſy; but the patient muſt beware of cold, damp, and moiſt air. He ought to wear flannel next his ſkin; and, if poſſible, ſhould remove into a warmer climate.

OF THE EPILEPSY, OR FALLING SICKNESS.

THE epilepſy is a ſudden deprivation of all the ſenſes, wherein the patient falls ſuddenly down, and is affected with violent convulſive motions. Children, eſpecially thoſe that are delicately brought up, are moſt ſubject to it. It more frequently attacks men than women, and is very difficult to cure. When the epilepſy attacks children, there is reaſon to hope it may go off about the time of puberty. When it attacks any perſon after twenty years of age, the cure is difficult; but when after forty, a cure is hardly to be expected. If the fit continues only for a ſhort ſpace, and returns ſeldom, there is reaſon to hope; but if it continues long and returns frequently, the proſpect is bad. It is a very

very unfavourable ſymptom, when the patient is ſeized with the fits in his ſleep.

CAUSES.——Sometimes the epilepſy is a hereditary diſeaſe. It may likewiſe proceed from a ſudden fright of the mother when with child of the patient; from blows, bruiſes, or wounds on the head; a collection of water, blood, or ſerous humours in the brain; a polypus; tumours or concretions within the ſkull; exceſſive drinking; intenſe ſtudy; exceſs of venery; worms; teething; ſuppreſſion of cuſtomary evacuations; too great emptineſs or repletion; violent paſſions or affections of the mind, as fear, joy, *&c.*; hyſteric affections; contagion received into the body, as the infection of the ſmall-pox, meaſles, *&c.*

SYMPTOMS.——An epileptic fit is generally preceded by unuſual wearineſs; pain of the head; dulneſs; giddineſs; noiſe in the ears; dimneſs of ſight; palpitation of the heart; diſturbed ſleep; difficult breathing; the bowels are inflated with wind; the urine is in great quantity, but thin; the complexion is pale; the extremities are cold, and the patient feels as it were a ſtream of cold air aſcending towards his head.

In the fit, the patient generally makes an unuſual noiſe; his thumbs are drawn in towards the palms of the hands; his eyes are diſtorted; he ſtarts, and foams at the mouth; his extremities are bent or twiſted various ways; he often diſcharges his ſeed, urine, and fœces involuntarily; and is quite deſtitute of all ſenſe and reaſon.

After

After the fit is over, his ſenſes gradually return, and he complains of a kind of ſtupor, wearineſs, and pain of his head; but has no remembrance of what happened to him during the fit.

Sometimes the fits return at ſtated periods, as at the full or change of the moon: at other times they are excited by violent affections of the mind, a debauch of liquor, exceſſive heat, cold, or the like.

This diſeaſe, from the difficulty of inveſtigating its cauſes, and its ſtrange ſymptoms, was formerly attributed to the wrath of the gods, or the agency of evil ſpirits. In modern times it has often, by the vulgar, been imputed to witchcraft or faſcination. It depends however as much upon natural cauſes as any other malady; and its cure can only be effected by perſiſting in the uſe of proper means.

REGIMEN.——Epileptic patients ought, if poſſible, to breathe a pure and free air. Their diet ſhould be nouriſhing, but of eaſy digeſtion. They ought to drink nothing ſtrong, to avoid ſwines fleſh, water fowl, and likewiſe all windy and oily vegetables, as cabbage, nuts, &c. They ought to keep themſelves cheerful, carefully avoiding all occaſions of violent paſſions, as anger, fear, &c*.

* It has already been obſerved that epileptic fits are often the effect of fear, and are occaſioned by that idle cuſtom among young people of frightening one another. Though this be generally done out of mere frolic, it has many dreadful conſequences, and ought by all means to be diſcouraged. It is ſurely a ſmaller crime to take away a perſon's life, than to render him at once miſerable in himſelf, and a burden to ſociety.

Exercise

EXERCISE is likewiſe of great uſe; but the patient muſt be careful to avoid all extremes either of heat or cold, all dangerous ſituations, as ſtanding upon precipices, riding deep waters, &c. Any thing that makes him giddy, is apt to occaſion a fit, as turning round, looking into a deep pit, or the like; all theſe ought therefore to be avoided with the utmoſt care.

MEDICINE——The intentions of cure muſt vary according to the cauſe of the diſeaſe. If the patient be of a ſanguine temperament, and there be reaſon to fear an inflammation in the brain, bleeding and other evacuations will be neceſſary. When the diſeaſe is occaſioned by the ſtoppage of cuſtomary evacuations, theſe, if poſſible, muſt be reſtored; if this cannot be done, others may be ſubſtituted in their place. Iſſues or ſetons, in this caſe, have often a very good effect When there is reaſon to believe that the diſeaſe proceeds from worms, proper medicines muſt be uſed to kill or carry off theſe vermin. When the diſeaſe proceeds from teething the belly ſhould be kept open by emollient clyſters, the feet frequently bathed in warm water, and, if the fits prove obſtinate, a bliſtering plaiſter may be put betwixt the ſhoulders. The ſame method is to be followed, when epileptic fits precede the eruption of the ſmall pox, or meaſles, &c.

WHEN the diſeaſe is hereditary, or proceeds from a wrong formation of the brain, a cure is not to be expected. When it is owing to ſome fault in the nervous ſyſtem, ſuch medicines as tend to brace and ſtrengthen the nerves may be uſed, as the Jeſuit's bark, Valerian root, miſletoe of the oak, ſnake-root, &c.

FULLER recommends the following electuary as a moſt excellent *anti-epileptic.* Take Jeſuits bark in powder three ounces, Virginian ſnake-root powdered one ounce, as much ſyrup of pæony or cloves as is ſufficient to form it into a ſoft electuary. The doſe to an adult is a dram, or about the ſize of a nutmeg, morning and evening. It muſt be continued for three or four months, and afterwards repeated, three or four days before the new and full moon, for ſome time.

MEAD recommends an electuary againſt the epilepſy much of the ſame nature, only he uſes Valerian root in place of the ſnake-root. It muſt be taken in the ſame manner as the above. The patient ought always to be bled, and to take a purge or two before he begins to uſe theſe medicines. They will likewiſe have a better effect if the patient drinks a tea-cupful of the decoction of *guaiacum* after each doſe. It may be made by boiling two ounces of guaiacum ſhavings, and one ounce of raiſins of the ſun ſtoned, in two Engliſh quarts of water to one. Strain the liquor, and afterwards let it ſtand to ſettle, then pour off the clear from the feces.

COLEBATCH ſays, that the miſletoe cures an epilepſy as certainly as the Jeſuits bark does an intermittent fever. The doſe to an adult is half a dram

dram of the powder, four times a-day, drinking after it a draught of a ſtrong infuſion of the ſame plant. Though this medecine has not been found to anſwer the high encomiums which have been paſſed upon it, yet in obſtinate epileptic caſes it deſerves a trial. It muſt be uſed for a conſiderable time, in order to produce any ſalutary effects.

MUSK has ſometimes been found to anſwer very well in the epilepſy. Ten or twelve grains of it, with the ſame quantity of factitious cinnabar, may be made up into a bolus and taken every night and morning.

SOMETIMES the epilepſy has been cured by electricity.

CONVULSION FITS proceed from the ſame cauſes, and muſt be treated in the ſame manner as the epilepſy.

THERE is one particular ſpecies of convulſions, which commonly goes by the name of St Vitus's dance, wherein the patient is agitated with ſtrange motions and geſticulations, which by the common people are generally believed to be the effects of witchcraft. This diſeaſe may be cured by repeated bleedings and purges; and afterwards uſing the medicines preſcribed above for the epilepſy, viz. the jeſuits-bark, and ſnake-root, &c. Chalybeate-waters, are found to be beneficial in this caſe. The cold bath is likewiſe of ſingular ſervice, and ought never to be neglected when the patient can bear it.

Of

Of NERVOUS, HYSTERIC, and HYPOCHONDRIAC Disorders.

Of all diseases incident to mankind, those of the nervous kind are the most complicated and difficult to cure. A volume would not be sufficient to point out their various symptoms. They imitate almost every disease; and are seldom alike in two different persons, or even in the same person at different times. Like Proteus, they are continually changing shape; and upon every fresh attack, the patient thinks he feels symptoms which he never experienced before. Nor do they only affect the body, the mind likewise suffers, and is often thereby rendered extremely weak and peevish. The low spirits, timorousness, melancholy, and fickleness of temper which generally attend nervous disorders, induce many people to believe, that they are entirely diseases of the mind; but this change of temper is rather a consequence, than the cause of nervous diseases.

CAUSES.——Every thing that tends to relax or weaken the body, predisposes it to nervous diseases, as indolence, excessive venery, drinking great quantities of tea, or other weak watery liquors, frequent bleeding, purging, vomiting, &c. Whatever hurts the digestion, or prevents the proper assimilation of the aliment, has likewise this effect, as long fasting, excess in eating

eating or drinking, the uſe of windy, crude, or unwholſome aliments, a bending poſture of the body, &c.

Nervous diſorders often proceed from affections of the mind, as grief, diſappointments, anxiety, intenſe ſtudy, &c. Few ſtudious perſons are free from nervous diſeaſes. Nor is this at all to be wondered at; intenſe thinking not only preys upon the ſpirits, but prevents the perſon from taking proper exerciſe, by which means the digeſtion is impaired, the nouriſhment prevented, the ſolids relaxed, and the whole maſs of humours vitiated. Grief and diſappointment likewiſe produce the ſame effects. I have known more hyſteric and hypochondriac patients, who dated the commencement of their diſorders from the loſs of a huſband, a favourite child, or from ſome diſappointment in life, than from any other cauſe. In a word, whatever weakens the body, or depreſſes the ſpirits, may occaſion nervous diſorders, as unwholeſome air, want of ſleep, great fatigue, &c.

SYMPTOMS.——We ſhall only mention ſome of the moſt general ſymptoms of theſe diſorders, as it would be both an uſeleſs and impracticable taſk to point out the whole. They generally begin with windy inflations or diſtenſions of the ſtomach and inteſtines, eſpecially under the falſe ribs of the left ſide, where a hard tumour may ſometimes be perceived.

The

The appetite and digeſtion are generally bad; yet ſometimes there is an uncommon craving for food, and a quick digeſtion. The food often turns ſour on the ſtomach; and the patient is troubled with vomiting of clear water, tough phlegm, or a blackiſh coloured liquor reſembling the grounds of coffee. Excrutiating pains are often felt about the navel, attended with a rumbling or murmuring noiſe in the bowels. The belly is ſometimes looſe, but more commonly bound, which occaſions a retention of wind and great uneaſineſs.

The urine is ſometimes in ſmall quantity, at other times very copious and quite clear. There is a great ſtraitneſs of the breaſt with difficulty of breathing; violent palpitations of the heart; ſudden fluſhings of heat in various parts of the body; at other times a ſenſe of cold, as if water were poured on them; flying pains in the arms and limbs; pains in the back and belly, reſembling thoſe occaſioned by gravel; the pulſe very variable, ſometimes uncommonly ſlow, and at other times very quick; yawning, the hiccup, frequent ſighings and a ſenſe of ſuffocation, as if from a ball or lump in the throat; alternate fits of crying and convulſive laughing; the ſleep is unſound, and ſeldom refreſhing; and the patient is often troubled with the night-mare.

As the diſeaſe increaſes, the patient is moleſted with headachs, cramps, and fixt pains in various parts of the body; the eyes are clouded, and often affected with pain and dryneſs; there is a noiſe in the ears, and often a dullneſs of hearing; in ſhort, the whole animal functions are impaired. The mind is diſturbed on the moſt trivial occaſions, and is hurried into the moſt perverſe commotions, inquietudes, terror, ſadneſs, anger, diffidence, &c. The patient is apt to entertain wild imaginations, and extravagant fancies; the memory becomes weak, and the reaſon fails. Nothing is more characteriſtic of this diſeaſe than a conſtant dread of death. This renders the patients peeviſh, fickle, impatient, and apt to run from one phyſician to another; which is one reaſon why they ſeldom reap any benefit from medicine, as they have not ſufficient reſolution to perſiſt in any one courſe till it has time to produce its proper effects. They are likewiſe apt to imagine that they labour under diſeaſes from which they are quite free, and are very angry if any one attempts to laugh them out of their ridiculous notions.

REGIMEN.——Hyſteric and hypochondriac perſons ought never to faſt long. Their food ſhould be ſolid and nouriſhing, but of eaſy digeſtion. Fat meats, and heavy ſauces, are hurtful. All exceſs ſhould be carefully avoided. They ought never to eat more at a time than they can eaſily digeſt. Heavy ſuppers are to be avoided. If the patient feels himſelf weak and faint between meals, he ought to eat a bit of bread, and drink a glaſs of wine. Tho' wine in exceſs enfeebles

feebles the body, and impairs the faculties of the mind, yet taken in moderation, it ſtrengthens the ſtomach, and promotes digeſtion. Wine and water is a very proper drink at meals. If wine ſours on the ſtomach, or the patient is much troubled with wind, brandy and water will anſwer better. Every thing that is windy, or hard of digeſtion, muſt be avoided. All weak and warm liquors are hurtful, as tea, coffee, punch, &c. People may find a temporary relief from theſe, but they always increaſe the malady, as they weaken the ſtomach, and hurt digeſtion. Above all things, drams are to be avoided. Whatever immediate eaſe the patient may feel from the uſe of ardent ſpirits, they are ſure to aggravate the malady, and prove certain poiſons at laſt. Theſe cautions are the more neceſſary here, as all hyſteric and hypochondriac perſons are peculiarly fond of tea and ardent ſpirits; to the uſe of which many of them fall a victim.

Exercise is of ſuch importance in nervous diſorders, that it is worth all other medicines. Riding on horſeback is generally eſteemed the beſt, as it gives motion to the whole body, without fatiguing it. I have known ſome patients, however, with whom walking agreed better, and others who were moſt benefited by riding in a machine. Every one ought to uſe that which he finds moſt beneficial. Long ſea voyages have an excellent effect; and to thoſe who can

can afford to take them, and have ſufficient reſolution, we would by all means recommend this courſe. Even change of place, and the ſight of new objects, by diverting the mind, have a great tendency to remove theſe complaints. For this reaſon a long journey, or a voyage, is of much more advantage than riding ſhort journeys near home.

A cool and dry air is the beſt, as it braces and imparts vigour to the whole body. Nothing tends more to relax and enervate than hot air, eſpecially that which is rendered ſo by great fires, or ſtoves in ſmall apartments. But when the ſtomach or bowels are weak, the body ought to be well guarded againſt cold, eſpecially in winter, by wearing a thin flannel waiſtcoat next the ſkin. This will keep up an equal perſpiration, and defend the alimentary canal from many impreſſions, to which it would otherwiſe be ſubject, upon every ſudden change from warm to cold weather. Rubbing the body frequently with a fleſh-bruſh, or a coarſe linen cloth, is likewiſe beneficial, as it promotes the circulation, perſpiration, &c. Perſons who have weak nerves ought to riſe early, and take exerciſe before breakfaſt, as lying too long a bed cannot fail to relax the ſolids. They ought likewiſe to be diverted, and to be kept as eaſy and cheerful as poſſible. Nothing hurts the nervous ſyſtem, or weakens the digeſtive powers more than fear, grief, or anxiety.

MEDICINES.— Tho' nervous diſeaſes

are ſeldom radically cured, yet their ſymptoms may ſometimes be alleviated, and the patient's life rendered, at leaſt, more comfortable, by proper medicines.

When the patient is coſtive, he ought to take a little rhubarb, or ſome other mild purgative, and ſhould never ſuffer his belly to be long bound. All ſtrong and violent purgatives are however to be avoided, as aloes, jalap, &c. I have generally ſeen an infuſion of ſenna and rhubarb in brandy anſwer very well. This may be made of any ſtrength, and taken in ſuch quantity as the patient finds neceſſary.

When the digeſtion is bad, and the ſtomach relaxed and weak, bitters will be of ſervice. The beſt of theſe are the jeſuits bark and gentian root, which may be prepared and uſed in the following manner. Take jeſuits bark in powder, an ounce and a half, gentian-root and orange-peel bruiſed, of each half an ounce. Infuſe theſe ingredients in a bottle of brandy or whiſky, for five or ſix days, then ſtrain the liquor, and take a table ſpoonful in half a glaſs of water an hour before breakfaſt, dinner, and ſupper.

Nothing tends more to ſtrengthen the nervous ſyſtem than cold bathing. This practice, if duly perſiſted in, will produce very extraordinary effects; but when the liver or other *viſcera* are obſtructed, or otherwiſe unſound, the cold bath is improper. The moſt proper ſeaſons for it are ſummer and autumn. It will be ſufficient, eſpecially for perſons of a ſpare habit,

to

to go into the cold bath three or four times a-week. If the patient be weakened by it, or feels chilly for a long time after coming out, it is improper.

In patients afflicted with wind, I have always observed the greatest benefit from the acid elixir of vitriol. It may be taken in the quantity of fifteen, twenty, or thirty drops, twice or thrice a-day, in a glass of water. This both expels wind, strengthens the stomach, and promotes digestion.

Opiates are greatly extolled in these maladies; but as they only palliate the symptoms, and generally afterwards increase the disease, we would advise people to be extremely cautious in the use of them, lest habit render them at last absolutely necessary.

It would be an easy matter to enumerate many medicines which have been extolled for relieving nervous disorders; but whoever wishes for a thorough cure must expect it from regimen alone; we shall therefore omit mentioning more medicines, and again recommend the strictest attention to DIET, AIR, EXERCISE, and AMUSEMENTS.

OF MELANCHOLY AND MADNESS.

Melancholy and madness are nearly allied. They both proceed from the same origin, and may be considered as only different degrees of of the ſame diſeaſe. *A delirium without a fever* is the common definition of madneſs: Indeed it is not a very accurate one; but there is no great occaſion to be ſolicitous about the definition of a diſeaſe which every body knows. It is of far greater importance to know how it is occaſioned, and by what means it may be cured.

CAUSES.—— It may proceed from a hereditary diſpoſition; intenſe thinking, eſpecially where the mind is long occupied about one object; violent paſſions or affections of the mind, as love, fear, joy, grief, over-weening pride, and ſuch like. It may alſo be occaſioned by exceſſive venery; narcotic or ſtupifactive poiſons; a ſedentary life; ſolitude; the ſuppreſſion of cuſtomary evacuations; accute fevers, or other diſeaſes. Violent anger will change melancholy into madneſs; and exceſſive cold, eſpecially of the lower extremities, will force the blood into the brain, and produce all the ſymptoms of madneſs. It may likewiſe proceed from the uſe of aliment that is hard of digeſtion, or which cannot be eaſily aſſimilated; from a callous ſtate of the integuments of the brain, or a dryneſs of the brain itſelf. To all which we may add gloomy or miſtaken notions of religion *.

SYMP-

* THE mind by dwelling too long upon the dark ſide of religion, is often, at length, overwhelmed with the deepeſt melancholy, which ends in madneſs. What a pity that *religion*, which was intended to alleviate the calamities of life, to keep the mind cheerful, and to raiſe it above diſappointments, ſhould ever be perverted into the means of producing theſe very evils it was deſigned to cure?

SYMPTOMS.—— When perſons begin to be melancholy, they are dull; dejected; timorous; watchful; fond of ſolitude; fretful; fickle; captious and inquiſitive; ſolicitous about trifles; ſometimes nigardly, and at other times prodigal. The belly is generally bound; the urine thin, and in ſmall quantity; the ſtomach and bowels inflated with wind; the complexion pale; the pulſe ſlow and weak. The functions of the mind are alſo greatly perverted, in ſo much that the patient often imagines himſelf dead, or changed into ſome other animal. Some have imagined, their bodies were made of glaſs, or other brittle ſubſtances, and were afraid to move leſt they ſhould be broken in pieces. The unhappy patient, in this caſe, unleſs carefully watched, is apt to put an end to his own miſerable life.

THE ſigns of approaching madneſs are: Redneſs of the eyes, with a tremulous and conſtant vibration of the eye lids; a change of diſpoſition and behaviour; ſupercilious looks; a haughty carriage; grinding of the teeth; unaccountable malice to particular perſons; exceſſive watchfulneſs; violent headachs; quickneſs of hearing; noiſe in the ears, &c.

PERSONS actually mad are in an exceſſive rage when provoked to anger. Some wander about, others make a hideous noiſe. Some ſhun the ſight of men; others, if permitted, would tear themſelves, or thoſe whom they meet, to pieces. Some

Some in the highest degree of the disorder see images before their eyes, and fancy themselves struck with lightening. To these we may add incredible strength, and great insensibity to hunger and cold.

WHEN the disease is owing to an obstruction of customary evacuations, or any bodily disorder, it is easier cured than when it proceeds from the mind. Madness attended with mirth is not so dangerous as that which is accompanied with sadness. A discharge of blood from the nose, a violent looseness, scabby eruptions, the bleeding piles, or the *menses*, sometimes carry off this disease.

DISEASES of the mind often intermit for several years, and return again. In some they return annually at the solstices; in others about the time of the equinoxes. Sometimes the raving fits observe the lunar periods; in which case the disease is thought to have some affinity with the epilepsy.

REGIMEN.—— The diet ought to consist chiefly of vegetables of a cooling and opening quality. Animal food, especially salted or smoke dried fish or flesh, ought to be avoided. All kinds of shell-fish are bad. Aliments prepared with onions, garlic, or any thing that generates thick blood, are likewise improper. All kind of fruits that are wholesome may be eat with advantage. Boerhaave gives an instance of a patient who by a long use of whey, water,

and

and garden-fruits, evacuated a great quantity of black matter, and recovered his ſenſes. This ſeems to have been the method of cure practiced at the Aſſyrian court; where we find the monarch himſelf, when ſeized with madneſs, was turned out to graze.

STRONG liquors of every kind ought to be avoided as poiſon. The moſt proper drink is water, whey, or very ſmall beer. Tea and coffee are improper. If honey agrees with the patient, it may be eat freely, or his drink ſweetened with it. Infuſions of balm leaves, pennyroyal, the roots of wild valerian, or the flowers of the lime-tree, may be drank freely, either by themſelves, or ſweetned with honey, as the patient ſhall chuſe.

THE patient ought to take as much exerciſe in the open air as he can bear. This helps to diſſolve the viſcid humours, it removes obſtructions, promotes the perſpiration, and all the other ſecretions. Every kind of madneſs is attended with a diminiſhed perſpiration; all means ought therefore to be uſed to promote that neceſſary and ſalutary diſcharge. Nothing can have a more direct tendency to increaſe the diſeaſe than the common method of confining the patient to a cloſe apartment. Were a proper ſpace allotted for him to run about in, where he could neither hurt himſelf nor others, it would contribute much to promote a cure. It would have

have ſtill a better effect, if he were obliged to labour a piece of ground. By digging, hoeing, planting, ſowing, &c. both the body and mind would be exerciſed.

A plan of this kind, with a ſtrict vegetable diet, would be a more rational method of cure than confining the patient in Bedlam, or ſending him to a private mad-houſe. Theſe inſtitutions, as they are generally managed, are far more likely to make a wiſe man mad than to reſtore a madman to his ſenſes. Even running about at large, tho' it may be attended with ſome bad conſequences, is more likely to reſtore the patient than confining him in a mad-houſe. I have known ſeveral inſtances of perſons cured by exerciſe, amuſements, and a vegetable diet, who, in all probability, had they been confined. would have continued lunatic for life. A long journey, or a voyage, eſpecially into a warmer climate, with agreeable companions, has often very happy effects.

MEDICINE.——In the cure of madneſs, great regard muſt be paid to the mind When the patient is in a low melancholy ſtate, his mind ought to be ſoothed and diverted with variety of amuſements, as entertaining ſtories, paſtimes, muſic, &c This ſeems to have been the method of curing melancholy among the Jews, as we learn from the ſtory of King Saul ; and indeed it is a very rational one. Nothing

Nothing can remove diseases of the mind so effectually as applications to the mind itself, the most efficacious of which is music. The patient's company ought likewise to consist of such persons as are agreeable to him. People in this state are apt to conceive unaccountable aversions against particular persons; and the very sight of such persons is sufficient to distract their minds, and throw them into the utmost perturbation. In all kinds of madness, it is better to sooth and calm the mind than to ruffle it by contradiction.

WHEN the patient is high, evacuations are necessary. In this case he must be bled, and have his belly kept open by purging medicines, as manna, rhubarb, cream of tartar, or the soluble tartar. I have seen the last have very good effects. It may be taken in the dose of half an ounce, dissolved in water gruel every day, for sundry weeks, or even for months, if necessary. More or less may be given according as it operates. Vomits have likewise a good effect; but they must be pretty strong, otherwise they will not operate.

MADNESS has sometimes been cured by camphire. Ten or twelve grains of it may be rubbed in a mortar with half a dram of nitre, and taken twice a day, or oftner if the stomach will bear it. If it will not sit upon the stomach in this form, it may be made into pills with gum asafætida and Russian castor, and taken in the quantity above directed. Musk has likewiſe been found efficacious in this caſe; but to have any effect, it muſt be given in large doſes. A ſcruple or twenty five grains may be made into a bolus with a little honey or ſyrup, and taken twice or thrice a day. The antimonial wine is by ſome extolled for the cure of madneſs. It may be taken in the doſe of forty or fifty drops, twice or thrice a day, in a cup of tea. The tincture of hellebore has likewiſe been in great eſteem; but I never ſaw any conſiderable effects from it. Each of the above medicines may be of ſervice in ſome particular caſe, provided it be duly perſiſted in, and where one fails, it may not be amiſs to try another.

As it is very difficult to induce patients in this diſeaſe to take medicines, we ſhall mention ſome outward applications which ſometimes do good; the principal of theſe are iſſues, ſetons, and cold bathing. Iſſues may be made in any part of the body, but they generally have the beſt effect near the ſpine of the back. The diſcharge from theſe may be greatly promoted by dreſſing them with the mild bliſtering ointment, and keeping what are commonly called the orrice peas in them. The ſalt water is moſt proper for bathing in; but when that cannot be obtained, the patient may be daily immerſed in freſh water. Some recommend bathing the body in warm water, and at the ſame time pouring cold water upon the head.

THAT

That kind of madneſs or delirium which proceeds from mere weakneſs, requires a quite different method of treatment. Is is often the effect of fevers injudiciouſly treated, wherein the patient's ſtrength has been exhauſted by frequent bleedings and purgings. This muſt be removed by nouriſhing diet, exerciſe proportioned to the patient's ſtrength, and cordial medicines. All vacuations are here carefully to be avoided. The patient may take frequently a glaſs of good wine, in which a little jeſuits bark has been infuſed.

OF POISONS.

EVERY perſon ought, in ſome meaſure, to be acquainted with the nature and cure of poiſons. They are generally taken unawares, and their effects are often ſo ſudden and violent, as not to admit of delay, or allow time to procure the aſſiſtance of phyſicians. Indeed no great degree of medical knowledge is here neceſſary, the remedies for moſt poiſons being generally at hand, or eaſily obtained, and nothing but common prudence needful in the application of them.

THE vulgar notion that every poiſon is cured by ſome counter poiſon, as a ſpecific, has done much hurt. People believe they can do nothing for the patient, unleſs they know the particular antidote to that kind of poiſon which he he has taken. Whereas the cure of all poisons taken into the stomach, without exception, depends on discharging them as soon as possible.

There is no case wherein nature points out the method of cure more clearly than in this. Poison is seldom long in the stomach before it occasions sickness with an inclination to vomit. This shews plainly what ought to be done. Indeed common sense dictates to every man, that, if any thing has been taken into the stomach which endangers life, it ought immediately to be discharged. Were this duly regarded, most of the mischief occasioned by poison might be prevented. The method of cure is obvious, and the means of performing it are in the hands of every man.

Poisons either belong to the animal, vegetable, or mineral kingdom.

Mineral poisons are commonly of an acrid or corrosive quality, as arsenic, the corrosive sublimate of mercury, &c.

Those of the vegetable kind are generally of a narcotic or stupifactive quality, as poppy, hemlock, henbane, berries of the deadly night-shade, &c.

Poisonous animals communicate their infection, either by the bite or sting. This poison is very different from the former, both in its symptoms and cure.

MINERAL POISONS.——Arsenic is the most common of this class; and, as the whole of them are pretty similar both in their effects and method

method of cure, what is ſaid with reſpect to it will be applicable to every other ſpecies of corroſive poiſon.

When a perſon has taken arſenic, he ſoon perceives a burning heat, and violent pricking pain in his ſtomach and bowels, with vomiting and intolerable thirſt. The tongue and throat feel rough and dry; and, if proper help be not ſoon adminiſtered, the patient is ſeized with great anxiety, hiccuping, faintings, and coldneſs of the extremities. To theſe ſucceed black vomits, fœtid ſtools, with a mortification of the ſtomach and inteſtines, which are the immediate forerunners of death.

On the firſt appearance of theſe ſymptoms, the patient ſhould drink large quantities of new milk and ſalad oil till he vomits; or he may drink warm water mixed with oil. Fat broths are alſo proper, provided they can be got ready in time. Where no oil is to be had, freſh butter may be melted and mixed with the milk or water. Theſe things are to be drank as long as the inclination to vomit continues. Some have drank eight or ten Engliſh quarts before the vomiting ceaſed; and it is never ſafe to leave off drinking while one particle of the poiſon remains in the ſtomach.

These oily or fat ſubſtances not only provoke vomiting, but likewiſe blunt the acrimony of the poiſon, and prevent its wounding the bowels; but if they ſhould not make the perſon vomit, half a dram or two ſcruples of the powder

der of ipecacoanha muſt be given, or a few ſpoonfuls of the oxymel of ſquils mixed with the water which he drinks. Vomiting may likewiſe be excited by tickling the inſide of the throat with a feather.

If the tormenting pains are felt in the lower belly, and there is reaſon to fear, that the inteſtines are attacked,. clyſters of milk and oil muſt be very frequently thrown up; and the patient muſt drink emolient decoctions of barley, oatmeal, marſhmallows, and ſuch like.

AFTER the poiſon has been evacuated, the patient ought, for ſome time, to live upon ſuch things as are of a healing and cooling quality. To abſtain from fleſh and all ſtrong liquors, and to live upon milk, broth, gruel, light puddings, and other ſpoon meats of eaſy digeſtion. His drink ſhould be barley water, linſeed tea, or infuſions of any of the mild mucilaginous vegetables.

VEGETABLE POISONS, beſides heat and pain of the ſtomach, commonly occaſion ſome degree of giddineſs, and often a kind of ſtupidity or folly. Perſons who have taken theſe muſt be treated in the ſame manner as for the mineral or corroſive.

Though the vegetable poiſons, when allowed to remain in the ſtomach, often prove fatal; yet the danger is generally over as ſoon as they are diſcharged. Not being of ſuch a cauſtic or corroſive nature, they are leſs apt to wound and inflame the bowels than mineral ſubſtances; no time however ought to be loſt in having them expelled the ſtomach.

Opium,

Opium, being frequently taken by miſtake, merits particular attention. It is uſed as a medicine both in a ſolid and liquid form, which latter commonly goes by the name of laudanum. It is indeed a valuable medicine when taken in proper quantity; but as an over doſe proves a ſtrong poiſon, we ſhall point out its common effects, together with the method of cure.

Too great a quantity of opium generally occaſions great drowſineſs, with ſtupor and other apoplectic ſymptoms. Sometimes the perſon has ſo great an inclination to ſleep, that it is almoſt impoſſible to keep him awake. Every method muſt however be tried for this purpoſe. He ſhould be toſſed, ſhaked, and moved about. Sharp bliſtering plaſters ſhould be applied to his legs or arms, and ſtimulating medicines, as ſalts of hartſhorn, &c. held under his noſe. It will alſo be proper to let blood. At the ſame time every method muſt be taken to make him diſcharge the poiſon. This may be done in the manner directed above, *viz.* by the uſe of ſtrong vomits, drinking plenty of warm water with oil, &c.

Mead, beſides vomits, in this caſe, recommends acid medicines with lixivial ſalts. He ſays, that he has often given ſalt of wormwood mixed with juice of lemon in repeated doſes with great ſucceſs.

If the body ſhould remain weak and languid after the poiſon has been diſcharged, nouriſhing diet and cordials will be neceſſary; but when there

there is reaſon to fear that the ſtomach or bowels are inflamed, the greateſt circumſpection is neceſſary both with regard to food and medicine.

ANIMAL POISONS.——We ſhall begin with the bite of a mad dog, as it is both the moſt common and dangerous animal poiſon in this country.

THE creatures naturally liable to contract the hydrophobia are, ſo far as we yet know, all of the dog kind, viz. dogs, foxes, and wolves. Of the laſt we have none in this iſland; and it ſo ſeldom happens that any perſon is bit by the ſecond, that they ſcarce deſerve to be taken notice of. It ſuch a thing ſhould happen, the method of treatment is preciſely the ſame as for the bite of a mad dog.

THE ſymptoms of madneſs in a dog are as follow. At firſt he looks dull, ſhews an averſion to food and company: He does not bark as uſual, but ſeems to murmur, is peeviſh, and apt to bite ſtrangers: His ears and tail droop more than uſual, and he appears drowſy. Afterwards he begins to loll out his tongue, and froth at the mouth, his eyes ſeeming heavy and watery. He now, if not confined, takes off, runs panting along with a kind of dejected air, and endeavours to bite every one he meets. Other dogs are ſaid to fly from him. Some think this a certain ſign of madneſs ſuppoſing that they know him by the ſmell; but it is not to be depended on. If he eſcapes being killed, he ſeldom runs

runs above two or three days, till he dies exhausted with heat, hunger, and fatigue.

This disease is most frequent after long dry hot seasons; and such dogs as live upon putrid stinking carrion, without having enough of fresh water, are most liable to it.

When any person is bit by a dog, the strictest inquiry ought to be made, whether the animal be really mad. Many disagreeable consequences arise from neglecting to ascertain this point. Some people have lived in continual anxiety for many years, because they had been bit by a dog which they believed to be mad; but, as he had been killed on the spot, it was impossible to ascertain the fact. This should induce us, instead of killing a dog the moment he has bit any person, to do all in our power to keep him alive, at least till we can be certain whether he be mad or not.

Many circumstances may contribute to make people imagine a dog mad. He loses his master, runs about in quest of him, is set upon by other dogs, and perhaps by men. The creature thus frightened, beat, and abused, looks wild, and lolls out his tongue as he runs along. Immediately a crowd is after him; while he, finding himself closely pursued, and taking every one he meets for an enemy, naturally attempts to bite in self-defence. He soon gets knocked on the head, and passes currently for a mad dog, as it is then impossible to prove the contrary.

This being the true hiſtory of, by far, the greater part of thoſe dogs which paſs for mad, is it any wonder that numberleſs whimſical medicines have been extolled for preventing the effects of their bite? This readily accounts for the great variety of infallible remedies for the bite of a mad dog, which are to be met with in almoſt every family. Though not one in a thouſand has any claim to merit, yet they are all ſupported by numberleſs vouchers. No wonder that imaginary diſeaſes ſhould be cured by imaginary remedies. In this way credulous people firſt impoſe upon themſelves, and then deceive others. The ſame medicine that was ſuppoſed to prevent the effects of the bite, when the dog was not mad, is recommended to a perſon who has had the misfortune to be bit by a dog that was really mad. He takes it, truſts to it, and is undone.

To theſe miſtakes we muſt impute the frequent ill ſucceſs in preventing the effects of the bite of a mad dog. It is not owing ſo much to a defect in medicine, as to wrong applications. I am perſuaded if proper medicines were taken immediately after the bite is received, and continued for a ſufficient length of time, we ſhould not loſe one in a thouſand of thoſe who have the misfortune to be bit by a mad dog.

This poiſon is generally communicated by a wound, which, nevertheleſs, heals as ſoon as a common wound: But afterwards it begins to feel painful, and as the pain ſpreads towards the

the neighbouring parts, the perſon becomes heavy and liſtleſs. His ſleep is unquiet with frightful dreams; he ſighs, looks dull, and loves ſolitude. Theſe are the forerunners, or rather the firſt ſymptoms, of that dreadful diſeaſe occaſioned by the bite of a mad dog. But as we do not propoſe to treat the diſeaſe itſelf, but to point out the method of preventing it, we ſhall not take up time in ſhewing its progreſs from the firſt invaſion to its commonly fatal end.

THE common notion, that this poiſon may lie in the body for many years, and afterwards prove fatal, ſeems not to be well founded. It muſt render ſuch perſons as have had the misfortune to be bit very unhappy, and can have no good effects. If the perſon takes proper medicines for forty days after being bit, and feels no ſymptoms of the diſeaſe, there is reaſon to believe him out of danger. Some indeed have gone mad twelve months after being bit; but I never knew it happen later; and of this I only remember to have ſeen one inſtance.

THE medicines recommended for preventing the effects of the bite of a mad dog, are chiefly ſuch as promote urine and perſpiration; to which may be added antiſpaſmodics.

DR Mead recommends a preventive medicine, which he ſays he never knew fail, though in the ſpace of thirty years he had uſed it a thouſand times.

THE medicine is as follows:

"TAKE aſh-coloured ground liver-wort, cleaned, dried, and powdered, half an ounce; of black pepper

pepper powdered, a quarter of an ounce. Mix these well together, and divide the powder into four doses; one of which must be taken every morning fasting, for four mornings successively, in half an English pint of cows milk warm.

After these four doses are taken, the patient must go into the cold bath, or a cold spring or river, every morning fasting, for a month; he must be dipped all over, but not stay in (with his head above water) longer than half a minute, if the water be very cold. After this he must go in three times a-week for a fortnight longer.

The person must be bled before he begins to use the medicine *."

* I was, some time ago, favoured with the following prescription for the bite of a mad dog, which had been long kept a secret in a gentleman's family in the north of England, and is said never to have failed, when given as a preventive either to man or beast.—"Take six ounces of Rue clean picked and bruised, four ounces of garlic pealed and bruised, four ounces of Venice-treacle, four ounces of scraped tin or pewter. Boil all these ingredients in two English quarts of the best ale, in a vessel close covered, over a slow fire, for the space of an hour; then strain the liquor, and give eight or nine spoonfuls of it warm to an adult person every morning fasting, for three or four mornings running. Less may be given to a young person, or one of a weak constitution. Some of the ingredients may be bound upon the wound, if it can be conveniently done.' This is ordered to be given within nine days after the bite. No doubt the sooner it is given the better.---The dose ordered for a horse is twelve spoonfuls, the same quantity for a bullock; and for a sheep, hog, or dog, four or five.

We

We shall next mention the famous East India specific, as it is called. This medicine is composed of cinnabar and musk. It is esteemed a great antispasmodic, and, by many, thought to be an infallible remedy for preventing the effects of the bite of a mad dog.

"Take native and factitious cinnabar, of each twenty-four grains, musk sixteen grains. Let these be made into a fine powder, and taken in a glass of arrack or brandy."

This single dose is said to secure the person for thirty days, at the end of which it must be repeated; but if he has any symptoms of the disease, it must be repeated in three hours.

The following is likewise a good antispasmodic medicine.

Take of Virginian snake-root in powder, half a dram, gum asafœtida twelve grains, gum Camphire seven grains; make these into a bolus with a little syrup of saffron.

Camphire may also be given in the following manner:

Take purified nitre half an ounce, Virginian snake-root in powder two drams, camphire one dram; rub them together in a mortar, and divide the whole into ten doses.

Mercury is another medicine of great efficacy, both in the prevention and cure of this kind of madness. When used as a preventive, it will be sufficient to rub daily a dram of the ointment into the parts about the wound.

Vinegar is likewise of considerable service, and

and ſhould be taken freely, either in the patient's food or drink.

THESE are the principal medicines recommended for preventing the effects of the bite of a mad dog. We would not however adviſe people to truſt to any one of them; but from a proper combination of their different powers, there is the greateſt reaſon to hope for ſucceſs.

THE great error in the uſe of theſe medicines lies in not taking them for a ſufficient length of time. They are uſed more like charms than medicines intended to produce any change in the body. To this, and not to the inſufficiency of the medicines, muſt we impute their frequent want of ſucceſs.

DR Mead ſays, that the virtue of his medicine conſiſts in promoting urine. But how a poiſon ſhould be expelled by urine, with only three or four doſes of any medicine, however powerful, is not eaſy to conceive. More time is certainly neceſſary; and here the defect of the Doctor's preſcription ſeems to lie.

THE Eaſt-India ſpecific is ſtill more exceptionable on this account.

As theſe and moſt other medicines, taken ſingly, have frequently been found to fail, we ſhall recommend the following courſe.

IF a perſon be bit in a fleſhly part, where there is no hazard of hurting any large blood-veſſel, the parts adjacent to the wound may be cut away. But if this be not done ſoon after receiving the bite, it will be better to omit it.

THE

The wound may be waſhed with ſalt and water, or a pickle made of vinegar and ſalt, and afterwards dreſſed twice a-day with yellow baſilicon mixed with ſome red precipitate.

The patient ſhould begin to uſe either Dr Mead's medicine, or ſome of the others mentioned above. If he takes Mead's medicine, he may uſe it as the Doctor directs for four days ſucceſſively. Let him then omit it for two or three days, and again repeat the ſame number of doſes as before.

During this courſe, he muſt rub into the parts about the wound, daily, one dram of the mercurial or blue ointment, as it is called. This may be done for ten or twelve days at leaſt.

When this courſe is over, he may take a purge or two, and then begin to uſe the cold bath. This muſt be uſed every morning for five or ſix weeks; but if the patient ſhould feel cold and chilly for a long time after coming out of the cold bath, it will be better to uſe a tepid one, or to have the water a little warmed.

In the mean time, we would adviſe him not to leave off all internal medicines, but to take either one of the boluſes of ſnake root, aſafœtida and camphire; or one of the powders of nitre, camphire, and ſnake root, twice a-day. Theſe may be continued for a fortnight or three weeks longer.

If the perſon has gone through the above courſe of medicine, and no ſymptoms of madneſs appear, he may be reckoned out of danger.

ger. It will neverthelefs be advifeable, for the greater fafety, to take a dofe or two of Dr Mead's medicine, at every full or change of the moon, for the three or four fucceeding months.

DURING the ufe of the mercurial ointment, the patient muft keep within doors, and take nothing cold.

A proper regimen muft be obferved during the whole courfe. The patient fhould abftain from flefh, and all falted and high-feafoned provifions. He muft avoid ftrong liquors, and live moftly upon a light and rather fpare diet. His mind fhould be kept as eafy and cheerful as poffible, and all exceffive heat and violent paffions avoided with the utmoft care.

I have never feen this courfe of medicine, with proper regimen fail to prevent the hydrophobia, and cannot help again obferving, that the want of fuccefs muft generally be owing either to the application of improper medicines, or not ufing proper ones for a fufficient length of time.

MANKIND are extremely fond of every thing that promifes a fudden or miraculous cure. By trufting to thefe they often lofe their lives, when a regular courfe of medicine would have rendered them abfolutely fafe. This holds remarkably in the prefent cafe: Numbers of people, for example, believe if they or their cattle be once dipped in the fea, it is fufficient; as if the falt water were a charm againft the effects of of the bite. This and ſuch like whims have proved fatal to many.

Some people believe, if a perſon be bit by a dog that is not mad, if he ſhould go mad afterwards, that the perſon will be ſeized with the diſorder at the ſame time. This notion is too ridiculous to deſerve a ſerious confutation *.

The next poiſonous animal that we ſhall mention is the VIPER. The greaſe of this animal rubbed into the wound is generally reckoned a cure for the bite. Though this is all that the viper catchers commonly do when they are bit, I ſhould hardly think it ſufficient for the bite of an *enraged* viper. It would ſurely be more ſafe to have the wound well ſucked, † and

 afterwards

* It is ſurpriſing that no proper inquiry has ever been made into the truth of the common opinion, that a dog which has been wormed cannot bite after he goes mad This circumſtance not only merits the attention of phyſicians, but of the legiſlature. If the fact could be aſcertained, and the practice rendered general, it would ſave both the lives and properties of many.

† The practice of ſucking out poiſons is very ancient; and indeed nothing can be more rational. It is the moſt likely method of extracting the poiſon where the bite cannot be cut out. There is no danger in performing this office; as the poiſon does no harm unleſs it be taken into the body by a wound. The perſon who ſucks the wound ought however to waſh his mouth frequently with ſalad-oil, which will ſecure him from even the leaſt inconveniency The ancient Pſylli in Africa, and the Marſi in Italy were famed for curing the bites of poiſonous animals by ſucking the wound; and we

afterwards rubbed with warm ſalad oil. A poultice of bread and milk, with plenty of ſalad oil in it, ſhould likewiſe be applied to the wound, and the patient ought to drink freely of wine whey with ſome ſpirits of hartſhorn; or, if that be not at hand, of water gruel with vinegar in it, to make him ſweat If the patient be ſick, he may take a vomit. This courſe will be ſufficient for the bite of any of the poiſonous animals of this country

WITH regard to poiſonous inſects, as the bee, waſp, hornet, &c. their ſtings are ſeldom attended with great danger, unleſs where a perſon happens to be ſtung by a number of them at once. In this caſe ſomething ſhould be done to abate the pain and inflammation. Some, for this purpoſe, apply honey, others lay pounded parſley to the part. Some recommend a mixture of vinegar and Venice-treacle; but I have always found rubbing the part with warm ſalad oil ſucceed very well. Indeed, if the ſtings be ſo numerous as to endanger the patient's life, which is ſometimes the caſe, he muſt not only have oily poultices applied to the part, but muſt likewiſe be bled and take ſome cooling medicines, as nitre, cream of tartar, &c. with plenty of diluting liquors.

IT is the happineſs of this iſland to have very few poiſonous animals, and even theſe are

we are told, that the Indians in North America practice the ſame at this day.

not

not of the moſt virulent kind. Nine tenths of the effects uſually attributed to poiſon or venom are really other diſeaſes, and depend upon quite different cauſes.

WE cannot however make the ſame obſervation with regard to poiſonous vegetables. Theſe abound every where, and prove often fatal to the ignorant and unwary *. This indeed is, in a great meaſure, owing to careleſſneſs. Children ought early to be cautioned againſt eating any ſort of roots or berries which they do not know. We would likewiſe adviſe parents to deſtroy all poiſonous plants in their gardens, &c. or elſe to keep them in places where their children can have no acceſs.

BUT it is not children alone who ſuffer by eating poiſonous plants: We have every year accounts of adults poiſoned by eating hemlock-roots inſtead of parſnips, or ſome fungus which they gather for muſhrooms, &c. Theſe examples ought to put people upon their guard with reſpect to the former, and to put the latter entirely out of uſe.

OF THE STONE AND GRAVEL.

WHEN ſmall ſtones are lodged in the kidneys, or diſcharged along with the urine, the patient is ſaid to be afflicted with gravel. If one of

* The principal of theſe are, hemlock, henbane, monkſhood, columbine, hellebore, berries of the deadly nightſhade, thorn-apple, all the ſpurges, and moſt muſhrooms, &c.

theſe ſtones happens to make a lodgement in the bladder for ſome time, it accumulates freſh matter, and at length becomes too large to paſs off with the urine. In this caſe the patient is ſaid to have the ſtone.

CAUSES.——This diſeaſe may be occaſioned by high living; the uſe of ſtrong aſtringent wines *; a ſedentary life; lying too hot, ſoft, or too much on the back; the conſtant uſe of water which is impregnated with earthy or ſtony particles, aliments of an aſtringent or windy nature, &c. It may likewiſe proceed from an hereditary diſpoſition Perſons in the decline of life, and thoſe who have been much afflicted with the gout or rheumatiſm are moſt ſubject to it.

SYMPTOMS.——Small ſtones or gravel in the kidneys occaſion pain in the loins; ſickneſs; vomiting; and ſometimes bloody urine. When the ſtone deſcends into the *ureter*, and is too large to paſs along with eaſe, all the above ſymptoms are increaſed; the pain extends towards the bladder; the thigh and leg of the affected ſide feel benumbed; the teſticles are drawn upwards, and the urine is obſtructed.

* It is a common notion that the tartar in wine generates the ſtone; but there is more reaſon to believe that its aſtringency, together with the fixed air contained in it, produce this effect. I know many perſons who never fail to paſs leſs urine and to complain of a pain in their kidneys for ſeveral days after drinking freely of red wine.

A

A STONE in the bladder is known from a pain at the time, as well as before and after making water; from the urine coming away by drops, or ſtopping ſuddenly when in a full ſtream; by a violent pain in the neck of the bladder upon motion, eſpecially on horſeback or in a coach on rough road; from a white, thick, copious, ſtinking, mucous ſediment in the urine; from an itching in the top of the *penis*; from an inclination to go to ſtool while the urine is diſcharged; from the patient's paſſing his urine more eaſily when lying than in an erect poſture; and from a kind of convulſive motion occaſioned by the ſharp pain in diſcharging the laſt drops of the urine.

REGIMEN.—— Perſons afflicted with the gravel or ſtone ſhould avoid aliments of a windy or heating nature, as ſalt-meats, ſour fruits, &c. Their diet ought chiefly to conſiſt of ſuch things as tend to promote the ſecretion of urine, and to keep the belly open. Artichoaks, aſparagus, ſpinnage, lettuces, ſuccory, parſley, purſlane, turnips, potatoes, carrots, and radiſhes may be ſafely eat. Onions, leeks, and cellery are, in this caſe, reckoned medicinal. The moſt proper drink is whey, butter-milk, milk and water, barley-water; decoctions of the roots of marſhmallows, parſley, liquorice; or of other mild mucilaginous vegetables, as linſeed, &c. If the patient has been accuſtomed to generous liquors, he may drink ſmall gin-punch without acid.

acid But ſpirits muſt be uſed very ſparingly, as every thing that heats is hurtful.

GENTLE exerciſe is proper; but if violent, it is apt to occaſion bloody urine. We would therefore adviſe that it ſhould be taken in moderation. Perſons afflicted with gravel often paſs a great number of ſtones after riding on horſeback, or in a machine; but thoſe who have a ſtone in the bladder are ſeldom able to bear theſe kinds of exerciſe. Where there is a hereditary tendency to this diſeaſe, a ſedentary life ought never to be indulged. Were people careful, upon the firſt ſymptoms of gravel, to obſerve a proper regimen of diet, and to take ſufficient exerciſe, it might often be carried off, or, at leaſt, prevented from increaſing; but if the ſame courſe which occaſioned the diſeaſe be perſiſted in, it cannot fail to become worſe.

MEDICINE—In what is called a fit of the gravel, which is commonly occaſioned by a ſtone ſticking in the *ureter* or ſome part of the urinary paſſages, the patient muſt be bled, warm fomentations applied to the parts, emolient clyſters adminiſtred, and deluting mucilaginous liquors drank, *&c.* The treatment of this caſe has been fully pointed out under the articles, *inflammation of the kidneys and bladder*, to which we refer the reader.

DR WHYTT adviſes patients who are ſubject to frequent fits of gravel in the kidneys, but have no ſtone in the bladder, to drink every morning, two or three hours before breakfaſt, an Engliſh pint of of oyſter or cockle-ſhell lime-water. The Doctor very juſtly obſerves, that though this quantity might be too ſmall to have any ſenſible effect in diſſolving a ſtone in the bladder; yet it may very probably prevent its growth.

When a ſtone is formed in the bladder, the Doctor recommends Alicant ſoap, and oyſter or cockle-ſhell lime-water * to be taken in the following manner. The patient muſt ſwallow every day, in any form that is leaſt diſagreeable, an ounce of the internal part of Alicant ſoap, and drink three or four Engliſh pints of oyſter or cockle-ſhell-lime water. The ſoap is to be divided into three doſes; the largeſt to be taken faſting in the morning early; the ſecond at noon; and the third at ſeven in the evening, drinking above each doſe a large draught of the lime-water; the remainder of which he may take any time betwixt dinner and ſupper, inſtead of other liquors.

The patient ſhould begin with a ſmaller quantity of the lime water and ſoap than what is mentioned above; at firſt an Engliſh pint of the former and three drams of the latter, taken daily, may be enough. This quantity, howe-

* Oyſter-ſhell lime-water is prepared by pouring an Engliſh gallon and a half of boiling water upon a pound of oyſter-ſhells reduced to quick-lime by being burnt. Where oyſter or cockle ſhells cannot be had, common quick lime may be uſed in their ſtead After the clear liquor has been poured off, the ſame quantity of lime will make a ſecond or third quantity of water of nearly the ſame ſtrength as the firſt.

ver,

ver, he may increaſe by degrees, and ought to perſevere in the uſe of theſe medicines, eſpecially if he finds any abatement of his complaints, for ſeveral months; nay, if the ſtone be very large, for years. It may likewiſe be proper for the patient, if he be ſeverely pained, not only to begin with the ſoap and lime-water in ſmall quantities, but to take the ſecond or third lime-water inſtead of the firſt. However, after he has been for ſome time accuſtomed to theſe medicines, he may not only take the firſt water, but, if he finds he can eaſily bear it, heighten its diſſolving power ſtill more by pouring it a ſecond time on freſh calcined ſhells.

THE only other medicine which we ſhall mention is the *uva urſi*. It has been greatly extolled of late years both for the gravel and ſtone. It ſeems, however, to be, in all reſpects, inferior to the ſoap and lime-water; but as it is leſs diſagreeable, and has frequently, to my knowledge, relieved gravelly complaints, it deſerves a trial. It is generally taken in powder from half a dram to a whole dram, two or three times a-day. It may be mixed in a cup of tea or gruel, or taken in any way that is moſt agreeable to the patient.

OF

OF THE HICCUP.

THE hiccup is a ſpaſmodic or convulſive affection of the ſtomach and midriff, ariſing from any cauſe that irritates their nervous fibres.

IT may proceed from exceſs in eating or drinking; from a hurt of the ſtomach; poiſons; inflammations of the ſtomach, inteſtines, bladder, midriff, or the reſt of the *viſcera*. In gangrenes, acute and malignant fevers, a hiccup is often the forerunner of death. I have known an obſtinate hiccup proceed from a ſchirrous tumour of the *pylorus*, or right orifice of the ſtomach.

WHEN the hiccup proceeds from exceſs, eſpecially from aliment that is flatulent, or hard of digeſtion, a draught of generous wine, or a dram of any ſpiritous liquor, will generally remove it. If poiſon be the cauſe, plenty of milk and oil muſt be drank, as has been formerly recommended. When it proceeds from an inflammation of the ſtomach, &c. it is very dangerous. In this caſe the cooling regimen muſt be obſerved. The patient muſt be bled, and take frequently a few drops of the ſweet ſpirits of nitre in a cup of wine-whey. His ſtomach muſt likewiſe be fomented with cloths dipped in warm water; or bladders filled with warm milk and water applied to it.

A hiccup proceeding from a gangrene, or mortification, is generally incurable. In this caſe the Peruvian bark, with other antiſeptic medicines, are moſt likely to ſucceed. If the hiccup be a primary diſeaſe, and proceeds from a foul ſtomach, loaded either with a pituitous or a bilious humour, a gentle vomit and purge, if the patient be able to bear them, will be of ſervice. If it ariſes from flatulencies, the carminatives directed for the heart-burn, page 434. muſt be uſed.

WHEN the hiccup proves very obſtinate, recourſe muſt be had to the moſt powerful aromatic and antiſpaſmodic medicines. The principal of theſe is muſk; fifteen or twenty grains of which may be made into a bolus, and repeated occaſionally. Opiates are likewiſe of ſervice; but they muſt be uſed with caution. A bit of ſugar dipped in compound ſpirits of lavender, or the volatile aromatic tincture, may be taken frequently. The Peruvian bark is likewiſe of uſe. External applications are ſometimes alſo beneficial; as the ſtomach plaſter, or a cataplaſm of the Venice treacle of the Edinburgh or London diſpenſatory, applied to the ſtomach.

I lately attended a patient who had almoſt a conſtant hiccup for above nine weeks. It was frequently ſtopped by the uſe of muſk, opium, wine, and other cordial and antiſpaſmodic medicines, but always returned. Nothing indeed, gave the patient ſo much eaſe as briſk ſmall beer. By drinking freely of this, the hiccup was often kept off for ſeveral days,

which

which was more than could be done by the moſt powerful medicines. He was at length ſeized with a vomiting of blood, which ſoon put an end to his life. Upon opening his body, a large ſchirrous tumour was found near the pylorus or right orifice of the ſtomach.

CRAMP OF THE STOMACH.

Tho' this, for the moſt part, is only a ſymptom of nervous or hyſteric diſorders, we thought proper to treat it ſeparately; as it often ſiezes people ſuddenly, is very dangerous, and requires immediate aſſiſtance.

If the patient has any inclination to vomit, he ought to take ſome draughts of warm water, or weak camomile tea, to clean his ſtomach. After this, if he has been coſtive, a laxative clyſter muſt be given. He ought then to take ſome doſes of laudanum. The beſt way of adminiſtering it is in a clyſter. Sixty or ſeventy drops of liquid laudanum may be given in a clyſter of warm water. This is much more certain than laudanum given by the mouth, which is often vomited, and in ſome caſes increaſes the pain and ſpaſms in the ſtomach.

If the pain and cramps return with great violence, after the effects of the anodyne clyſter are over, another with an equal or larger quantity of opium, may be given; and every four or five hours a bolus with ten or twelve grains

grains of muſk, and half a dram of the Venice treacle. In the mean time, the ſtomach ought to be fomented with cloths dipped in warm water; or bladders filled with warm milk and water, ſhould be conſtantly applied to it. I have often ſeen theſe produce the moſt happy effects. The anodyne balſam may alſo be rubbed into the ſtomach; and an antihyſteric plaſter worn upon it for ſome time after the cramps are removed, to prevent their return.

In very violent and laſting pains of the ſtomach, ſome blood ought to be let, unleſs the weakneſs of the patient makes it improper. When the pain or cramps of the ſtomach proceed from a ſuppreſſion of the *menſes*, bleeding is of great uſe. If they be owing to the gout, ſome of the warm cordial waters, or a large dram of good brandy or rum, will be neceſſary. Bliſtering plaſters ought likewiſe, in this caſe, to be applied to the ancles.

WANT OF APPETITE.

This may proceed from a foul ſtomach; indigeſtable food; the want of free air and exerciſe; grief; fear; anxiety; or any of the depreſſing paſſions; exceſſive heat; living much upon ſtrong broths, or fat meats; the immoderate uſe of ſtrong liquors, tea, tobacco, opium, &c.

The patient ought, if poſſible, to make choice of an open dry air; to take exerciſe daily on horſeback,

horſeback, or in a machine; to riſe betimes; and to avoid all intenſe thought. He ſhould uſe a diet of eaſy digeſtion, avoiding every thing that is fat and oily; he ought to chuſe agreeable company; and ſhould avoid intenſe heat and great fatigue.

If want of appetite proceeds from errors in diet, or any other part of the patient's regimen, it ought to be changed. If nauſea and reachings to vomit, ſhew that the ſtomach is loaded with crudities, a vomit will be of ſervice. After this a gentle purge or two of rhubarb, or any of the bitter purging ſalts, may be taken. The patient ought next to uſe an infuſion in wine of any of the ſtomachic bitters; as Gentian root, jeſuits bark, orange peel, &c. He may alſo eat orange peel or ginger candied.

Though gentle evacuations be neceſſary, all ſtrong purges and vomits are to be avoided, as they tend to weaken the ſtomach and hurt digeſtion. After proper evacuations, bitter elixirs and tinctures with aromatics may be uſed. The patient may take, twice a-day, a common ſpoonful of the ſtomachic tincture; or, if he be coſtive, the ſame quantity of the bitter tincture of rhubarb. Elixir of vitriol is an excellent medicine in moſt caſes of indigeſtion, weakneſs of the ſtomach, or want of appetite. Twenty or thirty drops of it may be taken twice or thrice a day in a glaſs of wine or water. It may likewiſe be mixed with the tincture of the bark, two drams of the former to an ounce of the latter,

latter, and a tea-ſpoonful of it taken in wine or water, as above.

THE chalybeate waters are of great ſervice in this caſe. I never knew theſe fail to ſharpen the appetite, if drank in moderation. The ſalt water has likewiſe this effect; but it muſt not be uſed, too freely. The waters of Harrowgate, Scarſborough, Moffat, and moſt other ſpaws in Britain, may be uſed with the ſame intention. We would adviſe all who are afflicted with indigeſtion and want of appetite, to repair to theſe places of public rendezvous. The very change of air, and the cheerful company will be of ſervice; not to mention the exerciſe, diſſipation, amuſements, &c.

OF DEAFNESS.

DEAFNESS is ſometimes owing to an original fault, or wrong formation of the ear itſelf. It may likewiſe be occaſioned by wounds, ulcers, or any thing that deſtroys the fabric of the ear. It is often the effect of old age; of violent colds in the head; of fevers; of exceſſive noiſe; of hard wax in the ear; of too great moiſture or dryneſs of the ear, &c.

PERSONS who are born deaf are ſeldom cured. When deafneſs is the effect of wounds or ulcers in the ear, or of old age, it is not eaſily removed. If it proceeds from cold of the head, the patient muſt be careful to keep his head warm,

warm, eſpecially in the night; he ſhould likewiſe take a purge or two, and ſhould keep his feet warm, and bathe them frequently in warm water. When deafneſs is the effect of fevers, it generally ceaſes of itſelf, after the patient recovers ſtrength. If it proceeds from dry wax ſticking in the ears, it muſt be ſoftened by dropping oil into them for a few nights, at bedtime; afterwards they muſt be ſyringed with warm milk and water, or milk and oil.

If deafneſs proceeds from dryneſs of the ears, which may be known by looking into them, half an ounce of the oil of almonds, and the ſame quantity of liquid opodeldoch, or tincture of aſafœtida, may be mixed together, and a few drops of it put into the ear every night at bedtime, ſtopping them afterwards with a little wool or cotten. I have often known this have good effects. When the ears abound with moiſture, it may be drained off by an iſſue or ſeton, which muſt be made as near the parts affected as poſſible.

Many medicines are recommended for the cure of deafneſs, ſome of which, in obſtinate caſes, at leaſt, deſerve a trial. Some recommend the gall of an eel mixed with ſpirit of wine, to be dropped into the ear; others equal parts of Hungary water and ſpirits of lavender. Etmuler recommends amber and muſk; and Brookes ſays he has often known hardneſs of hearing cured by putting a grain or two of muſk into the ear with cotton-wool. But theſe and

and other applications muſt be varied according to the cauſe. We cannot conclude this article without recommending the greateſt attention to *warmth*. From whatever cauſe deafneſs proceeds, the patient ought to keep his head warm. I have known more benefit from this alone, in the moſt obſtinate caſes of deafneſs, than from all the medicines I ever ſaw uſed.

OF THE NIGHT-MARE.

In this diſeaſe the patient, in time of ſleep, imagines he feels an uncommon oppreſſion or weight about his breaſt or ſtomach, which he can by no means ſhake off. He groans, and ſometimes cries out, tho' oftener he attempts to ſpeak in vain. Sometimes he imagines himſelf engaged with an enemy, and, in danger of being killed, attempts to run away, but finds he cannot. Sometimes he fancies himſelf in a houſe that is on fire, or that he is in danger of being drowned in a river. He often thinks he is falling over a precipice, and the dread of being daſhed to pieces ſuddenly awakes him.

This diſorder has been ſuppoſed to proceed from too much blood; from a ſtagnation of blood in the brain, lungs, &c. But its general cauſe is indigeſtion. Perſons of weak nerves, who lead a ſedentary life, and live full, are moſt commonly afflicted with the night mare. Nothing tends more to produce it than heavy ſuppers, eſpecially

eſpecially if eat late, or the patient goes to bed ſoon after. Wind is likewiſe a very frequent cauſe of this diſeaſe; for which reaſon thoſe who are afflicted with it ought to avoid all flatulent food. Deep thought, anxiety, or any thing that oppreſſes the mind, ought alſo to be avoided.

PERSONS afflicted with the night-mare ought to eat very light ſuppers. They ſhould never go to bed immediately after eating, nor lie upon their back with their head low. As they generally moan, or make ſome noiſe in the fit, they ſhould be waked, or ſpoken to by ſuch as hear them, as the uneaſineſs generally goes off as ſoon as the patient is awake. Dr Whytt ſays he generally found a dram of brandy, taken at bed-time, prevent this diſeaſe. That, however, is a bad cuſtom, and, in time, loſes its effect. We would rather have the patient depend upon cheerfulneſs, and exerciſe through the day, a light ſupper taken early, and the uſe of food of eaſy digeſtion, &c. than to accuſtom himſelf to drams. A draught of cold water will often promote digeſtion as much as a glaſs of brandy, and is much ſafer. After a perſon of weak digeſtion however has eat flatulent food, a dram may be neceſſary; in this caſe we would recommend it as the moſt proper medicine.

PERSONS who are young, and full of blood, if troubled with the night-mare, ought to purge, bleed, and uſe a ſpare diet.

OF SWOONINGS.

The principal caufes of fwooning are, fudden tranfitions from cold to heat; breathing air that is deprived of its proper fpring or elafticity; great fatigue; exceffive weaknefs; lofs of blood; long fafting; fear, grief, and other violent paffions or affections of the mind.

It is well known, that perfons who have been long expofed to cold, often faint or fall into a fwoon, upon coming into the houfe, efpecially if they drink hot liquor, or fit near a large fire. This might eafily be prevented by people taking care not to go into a warm room immediately after having been expofed to the cold air, to approach the fire gradually, and not to eat or drink any thing hot, till the body has been gradually brought into a warm temperature.

When any one, in confequence of neglecting thefe precautions, falls into a fwoon, he ought immediately to be removed to a cooler appartment, to have ligatures applied above his knees and elbows, and to have his hands and face fprinkled with vinegar. He fhould likewife be made to fmell to vinegar, and fhould have a fpoonful or two of water, if he can fwallow, with about a third part of vinegar mixed with it, poured into his mouth. If the fainting fits prove obftinate, it will be neceffary to bleed

bleed the patient, and afterwards to give him a clyſter.

As air that is breathed over and over loſes its elaſticity or ſpring, it is no wonder if perſons who reſpire in it often fall into ſwooning or fainting fits. They are, in this caſe, deprived of the very principle of life. Hence it is that fainting fits are ſo frequent in all crowded aſſemblies, eſpecially in hot ſeaſons. Such fits however muſt be conſidered as a kind of temporary death; and, to the weak and delicate, they ſometimes prove fatal in reality. They ought therefore to be avoided with the utmoſt care. The method of doing this is obvious. Let aſſembly rooms, and all other places of public reſort, be well ventilated; and let the weak and delicate avoid ſuch places, particularly in warm ſeaſons.

A perſon who faints, in ſuch a ſituation, ought immediately to be carried into the open air; his temples ſhould be rubbed with ſtrong vinegar or brandy, and volatile ſpirits or ſalts held to his noſe. He ſhould be laid upon his back with his head low, and have a little wine, or ſome other cordial, poured into his mouth, as ſoon as he is able to ſwallow it. If the perſon has been ſubject to hyſteric fits, caſtor or aſafætida ſhould be applied to the noſe, or burnt feathers, horn, or leather, &c.

When fainting fits proceed from mere weakneſs or exhauſtion, which is often the caſe after great fatigue, long faſting, loſs of blood, or the like,

like, the patient muſt be ſupported with generous cordials, as jellies, wines, ſpirituous liquors, &c. Theſe however muſt be given at firſt in very ſmall quantities, and increaſed gradually as the patient is able to bear them. He ought to be allowed to lie quite ſtill and eaſy upon his back, with his head low, and ſhould have freſh air admitted into his chamber. His food ſhould conſiſt of nouriſhing broths, ſago-gruel with wine, new milk, and other things of a light and cordial nature. Theſe things are to be given out of the fit. All that can be done while the perſon continues in the fit is, to let him ſmell to a bottle of Hungary water, *eau de luce*, or ſpirits of hartſhorn, and to rub his temples with warm brandy, or to lay a compreſs dipped in it to the pit of his ſtomach.

IN fainting fits that proceed from fear, grief, or other violent paſſions or affections of the mind, the patient muſt be very cautiouſly managed. He ſhould be ſuffered to remain at reſt, and only made to ſmell to ſome vinegar. After he is come to himſelf he may drink freely of warm lemonade, or balm tea, with ſome orange or lemon peel in it. It will likewiſe be proper, if the fainting fits have been long and ſevere, to clean the bowels by throwing in an emollient clyſter or two.

DIS-

DISEASES OF WOMEN.

THE diſeaſes peculiar to women ariſe chiefly from their monthly evacuations, pregnancy, and child-birth. Females generally begin to menſtruate about the age of fifteen, and leave it off about fifty, which renders theſe two periods the moſt critical of their lives. About the firſt appearance of this diſcharge the conſtitution undergoes a very conſiderable change, generally indeed for the better, but ſometimes for the worſe. The greateſt care is now neceſſary, as the future health and happineſs of the female depends, in a great meaſure, upon her conduct at this period. If a girl about this time of life be confined to the houſe, kept conſtantly ſitting, and neither allowed to romp about, nor employed in ſome active buſineſs, which gives exerciſe to the whole body, ſhe becomes weak, relaxed and puny; her blood not being duly prepared, ſhe looks pale and wan; her health, ſpirits, and vigor decline, and ſhe ſinks into a valetudinary for life. Such is the fate of numbers of thoſe unhappy females who either from the indulgence of mothers, or their own narrow circumſtances, are,

at

at this critical period of life, denied the benefit of exercise and free air.

A lazy indolent disposition proves very hurtful to girls at this period. One seldom meets with complaints from obstructions amongst the more active and laborious part of the sex; whereas the indolent and lazy are seldom free from them. These are, in a manner, eat up by the *chlorosis*, or green sickness, and other diseases of this nature. We would therefore recommend it to all who wish to escape these calamities, to avoid indolence and inactivity, as their greatest enemies, and to take as much exercise, especially in the open air, as possible.

ANOTHER thing that proves very hurtful to girls about this period of life, is unwholesome food. Fond of all manner of trash, they often eat every out-of-the-way thing they can get, till their blood and humours are quite vitiated. Hence ensue indigestions, want of appetite, and a whole train of evils. If the fluids be not duly prepared, it is utterly impossible that the secretions should be properly performed: Accordingly we find that such girls as lead an indolent life, and eat great quantities of trash, are not only subject to obstructions of the *menses*, but likewise to glandular obstructions; as the scrophula or King's evil, &c.

A dull disposition is likewise very hurtful to girls at this period. It is a rare thing to see a sprightly girl who does not enjoy good health, while

while the grave, moping, melancholy creature proves the very prey of vapours and hyſterics. Youth is the ſeaſon for mirth and cheerfulneſs. Let it therefore be indulged. It is an abſolute duty. To lay in a ſtock of health in time of youth is as neceſſary a piece of prudence as to make proviſion againſt the decays of ald age. While therefore wiſe Nature prompts the happy youth to join in ſprightly amuſements, let not the ſevere dictates of hoary age forbid the uſeful impulſe, nor damp with ſerious gloom the ſeaſons deſtined to mirth and innocent feſtivity.

ANOTHER thing very hurtful to females about this period of life is ſtrait cloaths. They are fond of a fine ſhape, and fooliſhly imagine, that this can be acquired by ſtrait cloaths. Hence by ſqueezing their ſtomach and bowels they hurt the digeſtion, and occaſion many incurable maladies. This error is not indeed ſo common as it has been; but, as faſhions change, it may come in again, we therefore think it not improper to mention it. I know many females who, to this day, feel the direful effects of that wretched cuſtom which prevailed ſome time ago, of ſqueezing every girl into as ſmall a ſize in the middle as poſſible. Human invention could not poſſibly have deviſed a practice more deſtructive to health.

AFTER a female has arrived at that period of life when the *menſes* uſually begin to flow, and they do not appear, but, on the contrary, her health

health and ſpirits begin to decline, we would adviſe, inſtead of ſhutting the poor girl up in the houſe, and doſing her with ſteel, aſafœtida, and other nauſeous drugs, to place her in a ſituation where ſhe can enjoy the benefit of free air and agreeable company. There let her eat wholeſome food, take plenty of exerciſe and amuſements, and we have little reaſon to fear but Nature, thus aſſiſted, will do her proper work. She ſeldom fails unleſs where the fault is on our ſide.

When the *menſes* have once begun to flow, the greateſt care ſhould be taken to avoid every thing that may tend to obſtruct them. Females ought to be exceeding careful of what they eat or drink at the time they are out of order. Every thing that is cold, or apt to ſour on the ſtomach, ought to be avoided; as fruit, butter-milk, and ſuch like. Fiſh, and all kinds of food that are hard of digeſtion, are alſo to be avoided. As it is impoſſible to mention every thing that may diſagree with individuals at this time, we would recommend it to every female to be very attentive to what diſagrees with her own ſtomach, and carefully to avoid it.

Cold is extremely hurtful to females at this particular period. More of the ſex date their diſorders from colds, caught while they were out of order, than from all other cauſes. This ought ſurely to put them upon their guard, and to make them very circumſpect in their conduct at ſuch times. A degree of cold that will

will not in the leaſt hurt them at another time, will, at this period, be ſufficient to ruin their health and conſtitution altogether.

THE greateſt attention ought at this time to be paid to the mind, which ſhould be kept as eaſy and cheerful as poſſible. Every part of the animal œconomy is influenced by the paſſions, but none more ſo than this Anger, fear, grief, and other affections of the mind, often occaſion obſtructions of the menſtrual flux, which prove abſolutely incurable.

FROM whatever cauſe this flux is obſtructed, unleſs the female be pregnant, proper means ſhould be uſed to reſtore it. For this purpoſe we would recommend plenty of exerciſe, in a dry, open, and rather cool air; wholeſome diet, and, if the body be weak and languid, generous liquors; alſo cheerful company, and all manner of amuſements. If theſe fail, the following medicines may be tried.

IF the obſtructions proceed from a weak relaxed ſtate of the ſolids, ſuch medicines as tend to promote digeſtion, to brace the ſolids, and aſſiſt the body in preparing good blood, ought to be uſed. The principal of theſe are iron, the jeſuits bark, and other bitter and aſtringent medicines. Filings of iron may be infuſed in wine or ale, two ounces to an Engliſh quart, and after it has ſtood in a warm place twenty-four hours, it may be ſtrained, and a ſmall cupful drank three or four times a-day; or they may be reduced to a fine powder, and taken in the doſe of half a dram, mixed with a little honey or treacle, three or four times a day. The bark and other bitters may either be taken in ſubſtance or infuſion, as is moſt agreeable to the patient.

WHEN obſtructions proceed from a viſcid ſtate of the blood, and the patient is of a groſs full habit, evacuations, and ſuch medicines as attenuate the humours, are neceſſary. The patient, in this caſe ought to be bled, to bathe her feet frequently in warm water, to take now and then a doſe of cooling phyſic, and to live upon a ſpare thin diet. Her drink ſhould be whey, water, or ſmall beer, and ſhe ought to take plenty of exerciſe.

WHEN obſtructions proceed from affections of the mind, every method ſhould be taken to amuſe and divert the patient. And that ſhe may the more readily forget the cauſe of her affliction, ſhe ought, if poſſible, to be removed from the place where it happened. A change of place, by preſenting the mind with a variety of new objects, has often a very happy influence in relieving it from the deepeſt diſtreſs. A ſoothing, kind, and affable behaviour to perſons in this ſituation is alſo of the laſt importance. This would often prevent the fatal conſequences which proceed from a *harſh* treatment of females, who are ſo unfortunate as to be croſſed in their inclinations; or who meet with diſappointments in love, &c.

THO' many diſeaſes proceed from obſtruction,

tion, it is not always to be conſidered as the cauſe, but often as the effect of other maladies. When that is the caſe, inſtead of giving medicines to force down the *menſes*, which might be dangerous, we ought, by all means, to endeavour to reſtore the patient's health and ſtrength. When that is effected, the other will return of courſe.

BUT the menſtrual flux may be too great as well as too ſmall. When that is the caſe, the patient becomes weak, the colour pale, the appetite and digeſtion are bad, and œdematous ſwellings of the feet, dropſies and conſumptions often enſue. This frequently happens to women about the age of forty five or fifty, and is very difficult to cure. It may proceed from a ſedentary life; a full diet, conſiſting chiefly of ſalted, high ſeaſoned, or acrid food; the exceſſive uſe of ſpiritous liquors; too much exerciſe; violent paſſions of the mind, &c.

To reſtrain this flux, the patient ought to be kept quiet and eaſy both in body and mind. If it be very violent, ſhe ought to lie in bed with her head low; to live upon a cool and ſlender diet, as veal or chicken broths with bread; and to drink decoctions of nettle-roots, or the greater comfrey. If theſe be not ſufficient to ſtop the flux, ſtronger aſtringents may be uſed, as allum, dragons blood, &c. As much powdered allum as will lie upon a ſixpence may be taken in a glaſs of red wine twice or thrice a-day, or oftener if the patient's ſtomach can bear it.

Such

Such as cannot take allum in ſubſtance may uſe the allum whey. Females who have frequent returns of this complaint, ought to uſe the jeſuits bark for a conſiderable time. Half a dram of bark may be mixed in a glaſs of red wine three or four times a-day, or it may be taken in common water, and ſharpened with ſpirits of vitriol.

But the *uterine flux* may offend in quality as well as in quantity. What is uſually called the *fluor albus* or whites, is a very common diſeaſe, and proves extremely hurtful to delicate women. This diſcharge is not always white, but ſometimes pale, yellow, green, or of a blackiſh colour; ſometimes it is ſharp and corroſive; ſometimes foul and fœtid, &c. It is attended with a pale complexion, pain in the ſpine of the back, loſs of appetite, ſwelling of the feet, &c. It generally proceeds from a relaxed and debilitated ſtate of the body, ariſing from indolence, the exceſſive uſe of tea, coffee, or other weak and watery diet.

To remove this diſeaſe, the patient muſt take as much exerciſe as ſhe can bear without fatigue. Her food muſt be ſolid and nouriſhing but of eaſy digeſtion; and her drink pretty generous, as red port or claret wine. Theſe may be drank pure or mixed with water, as the patient inclines Tea and coffee are to be avoided. I have often known ſtrong broths have an exceeding good effect in this caſe. The patient ought not to lie too long a bed. When medicine

dicine is wanted, we know none preferable to the jeſuits bark, which, in this caſe, ought always to be taken in ſubſtance.

THAT period of life at which the *menſes* ceaſe to flow is likewiſe very critical to the ſex. The ſtoppage of any cuſtomary evacuation, however ſmall, is ſufficient to diſorder the whole frame, and often to deſtroy life itſelf. Hence it comes to paſs that ſo many women either fall into chronic diſorders, or die about this time: Such of them however as ſurvive it, without contracting any chronic diſeaſe, often become more healthy and hardy than they were before, and enjoy ſtrength and vigour to a very great age.

IF the *menſes* ceaſe all of a ſudden, in women of a full habit, they ought to abate ſomewhat of their uſual quantity of food, eſpecially of the more nouriſhing kind, as fleſh, eggs, &c. They ought likewiſe to take plenty of exerciſe, and to keep the belly open. This may be done by taking, once or twice a week, a little rhubarb, or an infuſion of hiera picra in wine or brandy.

IT often happens that women of a groſs habit, at this period of life, have ulcerous ſores break out about their ancles, or in other parts of the body. Such ulcers ought to be conſidered as critical, and ſhould either be ſuffered to continue open, or artificial drains ſhould be opened in their ſtead. Women who will needs have ſuch ſores dried up, are often ſoon after ſeized with acute or chronic diſeaſes, of which they die.

PERSONS

Persons of either ſex ought to be very cautious in drying up ſores which break out towards the decline of life. We would lay it down as a rule, where-ever ſuch ſores appear, that before any attempts be made to heal them, an iſſue or ſeton ſhould be ſet in ſome part of the body. Few things bid fairer for preſerving health, or prolonging life, eſpecially in perſons who live full, than an iſſue, or ſome other drain conſtantly kept open in the decline of life. This is imitating Nature, who often, at this period, endeavours to relieve herſelf by a fiſtula, the hæmorrhoidal flux, &c.

OF PREGNANCY.

Pregnancy is not a diſeaſe, but as it ſubjects women to ſeveral ailments, it may not be improper to point out the methods of preventing or relieving them.

Pregnant women are often afflicted with the heart-burn. The method of treating this complaint has already been pointed out in page 432. and the two following. They are likewiſe, in the more early periods of pregnancy, often haraſſed with ſickneſs and vomiting, eſpecially in the morning. Theſe complaints may generally be relieved by carefully obſerving the directions contained in pages 416. and 417. The head ach and tooth-ach are alſo very troubleſome ſymptoms of pregnancy. The former may gene-

generally be removed by keeping the belly gently open, by the uſe of prunes, figs, roaſted apples, and ſuch like. When the pain is very violent, bleeding may be neceſſary. For the treatment of the latter, we muſt refer the reader to that article page 425.

Every pregnant woman is more or leſs in danger of abortion. This ſhould be guarded againſt with the greateſt care, as it not only weakens the conſtitution, but renders the woman liable to the ſame misfortune afterwards. Abortion may happen at any period of pregnancy, but it is moſt common in the ſecond or third month. Sometimes however it happens in the fourth or fifth. If it happens within the firſt month, it is uſually called a falſe conception; if after the ſeventh month, the child may often be kept alive by proper care.

The common cauſes of abortion are, the death of the child; weakneſs or relaxation of the mother; great evacuations; violent motion; raiſing great weights; reaching too high; vomiting; coughing; convulſion-fits; ſtrokes on the belly; falls; fevers; diſagreeable ſmells; exceſs of blood; indolence; high living; or the contrary; violent paſſions or affections of the mind, as fear, grief, &c.

The ſigns of approaching abortion are, a pain in the loins, or about the bottom of the belly; a dull heavy pain in the inſide of the thighs; a ſlight degree of coldneſs or ſhivering; ſickneſs; palpitation of the heart; the breaſts become

come flat and ſoft; the belly falls; and there is a diſcharge of blood or watery humours from the womb.

To prevent abortion, we would adviſe women of a weak or relaxed habit to uſe ſolid food, avoiding great quantities of tea, and other weak and watery liquors; to riſe early, and go ſoon to bed; to ſhun damp houſes; to take frequent exerciſe in the open air, but to avoid fatigue; and never to go abroad in damp foggy weather, if they can ſhun it. Women of a full habit ought to uſe a ſpare diet, avoiding ſtrong liquors, and every thing that may tend to heat the body, or increaſe the quantity of blood. Their diet ſhould be of an opening nature, conſiſting principally of vegetable ſubſtances. Every woman with child ought to be kept cheerful and eaſy in her mind. All violent paſſions hurt the *fœtus*, and endanger an abortion.

When any ſigns of abortion appear, the woman ought to be laid in bed on a mattreſs, with her head low. She ſhould be kept quiet, and her mind ſoothed and comforted. She ought not to be kept too warm, nor to take any thing of a heating nature. Her food ſhould conſiſt of broths, rice and milk, jellies, or gruels with a very little wine in them.

If ſhe be able to bear it, ſhe ſhould loſe, at leaſt, half a pound of blood from the arm. Her drink ought to be barley-water ſharpened with cream of tartar; or ſhe may take half a dram of of powdered nitre in a cup of water-gruel, every five or ſix hours. If the woman be ſeized with a violent looſeneſs, ſhe ought to drink the decoction of calcined hartſhorn prepared. If ſhe be affected with vomiting, let her take frequently one of the ſaline draughts recommended page 242.

SANGUINE robuſt women, who are liable to miſcarry at a certain time of pregnancy, ought always to be bled a few days before that period arrives. By this means, and obſerving the regimen above preſcribed, they may often eſcape that misfortune.

THO' we recommend due care for preventing abortion, we would not be underſtood as reſtraining pregnant women from their uſual exerciſes. This would operate the quite contrary way. Want of exerciſe not only relaxes the body, but induces a plethora, or too great a fulneſs of the veſſels, which are the two principal cauſes of abortion.

OF CHILD-BIRTH.

MANY diſeaſes proceed from the want of due care in child-bed. The more hardy part of the ſex are apt to deſpiſe the neceſſary precautions after delivery. They think, when the labour-pains are ended, the danger is over; but in truth it may only then be ſaid to be begun. Nature, if left to herſelf, will ſeldom fail to expel the *fœtus*; but proper care and management are certainly neceſſary for the recovery of the mother. No doubt, miſchief may be done by too much as well as by too little care. Hence it is that females who have the greateſt number of attendants in child-bed, generally recover worſt. But this is not peculiar to the ſtate of child-bed. Exceſſive care always defeats its own intention, and is generally more dangerous than none at all.

During actual labour, nothing of a heating nature muſt be given. The woman may, now and then, take a little panada, and her drink ought to be toaſt and water, or thin groat-gruel. Spirits, wines, cordial-waters, and other things, which are given with a view to ſtrengthen the mother, and promote the birth, for the moſt part tend only to increaſe the fever, inflame the womb, and retard the labour. Beſides, they endanger the woman afterwards, as they often occaſion violent and mortal hæmorrhages, or prediſpoſe her to eruptive and other fevers.

When the labour proves tedious and difficult, to prevent inflammations, it will be proper to bleed. An emolient clyſter ought likewiſe frequently to be adminiſtered; and the patient ſhould ſit over the ſteams of warm water. The paſſage ought to be gently rubbed with a little ſoft *pomatum* or freſh butter, and cloths wrung out of warm water applied over the belly. If Nature ſeems to ſink, and the woman

man be greatly exhausted with fatigue, a draught of generous wine, or some other cordial, may be given, but not otherwise. These directions are sufficient in natural labours, and in all preternatural cases, a skillful surgeon, or man-midwife, ought to be called as soon as as possible.

We cannot help taking notice of that ridiculous custom which still prevails in some country places, of collecting a number of women together upon such occasions. These, instead of being useful, serve only to crowd the house, and obstruct the necessary attendants. Besides, they hurt the patient with their noise ; and often by their untimely and impertinent advice, do much mischief.

After delivery, the woman ought to be kept as quiet and easy as possible. Her food should be light and thin ; as gruel, panada, &c. and her drink weak and diluting. To this rule however there are some exceptions. I have known several hysteric women, whose spirits could not be supported in child-bed without solid food and generous liquors ; to such a glass of wine and a bit of chicken must be allowed.

Sometimes an excessive hæmorrhage or flooding happens after delivery. In this case, the patient should be laid with her head low, have ligatures applied above her knees and elbows, and be in all respects treated as for an excessive flux of the *menses*. If the flooding proves violent, linen cloths, which have been wrung out of a mixture of equal parts of vinegar and water, should

ſhould be applied to the belly, the loins, and the thighs; Theſe muſt be changed as they grow dry; and may be diſcontinued as ſoon as the flooding abates.

If there be violent pains after delivery, the patient ought to drink plentifully of warm diluting liquors, as tea with a little ſaffron; or an infuſion of camomile flowers; and to take ſmall broths, with carroway ſeeds or a bit of orange-peel in them; an ounce of the oil of ſweet almonds may likewiſe be frequently taken in a cup of any of the above liquors; and if the patient be reſtleſs, a ſpoonful of the ſyrup of poppies may now and then be mixed with a cup of her drink. If ſhe be hot or feveriſh, one of the following powders may be taken in a cup of her uſual drink, every five or ſix hours. Take of crabs claws prepared half an ounce, purified nitre two drams, ſaffron powdered half a dram; rub them together in a mortar, and divide the whole into eight or nine doſes. When the patient is low ſpirited, or troubled with hyſterical complaints, ſhe ought to take frequently twelve or fifteen drops of the tincture of aſafœtida in a cup of penny-royal tea.

An inflammation of the womb is a dangerous and not unfrequent diſeaſe after delivery. It is known by pains in the lower part of the belly, which are greatly increaſed upon touching; by the tenſion or tightneſs of the parts; great weakneſs; change of countenance; a conſtant fever, with a weak and hard pulſe; a ſlight *deli-*

rium

rium or raving; ſometimes inceſſant vomiting; a hiccup; a diſcharge of rediſh ſtinking ſharp water from the womb; an inclination to go to ſtool; a heat, and ſometimes total ſuppreſſion of urine.

THIS muſt be treated like other inflammatory diſorders, by bleeding and plentiful dilution. The drink may be thin gruel or barley water; in a cup of which half a dram of nitre may be diſſolved, and taken three or four times a day. Clyſters of warm water muſt be frequently adminiſtred; and the belly ſhould be fomented by cloths wrung out of warm water, or by applying bladders filled with warm milk and water to it.

A ſuppreſſion of the *lochia*, or uſual diſcharges after delivery, and the milk-fever, muſt be treated nearly in the ſame manner as an inflammation of the womb. In all theſe caſes the ſafeſt courſe is plentiful dilution, gentle evacuations, and fomentations of the parts affected. In the milk-fever, the breaſts may be embrocated with a little warm linſeed oil, or the leaves of red cabbage may be applied to them. The child ſhould be often put to the breaſt, or it ſhould be drawn by ſome other perſon.

NOTHING would tend more to prevent the milk-fever than putting the child early to the breaſt. The cuſtom of not allowing children to ſuck for the firſt two or three days, is contrary to Nature and common ſenſe, and is very hurtful both to the mother and child. Every ry mother who has milk in her breaſts, ought either to ſuckle her own child, or to have her breaſts frequently drawn, at leaſt for the firſt month. This would prevent many of the diſeaſes which prove fatal to women in child-bed.

When an inflammation happens in the breaſt, attended with redneſs, hardneſs, and other ſymptoms of ſuppuration, the ſafeſt application is a poultice of bread and milk, ſoftened with oil or freſh butter. This may be renewed twice a-day, till the tumour be either diſcuſſed or brought to ſuppuration. Afterwards it may be dreſſed with yellow baſilicon, or any other digeſtive ointment. The uſe of repellants, in this caſe, is very dangerous; they often occaſion fevers, and ſometimes cancers: Whereas a ſuppuration is ſeldom attended with any danger, and has often the moſt ſalutary effects.

When the nipples are fretted or chapt, they may be anointed with a mixture of oil and bees-wax, or a little gum-arabic may be ſprinkled on them. I have ſeen Hungary-water applied to the nipples have a very good effect. Should the complaint prove obſtinate, the nurſe ought to be purged, which generally removes it.

The miliary fever is a diſeaſe very incident to women in child-bed. But as it has been treated of already, we ſhall take no farther notice of it here than only, with the celebrated Hoffman, to obſerve, that this fever of child-bed women might generally be prevented, if they, during their pregnancy, were regular in their diet, uſed moderate

moderate exercise, took now and then a gentle laxative of manna, rhubarb, or cream of tartar; not forgetting to bleed in the first months, and avoid all sharp air. When the labour is coming on, it is not to be hastened with forcing medicines, which inflame the blood and humours, or put them into unnatural commotions. Care should be taken, after the birth, that the natural excretions proceed regularly; and if the pulse be quick, a little nitrous powder should be given, &c.

We shall conclude our observations on child-bed women by recommending it to them, above all things, to beware of cold. Poor women, whose circumstances oblige them to quit their bed too soon, often contract diseases from cold, of which they never recover. It is pity the poor are not better taken care of in this situation. But the better sort of women run the greatest hazard from being kept too hot. They are generally kept in a sort of bagnio for the first eight or ten days, and then dressed out to see company. The danger of this conduct must be obvious to every one. The superstitious custom of obliging women to keep the house till they go to church, is likewise a very common cause of catching cold. All churches are damp, and most of them cold; consequently they are the very worst places to which a woman can go to make her first visit, after being confined in a warm room for a month. We make this observation from experience, having often had occasion to attend

attend women whoſe diſorders were the effect of cold caught in this way.

OF BARRENNESS.

Barrenness may be very properly reckoned among the diſeaſes of females, as few married women who have not children enjoy a good ſtate of health. It may proceed from various cauſes; but we ſhall only take notice of two, viz. high living and relaxation. It is very certain that high living vitiates the humours, and prevents fecundity. We ſeldom find a barren woman among the labouring poor, while nothing is more common amongſt the rich and affluent. The inhabitants of every country are prolific in proportion to their poverty, and it would be an eaſy matter to adduce many inſtances of women who, by being reduced to live intirely upon a milk and vegetable diet, have conceived and brought forth children, though they never had any before. Would the rich uſe the ſame ſort of food and exercife as the better ſort of peaſants, they would ſeldom have cauſe to envy their poor vaſſals and dependents the bleſſing of a numerous and healthy offspring, while they pine in ſorrow for the want of even a ſingle heir to their extenſive dominions.

Affluence begets indolence, which not only vitiates the humours, but induces a general relaxation

relaxation of the ſolids; a ſtate highly unfavourable to procreation. As we have the greateſt reaſon to believe, that relaxation is one of the moſt common cauſes of barrenneſs, we would recommend the following courſe for removing it. Firſt, plenty of exerciſe in the open air; ſecondly, the uſe of the cold bath; and laſtly, aſtringent medicines. It is well known, that many women who had been long barren, have, by the uſe of the cold bath not only become mothers, but have afterwards enjoyed a much better ſtate of health. This ſhould induce all barren women not only to try the cold bath, but to perſiſt in the uſe of it for a long time, otherwiſe it cannot be expected to produce any conſiderable effects.

THO' a vegetable diet, plenty of exerciſe, and the cold bath, are the medicines moſt to be relied upon, we ſhall mention one more, which has ſometimes proved effectual, viz. common *allum*. About the third or fourth day of the menſtrual flux the woman muſt take as much powdered allum at bed time, in a cup of wine or negas, as will lie upon ſixpence. This muſt be repeated for three or four nights running. If it has not the deſired effect, it may be taken in the ſame manner next time the *menſes* return. I have known ſeveral women who always conceived after taking this medicine, and never without it.

THE above obſervations on diet, air, and exerciſe, are applicable to men as well as to women.

men. Dr Chyne avers, that want of children is oftener the fault of the male than of the female, and ſtrongly recommends a milk and vegetable diet to the former as well as the latter; adding, that his friend Dr Taylor, whom he calls the milk Doctor of Croyden, had brought ſundry opulent families in his neighbourhood, who had continued ſome years after marriage without progeny, to have ſeveral fine children, by keeping both parents, for a conſiderable time, to a milk and vegetable diet.

DISEASES OF CHILDREN.

The nurſing and management of children having been pretty fully treated of in the firſt part of this book, we ſhall only here take notice of ſuch of their diſeaſes as have not been already mentioned.

RETENTION of the MECONIUM.

The ſtomach and bowels of a new-born infant are filled with a blackiſh-coloured matter of the conſiſtence of ſyrup, commonly called the *meconium.* This is generally paſſed ſoon after the birth by the mere effort of nature, in which caſe it is not neceſſary to give the infant any kind of medicine. But if it ſhould be retained, or not ſufficiently carried off, it may occaſion wind, gripes, jaundice, reſtleſſneſs, convulſions, &c.

The

THE moſt proper medicine for expelling the *meconium* is the mother's milk, which is always, at firſt, of a purgative quality. But, if the mother does not give ſuck, or, if her milk happens not to be ſufficiently purgative, a little of the ſyrup of pale roſes may be given, or a ſmall quantity of the ſyrup of rhubarb diluted with water, and ſweetened with honey or coarſe ſugar. If theſe are not at hand, a common ſpoonful of whey ſweetened with a tea-ſpoonful of honey may be given.

ALL kind of oils are to be avoided; they are quite indigeſtible by infants, and tend only to load their ſtomachs and make them ſick.

THE APHTHÆ OR THRUSH.

THE aphthæ are little whitiſh ulcers affecting the whole inſide of the mouth, tongue, throat, and ſtomach of infants. Sometimes they reach through the whole inteſtinal canal; in which caſe they are very dangerous, and often put an end to the infant's life.

IF the aphthæ are of a pale colour, pellucid, few in number, ſoft, ſuperficial, and fall eaſily off, they are not dangerous; but if opake, yellow, brown, black, thick, or running together, they are bad.

IT is generally thought that the aphthæ owe their origin to acid humours; but we have reaſon to believe that theſe, and ſeveral other eruptive diſeaſes of infants, are, in a great meaſure,

ſure, owing to too hot a regimen both of the mother and child. It is a rare thing to find a child who is not doſed with wine, punch, cinnamon waters, or ſome other hot and inflaming liquors, almoſt as ſoon as it is born. It is well known that theſe will occaſion inflammatory diſorders even in adults; is it any wonder then that they ſhould heat and inflame the tender bodies of infants, and ſet, as it were, the whole conſtitution on a blaze?

THE moſt proper medicines for the aphthæ are thoſe of a cooling and gently opening nature. Five grains of rhubarb and a dram of *magneſia alba* may be rubbed together, and divided into ſix doſes, one of which may be given to the child every five or ſix hours. Theſe powders may either be given in the child's food or a little of the ſyrup of pale roſes, and may be repeated as often as is found neceſſary to keep the belly open.

MANY things have been recommended for gargling the mouth and throat in this diſeaſe; but it is not eaſy to apply theſe in very young infants; we would therefore recommend it to the nurſe to rub the child's mouth frequently with a little borax and honey; or with the following mixture. Take fine honey an ounce, borax a dram, burnt allum half a dram, roſe-water two drams; mix them together. Theſe may be applied with the finger, or by means of a bit of ſoft rag tied to the end of a probe.

OF

OF ACIDITIES.

The food of children being, for the moſt part, of an aceſcent nature, it readily turns ſour upon the ſtomach, eſpecially if the body be any how diſordered. Hence it comes to paſs, that moſt diſeaſes of children are accompanied with evident ſigns of acidity, as green ſtools, gripes, &c. Theſe appearances have induced many to believe, that all the diſeaſes of children were owing to an acid abounding in the ſtomach and bowels; but whoever conſiders the matter attentively, will find, that theſe ſymptoms of acidity are oftener the effect than the cauſe of diſeaſes.

Nature evidently intended, that the food of children ſhould be aceſcent; and until the body be diſordered, or the digeſtion hurt, from ſome other cauſe, we will venture to ſay, that the aceſcent quality of their food is ſeldom injurious to them. Acidity however is often a ſymptom of infantile diſorders, and, as it is a very troubleſome one, we ſhall point out the method of relieving it.

When green ſtools, gripes, purgings, &c. ſhew, that the bowels abound with an acid, the child ſhould have a little ſmall broth inſtead of milk, with light white bread in it; and ſhould have plenty of exerciſe in order to promote the digeſtion. It has been cuſtomary in this

this caſe to give the pearl-julep, chalk, crabs eyes, and other teſtaceous powders. Theſe indeed, by their abſorbent quality, may correct the acidity; but they are attended with this inconveniency, that they are apt to lodge in the bowels, and occaſion a coſtiveneſs, which may prove very hurtful to the infant. For this reaſon they ſhould never be given unleſs mixed with purgative medicines; as rhubarb, manna, or ſuch like.

THE beſt medicine which we know, in all caſes of acidity, is that fine inſipid powder called *magneſia alba*. It purges, and, at the ſame time, corrects the acidity; by which means it not only removes the diſeaſe, but carries off its cauſe. It may be given in any kind of food, from ten grains to a tea-ſpoonful, according to the age of the patient. I have often known it have good effects when given in the following manner. Take of *magneſia alba* two drams, fine rhubarb in powder half a dram, peppermint water and common water, of each two ounces, as much ſyrup of ſugar as will make it agreeable. Shake the bottle, and give the child a table-ſpoonful three or four times a-day.

WHEN an infant is troubled with gripes, it ought not to be doſed with brandy, ſpiceries, and other hot things, but ſhould have its belly opened with an emollient clyſter, or the medicine mentioned above; and at the ſame time a little brandy may be rubbed on its belly with a warm a warm hand before the fire. I have ſeldom ſeen this fail to eaſe the gripes of infants. It is often more effectual, and always more ſafe than brandy taken inwardly.

GALLING AND EXCORIATION.

THESE are very troubleſome to children. They happen chiefly about the groin and wrinkles of the neck, under the arms, behind the ears, and in other parts that are moiſtened by the ſweat or urine.

As theſe complaints are, in a great meaſure, owing to want of cleanlineſs, the moſt effectual means of preventing them are, to waſh the parts frequently with water, to change the linen often, and, in a word, to keep the child, in all reſpects, thoroughly clean. When this is not ſufficient, the excoriated parts may be ſprinkled with abſorbent or drying powders; ſuch as burnt hartſhorn, tutty, chalk, crabs claws prepared, &c. Any of theſe may be tied in a rag, and the powder ſhook out on the diſordered places.

WHEN the parts affected are very ſore, and tend to a real ulceration, it will be proper to add a little ſugar of lead to the powders; or to anoint the place with a little camphorated ointment. If the parts be waſhed with ſpring-water, in which a little white vitriol has been diſſolved, it will dry and heal them very powerfully.

STOP-

STOPPAGE OF THE NOSE.

THE noſtrils of infants are often plugged up with a groſs *mucus*, which prevents their breathing freely, and likewiſe renders it difficult for them to ſuck or ſwallow.

SOME, in this caſe, order, after a ſuitable purge, two or three grains of white vitriol diſſolved in half an ounce of marjoram water and filtred, to be applied now and then to the noſtrils with a linen rag. Wedelius ſays, If two grains of white vitriol, and the ſame quantity of *elaterium*, be diſſolved in half an ounce of marjoram water, and applied to the noſe, as above directed, that it brings away the *mucus* without ſneezing.

IN obſtinate caſes theſe things may be tried; but we have never found any thing elſe neceſſary, than to rub the noſe at bed-time with a little oil of ſweet almonds, or a bit of freſh butter. This reſolves the filth, and renders the breathing more free.

Of ERUPTIONS.

CHILDREN, while on the breaſt, are ſeldom free from eruptions of one kind or other. Theſe however are not often dangerous, and ought never to be ſtopped but with the greateſt caution. They tend to free the bodies of infants from

from hot and acrid humours, which, if retained, might produce fatal diſorders.

The eruptions of children are chiefly owing to the following cauſes, viz. improper food, and neglect of cleanlineſs. If a child be ſtuffed at all hours with food that his ſtomach is not able to digeſt, ſuch food, not being properly aſſimilated, inſtead of nouriſhing the body, fills it with groſs humours. Theſe muſt either break out in form of eruptions upon the ſkin, or remain in the body, and occaſion fevers and other internal diſorders. That neglect of cleanlineſs is a very general cauſe of eruptive diſorders, muſt be obvious to every one. The children of the poor, and of all who deſpiſe cleanlineſs, are almoſt conſtantly found to ſwarm with vermin, and are generally covered over with the ſcab, itch, and other eruptions.

When eruptions are the effect of improper food, or want of cleanlineſs, a proper attention to theſe alone will generally be ſufficient to remove them. If this ſhould not be the caſe, ſome drying medicines will be neceſſary; but they ſhould never be applied without the greateſt caution. If drying medicines are applied, the belly ought at the ſame time to be kept open, and cold is carefully to be avoided. We know no medicine that is more ſafe for drying up cutaneous eruptions than ſulphur, provided it be ſparingly uſed. A little of the flowers of ſulphur may be mixed with the white ointment, or hog's lard, and the parts affected frequently touched with it.

The most obstinate of all the eruptions incident to children are, the *tinea capitis*, or scabbed head, and chilblains. The scabbed head is often exceeding difficult to cure, and sometimes indeed the cure proves worse than the disease. I have frequently known children seized with internal disorders, of which they died soon after their scabbed heads had been healed by the application of drying medicines *. The cure ought always first to be attempted by keeping the head very clean, cutting off the hair, combing and brushing away the scabs, &c. If this be not sufficient, let the head be shaved once a-week, and washed daily with soap and warm water, or with lime water. Should these fail, a plaster of black pitch may be applied, in order to pull out the hair

* I some time ago saw a very striking instance of the danger of substituting drying medicines in the place of cleanliness and wholesome food.

Being consulted for the children of a certain Hospital in England, who were grievously afflicted with scabbed heads, and other cutaneous disorders. I found, upon inquiry, that the children were fed upon potatoes, and other crude vegetables, thro'the whole year, and that cleanliness was totally neglected. My advice was to give them more wholesome food, and to keep them thoroughly clean. This advice however was not followed. It was too troublesome to the servants, superintendents, &c. The business was to be done by medicine; which was accordingly attempted, but had like to have proved fatal to the whole house. Fevers and other internal disorders immediately appeared, and, at length, a putrid dysentery broke out which carried off a great many of the children.

hair by the roots. And if there be proud flesh, it should be touched with a bit of blue vitriol, or sprinkled with a little burnt allum. While these things are doing, the patient must be kept to a regular light diet, his belly should be kept gently open; and cold, as far as possible, ought to be avoided. To prevent any bad consequences from stopping this discharge, it will be proper, especially in children of a delicate habit, to make an issue in the neck or arm, which may be kept open till the patient becomes more strong, and the constitution be somewhat confirmed.

CHILBLAINS commonly attack children in cold weather. They are generally occasioned by the feet or hands being kept long wet or cold, and afterwards suddenly heated. When children are cold, instead of taking exercise to warm themselves gradually, they run to the fire. This occasions a sudden rarefaction of the humours, and an infarction of the vessels; which being often repeated, the vessels are, at last, over-distended, and forced to give way.

To prevent it, violent cold and sudden heat must be equally avoided. When the parts begin to look red and swell, the patient ought to be purged, and to have the affected parts frequently rubbed with mustard and brandy, or something of a warm nature. They ought likewise to be covered with flannel, and kept warm and dry. Some apply warm ashes betwixt cloths

cloths to the ſwelled parts, which frequently help to reduce them. When there is a ſore, it muſt be dreſſed with Turner's cerate, or ſome other drying ointment; as the ointment of tutty, the plaſter of ceruſs, &c. Theſe ſores are indeed troubleſome, but ſeldom dangerous. They generally heal as ſoon as the warm weather ſets in

OF DIFFICULT BREATHING.

CHILDREN are often ſeized very ſuddenly with a great difficulty of breathing, which, if not quickly relieved, proves mortal. This diſeaſe is known by various names in different parts of the country. In the Eaſt coaſt of Scotland it is called the *croup*. On the Weſt they call it the *chock* or *ſtuffing*. In ſome parts of England, where I have met with it, the good women call it the riſing of the lights. It ſeems to be a ſpecies of *aſthma*. attended with very acute and violent ſymptoms.

THIS diſeaſe generally prevails in cold and wet ſeaſons. It is moſt common upon the ſea-coaſt, and in low marſhy countries. Children of a groſs and lax habit are moſt liable to it. I have ſometimes known it hereditary. It generally attacks children in the night, after having been much expoſed to damp cold eaſterly winds through the day. Damp houſes, wet feet, thin ſhoes,

ſhoes, wet cloaths, or any thing that obſtructs the perſpiration, may occaſion this diſeaſe.

It is attended with a frequent pulſe, quick and laborious breathing, which is performed with a peculiar kind of croaking noiſe that may be beard at a conſiderable diſtance. The voice is ſharp and ſhrill and the face is generally much fluſhed, tho' ſometimes it is of a livid colour.

When a child is ſeized with the above ſymptoms, his feet ſhould be put into warm water. He ought likewiſe to be bled, and to have a laxative clyſter adminiſtered as ſoon as poſſible. He ſhould be made to breathe over the ſteams of warm water, or an emollient decoction, and emollient cataplaſms or fomentations may be applied round his neck. If the ſymptoms do not abate, a bliſtering plaſter muſt be applied round the neck, or betwixt the ſhoulders, and the child may take frequently a table ſpoonful of the following julep. Take penny-royal water three ounces, ſyrup of althea and balſamic ſyrup, each one ounce, mix them together.

Some, in this caſe, recommend aſafœtida. It may both be given in form of clyſter, and taken by the mouth. Two drams of aſafœtida may be diſſolved in one ounce of Mindererus's ſpirit, and three ounces of penny royal water. A table-ſpoonful of this mixture may be given every hour, or oftener if the patient's ſtomach be able to bear it. If the patient cannot be brought to take this medicine, two drams of the aſafœtida asafœdita may be dissolved in a common clyster, and administered every six or eight hours, till the violence of the disease abates.

To prevent a return of this disease, all those things which occasion it must be carefully avoided; as wet feet, cold, damp easterly winds, &c. Children who have had frequent returns of this disease, or whose constitution seems to predispose them to it, ought to have their diet properly regulated; all food that is viscid or hard of digestion, and all crude, raw, trashy fruits, are to be avoided. They ought likewise to have a drain constantly kept open in some part of their body, by means of a seton or issue. I have sometimes known a Burgundy pitch plaster, worn continually betwixt the shoulders for several years, have a very happy effect in preventing the return of this dreadful disorder.

OF TEETHING.

Dr Arbuthnot observes, that above a tenth part of infants die in teething, by symptoms proceeding from the irritation of the tender nervous parts of the jaws, occasioning inflammations, fevers, convulsions, gangrenes, &c. These symptoms are, in a great measure, owing to the great delicacy and exquisite sensibility of the nervous system at this time of life. But this natural sensibility of the nerves in infancy is too often increased by an effeminate education.

tion. Hence it comes to paſs, that children who are delicately brought up always ſuffer moſt in teething, and often fall by convulſive diſorders.

About the ſixth or ſeventh month the teeth generally begin to make their appearance; firſt the *inciſores*, or foreteeth; next the *canini*, or dog-teeth; and laſtly, the *molares*, or grinders. About the ſeventh year there comes a new ſet; and about the twentieth the two inner grinders, called *dentes ſapientiæ*, the teeth of wiſdom.

Children, about the time of cutting their teeth, ſlaver much, and have generally a looſeneſs, which is no bad ſign; but when the teething is difficult, eſpecially when the dog-teeth begin to make their way through the gums, the child has ſtartings in his ſleep, tumours of the gums, inquietude, watchings, gripes, green ſtools, the thruſh, fever, difficult breathing, convulſions, and epilepſies, which often end in death.

Difficult teething is, in all reſpects, to be treated as an inflammatory diſeaſe. If the belly be bound, it muſt be opened either by emollient clyſters or gentle purgatives; as manna, *magneſia alba*, rhubarb, ſenna, &c. The food ſhould be light, and in ſmall quantity; the drink plentiful, but weak and diluting, as infuſions of balm, or of the lime-tree flowers; to which about a third or fourth part of milk may be added.

If the fever be very high, bleeding will be neceſſary; but this, in very young children, ought

ought always to be ſparingly performed. It is an evacuation which they bear the worſt of any. Purging, vomiting, or ſweating, agree much better with them, and are generally more beneficial. Harris however obſerves, that, when an inflammation appears, the phyſician will labour in vain, if the *cure* be not begun with applying a leech under each ear. If the child be ſeized with convulſion fits, a bliſtering plaſter may be applied betwixt the ſhoulders, or one behind each ear.

Dr Sydenham ſays, that in fevers occaſioned by teething, he never could find any remedy ſo effectual as two, three, or four drops of ſpirits of hartſhorn in a ſpoonful of ſimple water, or other convenient vehicle, given every four hours. The number of doſes may be four, five, or ſix. I have often preſcribed this medicine with ſucceſs, but always found a larger doſe neceſſary. It may be given from five drops to fifteen or twenty, according to the age of the child.

In Scotland, it is very common, when children are cutting their teeth, to put a ſmall Burgundy pitch plaſter between their ſhoulders. This generally eaſes the tickling cough which attends teething, and is by no means an uſeleſs application. When the teeth are bred with difficulty, it ought to be kept on during the whole time of teething. It may be enlarged as occaſion requires, and ought to be renewed, at leaſt, once a month.

SEVE-

Several things have been recommended for rubbing the gums, as oils, mucilages, &c.; but from these much is not to be expected. What we would recommend for this purpose is virgin-honey. A little of this may be rubbed on with the finger three or four times a day. Children are generally at this time disposed to chew whatever they get into their hands. For this reason they ought never to be without somewhat that will yield a little to the pressure of their gums, as a crust of bread, a wax-candle, a bit of liquorice-root, or such like. These are far more proper than corral, ivory, silver, or any other impenetrable substance.

With regard to cutting the gums, we have seldom known it of any real advantage. In obstinate cases it ought however to be tried; but as it is generally performed by a surgeon, we shall not spend time in describing the operation.

In order to render the teething less difficult, parents ought to take care that their childrens food be light and wholesome, and that their nerves be braced by plenty of exercise without doors, and the use of the cold bath, &c. Were these things duly regarded, few children would die of teething.

As the limits of this performance will not permit us to treat the diseases of infants at more length, we shall only observe, that, if properly nursed, their diseases would be very few, and would seldom prove fatal. The nurse may,

 for

for the moſt part, do the buſineſs of the phyſician; but the phyſician can never do that of the nurſe.

The diſeaſes of children are far leſs complicated than thoſe of adults, and conſequently much eaſier underſtood; the method of curing them is likewiſe very ſimple, and cannot readily be miſtaken. In all the acute diſeaſes of children, cool air, diluting liquors, and gentle evacuations, are almoſt the only things needful; and in their chronic diſeaſes, reſtorative diet, free air, and proper exerciſe, are what the cure muſt chiefly depend upon.

OF WOUNDS.

No part of medicine has been more miſtaken than the treatment and cure of wounds. Mankind in general believe, that certain herbs, ointments, and ſalves are poſſeſſed of wonderful healing virtues, and imagine that no wound can be cured without the application of them. It is however a fact, that no external application whatever contributes towards the cure of a wound, any other way than by keeping the parts ſoft, and defending them from the external air, which may be as effectually done by ſoft lint as by the moſt pompous applications, while it is exempt from many of the bad conſequences attending them.

The ſame obſervation holds with reſpect to internal applications. Theſe only promote the

the cure of wounds in ſo far as they tend to prevent a fever, or to remove any cauſe that might obſtruct or impede the operations of Nature. It is Nature alone that cures wounds; all that art can do is to remove obſtacles, and to put the parts in ſuch a condition as is the moſt favourable to Nature's efforts.

WITH this ſimple view, we ſhall conſider the treatment of wounds, and endeavour to point out ſuch ſteps as ought to be taken to facilitate their cure.

THE firſt thing to be done when any perſon has received a wound is to examine whether any foreign body be lodged in it, as wood, ſtone, iron, lead, glaſs, dirt, bits of cloth, &c. Theſe, if it can be eaſily done, ought to be extracted, and the wound cleaned, before any dreſſings be applied. When that cannot be effected with ſafety, on account of the patient's weakneſs, or loſs of blood, &c. they muſt be ſuffered to remain in the wound, and be afterwards extracted when the patient is more able to bear it.

WHEN a wound penetrates into any of the cavities of the body, as the breaſt, the bowels, &c. or where any conſiderable blood-veſſel is cut, a ſkilful ſurgeon ought immediately to be called, otherwiſe the patient may loſe his life. But ſometimes the diſcharge of blood is ſo great, that if it be not ſtopt, the patient may die even before a ſurgeon, tho' at no great diſtance, can arrive. In this caſe, ſomething muſt be done

by

by thoſe who are preſent. If the wound be in any of the limbs, the bleeding may generally be ſtopt by applying a tight ligature or bandage round the member a little above the wound. The beſt method of doing this is to put a ſtrong broad garter round the part, but ſo ſlack as eaſily to admit a ſmall piece of ſtick to be put under it. which muſt be twiſted, in the ſame manner as a country man does a cart-rope to ſecure his loading, till the bleeding ſtops. Whenever this is the caſe, he muſt take care to twiſt it no longer, as ſtraining too tight might occaſion an inflammation of the parts and endanger a gangrene.

In parts where this bandage cannot be applied, various other methods may be tried to ſtop the bleeding, as the application of ſtyptics, aſtringents, &c. Cloths dipped in a ſolution of blue vitriol in water, or the *ſtyptic water* of the Diſpenſatories, may be applied to the wound. When theſe cannot be obtained, ſtrong ſpirits of wine may be uſed. Some recommend the *Agaric* * of the oak as preferable to any of the other

* Dr Tiſſot, in his *Advice to the people*, gives the following directions for gathering, preparing, and applying the agaric.——"Gather in autumn, while the fine weather laſts, the agaric of the oak, which is a kind of fungus or excreſcence iſſuing from the wood of that tree It conſiſts at firſt of four parts, which preſent themſelves ſucceſſively: 1 he outward rind or ſkin, which may be thrown away. 2. The part immediately under this rind, which is the beſt of all. This is to be beat well with a hammer, till it becomes ſoft and very pliable.

other ſtyptics; and indeed it deſerves conſiderable encomiums. It is eaſily obtained, and ought to be kept in every family, in caſe of accidents. A piece of it muſt be laid upon the wound and covered with a good deal of lint, above which a bandage muſt be applied ſo tight as to keep it firmly on.

THO' ſpirits, tinctures, and hot balſams may be uſed in order to ſtop the bleeding when it is exceſſive, they are improper at other times. They do not promote but retard the cure, and often change a ſimple wound into an ulcer. People imagine, becauſe hot balſams congeal the blood, and ſeem, as it were, to ſolder up the wound, that they therefore heal it; but this is only a deception. They may indeed ſtop the flowing blood, by ſearing the mouths of the veſſels; but, by rendering the parts callous, they obſtruct the cure.

IN ſlight wounds which do not penetrate much deeper than the ſkin, the beſt application is a bit of the common black ſticking plaſter. This keeps the ſides of the wound together, and prevents the

pliable. This is the only preparation it requires, and a ſlice of it of a proper ſize is to be applied directly over the burſting open blood veſſels. It conſtringes and brings them cloſe together, ſtops the bleeding, and generally falls off at the end of two days. 3 The third part adhering to the ſecond may ſerve to ſtop the bleeding from the ſmaller veſſels: and the fourth and laſt part may be reduced to powder as conducing to the ſame purpoſe ——That agaric which ſprings from thoſe parts of the tree from whence large boughs have been lopped, is generally reckoned the beſt."

the air from getting into it, which is all that is neceſſary. When a wound penetrates deep, it is not ſafe to keep its lips quite cloſe; this keeps in the matter, and is apt to make the wound feſter. In this caſe the beſt way is to fill the wound with ſoft lint, commonly called *caddis*. This however muſt not be ſtuffed in too hard, otherwiſe it will do hurt. It may be covered over with a cloth dipped in oil, or ſpread with the common wax * plaſter; and the whole muſt be kept on by a proper bandage.

We ſhall not ſpend time in deſcribing the different bandages that may be proper for wounds in different parts of the body; common ſenſe will generally ſuggeſt the moſt commodious method of applying a bandage; beſides deſcriptions of this kind are not eaſily remembered.

The firſt dreſſing ought to continue on for at leaſt two days; after which it may be removed, and freſh lint applied as before. If any part of the firſt dreſſing ſticks ſo cloſe that it cannot be removed with eaſe or ſafety to the patient, it may be allowed to continue, and freſh lint dipped in ſweet oil laid above it. This will ſoften it ſo as to make it come off eaſily at next dreſſing.

After-

* The wax plaſter is made by melting together over a ſlow fire, a pound of yellow wax; white reſin, and mutton ſuet, of each half a pound. This not only ſupplies the place of melilot plaſter, formerly ſo much in vogue, but makes a very proper application to ſlight wounds, and to large ones after they are nearly heal.

Afterwards the wound may be dreſſed every day in the ſame manner till it be quite heal. Thoſe who are fond of ſalves or ointments, may, after the wound is become very ſuperficial, dreſs it, twice a-day, with the yellow *baſilicum* ointment*; and if fungous, or what is called *proud fleſh*, ſhould riſe in the wound, it may be checked, by mixing with the ointment, a little burnt allum or red precipitate.

When a wound is greatly inflamed, the moſt proper application is a pultice of bread and milk, ſoftened with a little ſweet oil or freſh butter. This muſt be applied inſtead of the plaſter, and ſhould be changed two or three times a-day.

If the wound be large, and there is reaſon to fear an inflammation, the patient muſt be kept on a very low diet. He muſt abſtain from fleſh, ſtrong liquors, and every thing that is of a heating nature. If he be of a full habit, and has loſt but little blood from the wound, he muſt be bled; and, if the ſymptoms be urgent, the operation may be repeated. But when the patient has been greatly weakened by loſs of blood from the wound, it will be dangerous to bleed

* The yellow baſilicum ointment is prepared in the following manner. Take of olive oil an Engliſh pint, yellow wax, yellow reſin, and Burgundy pitch, of each one pound; common turpentine three ounces. Melt the wax, reſin, and pitch, along with the oil over a ſlow fire; after taking them from the fire, add the turpentine, and, whilſt the mixture remains hot, ſtrain it.

bleed him, even tho a fever ſhould enſue. Nature ſhould never be too far exhauſted. It is always more ſafe to allow her to ſtruggle with the diſeaſe in her own way, than to ſink the patient's ſtrength by exceſſive evacuations.

WOUNDED perſons ought to be kept very quiet and eaſy. Every thing that ruffles the mind, or moves the paſſions, as love, anger, fear, exceſſive joy, &c. are very hurtful. They ought, above all things to abſtain from venery. The belly ſhould be kept gently open either by laxative clyſters or by cool vegetable diet, as roaſted apples, ſtewed prunes, boiled ſpinnage, &c.

OF BURNS.

IN ſlight burns which do not break the ſkin, it is cuſtomary to hold the part near the fire for a competent time, to rub it with ſalt, or to lay a compreſs upon it dipped in ſpirits of wine or brandy. But when the burn has penetrated ſo deep as to bliſter or break the ſkin, it muſt be dreſſed with ſome emollient and gently drying ointment, as the ointment of calamine, commonly called *Turner's cerate* *. This may be

* Turner's cerate may be prepared by diſſolving half a pound of yellow wax in an Engliſh pint of olive-oil over a gentle fire. As the mixture cools, and begins to grow ſtiff, half a pound of calamine prepared muſt be ſprinkled into it, keeping conſtantly ſtirring them together till the cerate is grown quite cold.

be mixed with an equal quantity of fresh olive-oil, and spread upon a soft rag, and applied to the part affected. When this ointment cannot be had, an egg may be beat up with about an equal quantity of the sweetest salad oil. This will serve very well till a proper ointment can be prepared. When the burning is very deep, after the first two or three days, it should be dressed with equal parts of yellow *basilicum* ointment and Turner's cerate mixed together.

When the burn is violent, or has occasioned a high degree of inflammation, and there is reason to fear a gangrene or mortification will ensue, the same means must be used to prevent it as are recommended in other violent inflammations. The patient, in this case, must live low, and drink freely of weak diluting liquors He must likewise be bled once, and, if occasion requires, a second time. His belly should be kept open; and, if the burnt parts become livid or black, with other symptoms of mortification, it will be necessary to bathe them frequently with warm camphorated spirits of wine, tincture of myrrh, or other antiseptics mixed with a decoction of the bark. In this case the bark must likewise be taken internally.

OF BRUISES.

Bruises are generally productive of worse consequences than wounds. The danger from them does not appear immediately, by which means it often happens that they are neglected till paſt cure. It is needleſs to give any definition of a diſeaſe ſo univerſally known; we ſhall therefore proceed to point out the method of treating it.

In ſlight bruiſes it will be ſufficient to bathe the part with a mixture of equal quantities of vinegar and water, and to keep cloths wet with this mixture conſtantly applied to it. This is far more proper than rubbing it with brandy, ſpirits of wine, or other ardent ſpirits, which are commonly uſed in ſuch caſes.

In ſome parts of the country the peaſants apply to a recent bruiſe a poultice of freſh cow's dung, with very happy effects.

When a bruiſe is very violent, the patient ought immediately to be bled, and put upon a proper regimen. His food ſhould be light and cool, and his drink weak, and of an opening nature; as whey ſweetened with honey, decoctions of tamarinds, barley, cream-tartar-whey, and ſuch like. The bruiſed part muſt be bathed with vinegar and water, as directed above; and a poultice made by boiling crumbs of bread, elder flowers, and camomile flowers, in equal quantities of vinegar and water, applied to it. This poultice is peculiarly proper when a wound is joined to the bruiſe. It may be renewed two or three times a day.

As the ſtructure of the veſſels is totally deſtroyed by a violent bruiſe, there often enſues a great loſs of ſubſtance, which produces an ulcerous

cerous ſore very difficult to cure. If the bone be affected, the ſore will not heal before an exfoliation takes place, that is, before the diſeaſed part of the bone ſeparates, and comes out through the wound. This is often a very ſlow operation, and may even require ſeveral years to be compleated. Hence it happens, that theſe ſores are frequently miſtaken for the King's evil, and treated as ſuch, though, in fact, they proceed ſolely from the injury which the ſolid parts received from the blow.

PATIENTS in this ſituation are peſtered with different advices. Every perſon who ſees them propoſes a new remedy, till the ſore is, in a manner, poiſoned with various and oppoſite applications, and is often at length rendered abſolutely incurable. The beſt method of managing ſuch ſores is, to take care that the patient's conſtitution does not ſuffer by confinement, or improper medicine, and to apply nothing to them but ſome ſimple ointment ſpread upon ſoft lint, over which a poultice of bread and milk, with boiled camomile flowers, or the like, may be put to nouriſh the part, and keep it ſoft and warm. Nature, thus aſſiſted, will generally in time operate a cure, by throwing off the diſeaſed parts of the bone, after which the ſore ſoon heals.

OF

OF DISLOCATIONS.

Dislocations are generally occaſioned by falls, blows, or the like. They are always dangerous, and ſometimes, unleſs immediately reduced, they prove fatal. A perſon who has the misfortune, by a fall from his horſe, or the like, to diſlocate his neck is often left to periſh, while it is in the power of every perſon preſent to do all that is neceſſary for his recovery. But people are ſeized with a kind of panic upon theſe occaſions, and are often ſo much afraid of doing wrong, that they do nothing at all. This is, in fact, allowing a perſon to die for fear of hurting him.

When the neck is diſlocated, or put out of joint, the patient is immediately deprived of all ſenſe and motion; his countenance ſoon turns bloated and blackiſh; his neck ſwells; and his face is generally turned towards one ſhoulder. He ſhould immediately be laid upon his back on the ground, and the operator muſt place himſelf behind him in ſuch a manner, as to be able to lay hold of his head with both his hands, while he makes a reſiſtance by placing his knees againſt the patient's ſhoulders. In this poſition, with one hand under the chin, and the other under the hinder part of the head, he muſt pull with conſiderable force, gently twiſting it at the ſame time, if the face be turned ed to one ſide, till he perceives that the joint is replaced. This is eaſily known from the noiſe which the bones generally make upon one another in the very act of reduction, from the patient's beginning ſoon after to breathe, and from the head continuing in its proper poſition, &c. This operation, like many others, is eaſier performed than deſcribed, and requires only common prudence and ſufficient reſolution in the operator. I have known inſtances of its being happily performed even by women, and frequently by men of no medical education.

THO' diſlocations of the limbs are leſs dangerous, they ought nevertheleſs to be reduced as ſoon as poſſible. When the operation is long delayed it becomes very difficult, and ſometimes even impracticable. Beſides, when a bone has been diſlocated for a conſiderable time, it can ſeldom be kept in its place after it has been reduced. A mechanical genius, with a very ſlight notion of the ſtructure of the human body, will enable any perſon to reduce a diſlocated bone. All that is neceſſary is to make a proper extenſion, and, at the ſame time to puſh the head of the bone towards the ſocket *.

AFTER the bone has been reduced, a roller wet with equal parts of vinegar and water may be applied round the joint. The member ought to

* WE intended here to have treated of the various kinds of diſlocations, and to have ſhewn the method of reducing them; but this the limits of our performance will not permit.

to be placed in the moſt natural and eaſy poſture, and kept ſo for ſome time, till the parts recover their wonted ſtrength and tone.

OF BROKEN BONES.

THERE are in moſt country villages ſome perſon who pretends to the art of reducing fractures. Tho in general ſuch perſons are very ignorant, yet ſome of them are very ſucceſsful; which evidently proves, that a ſmall degree of learning, with a ſufficient ſhare of common ſenſe, will enable a man to be uſeful in this way. We would however adviſe people never to truſt ſuch operators when an expert and ſkilful ſurgeon can be had; but when that is impracticable, they muſt be employed; we ſhall therefore recommend the following hints to their conſideration.

WHEN a large bone is broken, the patient's diet ought, in all reſpects, to be the ſame as that of a perſon in a fever. He ſhould likewiſe be kept quiet and cool, and his belly ſhould be kept gently open either by emollient clyſters, or, if theſe cannot be conveniently adminiſtered, by food that is of an opening quality; as ſtewed prunes, apples boiled in milk, boiled ſpinnage, &c. It ought however to be here remarked, that perſons who have been accuſtomed to live high, are not all of a ſudden to be reduced to a very low diet.

diet. This might have fatal consequences. There is often a necessity of indulging bad habits, in some measure even where the nature of the disease might require a different treatment.

It will generally be necessary to bleed the patient after a fracture, especially if he be young, of a full habit, or has, at the same time, received any bruise or contusion. This operation should be performed as soon after the accident happens as possible, and if the patient be very feverish, it may be repeated next day. When several of the ribs are broken, bleeding is peculiarly necessary.

If any of the large bones which support the weight of the body be broken, the patient must keep his bed for several weeks. It is by no means however necessary that he should lie all this while as is customary, upon his back. This situation sinks the spirits, galls and frets the patient's skin, and renders him very uneasy. After the second week he may be gently raised up, and may sit several hours, supported by a bed-chair or the like, which will greatly relieve him. Great care however must be taken in raising him up, and laying him down, that he exert no strength of his own, otherwise the action of the muscles may pull the bone out of its place.

It is of great importance to keep the patient dry and clean while in this situation. By neglecting this he is often so galled and excoriated that he is forced to keep shifting places for ease. I have some-

ſometimes known a fractured thigh bone, after it had lain ſtrait for above a fortnight, diſplaced by this means, and continue bent for life, in ſpite of all that could be done.

Bone-setters ought carefully to examine whether the bone be not ſhattered, or broken into a great many pieces. In this caſe it will generally be neceſſary to have the limb taken off, otherwiſe a gangrene or mortification may enſue. The horror which attends the very idea of an amputation often occaſions its being delayed in ſuch caſes till too late. I, ſome time ago, ſaw a ſhocking inſtance of this in a maſon, who had the misfortune to fall from the third ſtory of a houſe. In one of his legs, which had ſtruck a beam, the bones were ſo ſhattered and ſplit near the ancle, that they felt almoſt like a bag of ſmall ſtones. Some of their ſharp points had likewiſe penetrated the ſkin. It was adviſed that the leg ſhould immediately be taken off; but to this the patient's friends would not conſent. After taking three or four days to conſider of it, the operation was at laſt determined upon, and was accordingly performed; but alas, it was in vain! The mortification had already proceeded too far to be ſtopped, and the miſerable patient died in two days.

When a fracture is accompanied with a wound, it muſt be dreſſed in all reſpects as a common wound.

All that art can do towards the cure of a broken

broken bone, is to lay it perfectly ſtraight, and to keep it quite eaſy. All tight bandages do hurt. They had much better be wanting altogether. A great many of the bad conſequences which proceed from fractured bones are owing to tight bandages. This is one of the ways in which the exceſs of art, or rather the abuſe of art, does more miſchief than would be occaſioned by the want of it. Some of the moſt ſudden cures of broken bones which were ever known, happened when no bandages were applied at all. Some method however muſt be taken to keep the member ſteady; but this may be done many ways without bracing it with a tight bandage. We are not however againſt the uſe of bandages altogether. It is only the wrong application of them which we find fault with.

In fractures of the ribs, where a bandage cannot be properly uſed, an adheſive plaſter may be applied over the part. The patient in this caſe ought to keep himſelf quite eaſy, avoiding every thing that may occaſion ſneezing, laughing, coughing, or the like. He ought to keep his body in a ſtraight poſture and ſhould take care that his ſtomach be conſtantly diſtended, by taking frequently ſome light food, and drinking freely of weak watery liquors.

The moſt proper external application for a fracture is *oxycrate*, or a mixture of vinegar and water. The bandages ſhould be wet with this a every dreſſing before they be applied, and the part may be frequently ſprinkled with it.

OF STRAINS.

STRAINS are often attended with worſe conſequences than broken bones. The reaſon is obvious; they are generally neglected. When a bone is broken, the patient is under a neceſſity of keeping it eaſy, becauſe he cannot make uſe of it; but when a joint is only ſtrained, the perſon, finding he can ſtill make a ſhift to move it, is ſorry to loſe his time for ſo trifling an ailment In this way he deceives himſelf, and converts into an incurable malady what might have been removed by only keeping the part eaſy for a few days.

COUNTRY people generally immerſe a ſtrained limb in cold water. This is very proper, provided it be done immediately and not kept in too long. But the cuſtom of keeping the part immerſed in cold water for many hours together, is certainly dangerous. This relaxes inſtead of bracing the part, and is more likely to produce a diſeaſe than remove one.

WRAPPING a garter, or ſome other bandage, pretty tight about the ſtrained part, is likewiſe of uſe. It helps to reſtore the proper tone of the veſſels, and prevents the action of the parts from encreaſing the diſeaſe. It ſhould not however be applied too tight. I have frequently known

known bleeding near the affected part, in violent ſtrains, have a very good effect.

But what we would recommend above all things for a ſtrain is *eaſe*. It is more to be depended upon than any medicine, and ſeldom fails to remove the complaint.

OF ULCERS.

Ulcers may be the conſequence of wounds, bruiſes, or tumours, improperly treated; but they generally proceed from an ill ſtate of the humours, or what may be called a bad habit of body.

When this is the caſe, they ought not to be haſtily dried up, otherwiſe it may prove fatal to the patient. Ulcers happen moſt commonly in the decline of life; and perſons who neglect exerciſe, and live full, are moſt liable to them. They might often be prevented by retrenching ſome part of the ſolid food, or by opening artificial drains, as iſſues, ſetons, or the like.

An ulcer may be known from a wound by its diſcharging a thin watery humour, which is often ſo acrid as to inflame and corrode the ſkin; by the hardneſs and perpendicular ſituation of its ſides or edges, and by the time of its duration, &c.

It requires conſiderable ſkill to be able to judge when an ulcer ought to be healed, and when not. In general, all ulcers which proceed from a bad habit of body ſhould be ſuffered

fered to continue open at leaſt till the conſtitution be ſo far changed by proper regimen, or the uſe of medicine, that they ſeem diſpoſed to heal of their own accord. Ulcers which are the effect of malignant fevers, or other acute diſeaſes, may generally be healed with ſafety after the health has been reſtored for ſome time. The cure ought not however to be attempted too ſoon, nor at any time without the uſe of purging medicines and a proper regimen. When wounds or bruiſes have, by wrong treatment, degenerated into ulcers, if the conſtitution be good, they may generally be healed with ſafety. When ulcers either accompany chronical diſeaſes, or come in their ſtead, they muſt be cautiouſly healed. If an ulcer conduces to the patient's health, it ought never to be healed; but if, on the contrary, it waſtes the ſtrength, and conſumes the patient by a ſlow fever, it ſhould be healed as ſoon as poſſible.

We would earneſtly recommend a ſtrict attention to theſe particulars, to all who have the misfortune to labour under this diſorder, as we have frequently known people throw away their lives by the want of it, while they were extolling and generouſly rewarding thoſe whom they ought to have looked upon as their murderers.

The moſt proper regimen for promoting the cure of ulcers, is to avoid all ſpices, all ſalted and high ſeaſoned food, all ſtrong liquors, and to leſſen the uſual quantity of fleſh meat The belly ought to be kept gently open by a diet

diet consisting chiefly of cooling laxative vegetables, and by drinking butter-milk, or whey sweetened with honey, or the like. The patient ought to be constantly cheerful, and should take as much exercise as he can easily bear.

WHEN the bottom and sides of an ulcer seem hard and callous, they may be sprinkled twice a-day with a little red precipitate of mercury, and afterwards dressed with the yellow *basilicum* ointment. Some chuse to have the edges of the ulcer scarified with a lancet; but this operation ought to be performed by a surgeon.

LIME-WATER has frequently been known to have very happy effects in the cure of obstinate ulcers. It may be used in the same manner as directed for the stone and gravel.

MY late learned and ingenious friend, Dr Whytt, strongly recommends the use of a solution of the corrosive sublimate of mercury in brandy, for the cure of obstinate ill-conditioned ulcers. I have frequently found this medicine, when given according to the Doctor's directions, prove very successful; but it should never be administered without the greatest care. It is made by dissolving four grains of the corrosive sublimate of mercury in eight ounces of the best French brandy. The dose is a table-spoonful night and morning; at the same time washing the sore twice or thrice a-day with it. In a letter which I had from the Doctor a little before his death, he informs me, "That he observed washing the sore thrice a-day with a solua ſolution of a triple ſtrength was very uſeful.' This medicine ought always to be prepared with the greateſt care, and ought never to be adminiſtered but under the eye of ſome perſon of ſkill in phyſic.

Of IMPOSTHUMES or BOILS.

Boils are generally the efforts of Nature to expel noxious humours out of the body. Their ſuppuration ought therefore by all means to be promoted. I do not remember ever to have ſeen one inſtance of the conſtitution being hurt by them, but have often known it greatly mended, eſpecially when care was taken to promote a full and free ſuppuration.

Imposthumes may proceed from the uſe of traſhy fruits, or any other unwholeſome food, from hunger, exceſſive labour, or the like. They are attended with acute pain, hardneſs, redneſs of the part, and all the ſymptoms of inflammation.

Bleeding and purging will ſometimes diſcuſs theſe tumours at the beginning; but as ſoon as it is evident that matter is collecting, it will be proper to apply a poultice of bread and and milk, with a little oil or freſh butter. This may be renewed twice a day; and if the ſuppuration goes ſlowly on, a raw onion may be cut into ſmall pieces, or bruiſed in a mortar, and ſpread

ſpread upon the top of the poultice. This will promote the ſuppuration more in one day than a ſimple poultice will do in three or four.

WHEN the boil turns ſoft, appears of a white or yellowiſh colour, and is quite full of matter, if it does not break of itſelf, it ſhould be opened with a lancet. This operation is noways dangerous, and is very little painful, as the ſkin is very thin and greatly diſtended. If no other inſtrument be at hand, it may be opened with a large needle; but it is always better to make uſe of a lancet, or ſome inſtrument that will make a pretty large wound, in order that the matter may be diſcharged freely.

AFTER the impoſthume has broke, or been opened, it may be dreſſed twice a-day with yellow *baſilicum* ointment, ſpread upon lint, or a bit of ſoft rag. It will ſtill however be proper to keep the poultice applied to it, till ſuch time as the matter be entirely diſcharged. After the matter has been diſcharged, the patient ought to be purged.

WHEN boils return frequently, it ſhews a bad ſtate of the humours, and merits particular attention. The patient ought to be peculiarly attentive to his diet, and, if the diſeaſe proceeds from any error in it, it ſhould be changed as ſoon as poſſible. Repeated purges are generally neceſſary in this caſe; and infuſions of the bitter plants, as water-trefoil, camomile-flowers, &c. ought to be drank freely. Thoſe who

who are able to afford it, ſhould take a courſe of the purging mineral waters.

OF WHITLOWS.

A *whitlow* is a painful tumour appearing near the end of a finger, the humour of which is often ſo ſharp as to corrode the tendons and nerves, and ſometimes even the bone itſelf.

THESE tumours ſometimes proceed from the puncture of a ſharp body, as a thorn, a pin, a ſplinter, or the like. But their moſt general cauſes, as was formerly obſerved, are ſudden changes from cold to heat, or the contrary. Hence the diſeaſe is very common among milk-maids, eſpecially at that ſeaſon of the year when they go a milking in a cold nipping froſty morning, and, as ſoon as they get home, plunge their hands into warm water, or hold them near the fire.

THE pain of a whitlow is commonly ſo great, as to render the patient exceeding reſtleſs. It is attended with an inflammation and often with an evident pulſation. When the humour lies deep, the inflammation ſpreads over the whole hand, and ſometimes it extends up the arm even to the ſhoulder. The pain, inflammation, and fever have ſometimes been ſo violent, in this caſe, as to prove mortal.

MANY things are recommended for diſcuſſing the inflammation; as bleeding, bliſtering, the

the patient, the holding the part in diſtilled vinegar, dipping it frequently in ſcalding-hot water, and ſuch like. Theſe may ſometimes ſucceed at the beginning, but they do no good afterwards. The ſafeſt courſe is to promote the ſuppuration, by applying cataplaſms, or poultices of bread and milk, with boiled camomile flowers. Or, if a more active and ripening poultice be neceſſary, the white lilly root, or a little honey may be added; but theſe ſhould not be applied till there be evident ſigns of a ſuppuration.

WHEN the inflammation and fever run very high, it will be neceſſary to bleed the patient, and to keep him upon a low diet, allowing him to drink freely of diluting liquors.

WHEN the matter is lodged deep, it is not ſafe to wait till the tumour breaks and diſcharges itſelf. In this caſe the matter muſt be let out by making a deep inciſion, otherwiſe it will corrode and deſtroy the bone. This operation ſhould always be performed by a ſurgeon, if one can be had. I have frequently ſeen one bone of the finger loſt by the matter remaining too long in contact with it. Indeed whenever the inflammation begins very deep, it is hardly poſſible to ſave the bone.

AFTER the tumour has burſt, or been laid open, it may be dreſſed with the yellow *baſilicum* ointment, or ſome other digeſtive, and a poultice applied over it. If proud fleſh appears, it may be kept down by ſprinkling a little burnt allum over it.

If any ſymptoms of a gangrene or mortification appear, as a black, pale, or livid colour of the parts, &c the patient muſt have immediate recourſe to the bark, a dram of which muſt be taken every two or three hours. The part muſt alſo be ſcarified, and fomented with a ſtrong decoction of the bark, or camomile flowers; to which ſome ſpirit of ſea-ſalt, or ſtrong vinegar, may be added.

As whitlows and mortifications of the extremities are often the effects of violent cold, we would adviſe people who have been expoſed to an exceſſive degree of it, if their hands or feet are greatly benumbed, to waſh them in cold water, or rub them, for ſome time with ſnow, and to keep at a diſtance from the fire. This would not only prevent whitlows, but is the only method of reſtoring frozen limbs, and of preventing a mortification from extreme cold.

OF RUPTURES.

This diſeaſe happens moſt frequently to children and old people. Men are greatly more liable to it than women, eſpecially thoſe who are naturally of a weak and relaxed habit. In infants it is generally occaſioned by exceſſive crying, violent coughing, repeated efforts to vomit, &c. In adults it is commonly the effect of blows, violent exertions of the ſtrength, as leaping, carrying great weights, &c. An oily or very moiſt diet, by inducing a general relaxation of of the ſolids, is commonly thought to prediſpoſe the body to ruptures.

On the firſt appearance of a rupture in an infant it ought to be laid upon its back, with its head very low. While in this poſture, if the gut does not return of itſelf, it may eaſily be put up by gentle preſſure. After it is returned, a piece of ſticking plaſter may be applied over the part, and a proper truſs or bandage muſt be conſtantly worn for a conſiderable time. The method of making and applying theſe rupture bandages for children is pretty well known. The child muſt, as far as poſſible, be kept from crying, and from all violent motion, till the rupture is quite healed.

In adults, when the gut has been forced down with great violence, or happens, from any cauſe, to be inflamed, it is often very difficult to return it, and ſometimes quite impracticable without an operation which it is not our buſineſs to deſcribe. As I have been fortunate enough however always to ſucceed in my attempts to return the gut, without having recourſe to any other means than what are in the power of every man, I ſhall very briefly mention the method which I generally purſue. After the patient has been bled, he muſt be laid upon his back, with his head very low, and his breech raiſed high with pillows. In this ſituation flannel-cloths wrung out of a decoction of mallows and camomile-flowers, or, if theſe are not at hand, of warm water, muſt be applied for a conſiderable time. A clyſter made of this de-

decoction, with a large ſpoonful of butter and a little ſalt, may be afterwards thrown up. If theſe ſhould not prove ſucceſsful, recourſe muſt be had to preſſure. If the tumour be very hard, conſiderable force will be neceſſary; but it is not force alone which ſucceeds here. The operator, at the ſame time that he makes a preſſure with the palms of his hands, muſt with his fingers conduct the gut in by the ſame aperture thro' which it came out. The manner of doing this can be much eaſier conceived than deſcribed. Should all theſe endeavours prove ineffectual, clyſters of the ſmoke of tobacco muſt be tried These have been often known to ſucceed where every other method failed.

An adult, after the gut has been returned, muſt wear a ſteel bandage. It is needleſs to deſcribe theſe, as they are only to be had from the artiſts who make them. They are generally uneaſy to the wearer for ſome time, but by cuſtom they become quite eaſy. No perſon who has had a rupture after he arrived at man's eſtate, ſhould ever be without one of theſe bandages.

Persons who have a rupture ought carefully to avoid all violent exerciſe, carrying great weights leaping, running, and the like. They ſhould likewiſe avoid windy aliment and ſtrong liquors; and ſhould carefully guard againſt catching cold.

Of

OF CASUALTIES.

As it is often impracticable to obtain even the ſmalleſt degree of medical aſſiſtance in many of thoſe accidents which endanger life, we ſhall conclude with a few obſervations upon ſome of the moſt common and hazardous of them.

THE firſt we ſhall name is *the ſtoppage of ſubſtances between the mouth and the ſtomach.* Though accidents of this kind are unavoidable, yet, generally ſpeaking, they are the effect of careleſſneſs. Children have a ſtrong inclination to put every thing in their mouths which they get hold of. This ought to make nurſes careful in keeping every thing from them that they can ſwallow, which would be hurtful. Even adults are far leſs careful in this reſpect than they ought to be. Nothing ſhould ever be held in the mouth which it would be dangerous to ſwallow, as a fit of coughing, or ſome other accident, may force it over. Notwithſtanding the numberleſs accidents which are daily occaſioned by holding pins in the mouth, many women have their mouths, for the moſt part, full of them through the day; and ſome of them even ſleep with them there all night.

WHEN a pin, or any other ſharp body is ſwallowed, it will generally deſcend into the ſtomach, if its head, or blunt end goes foremoſt; but if the point goes foremoſt, it is apt to ſtop, and when that happens, every effort to force it down

down will only ſerve to fix it faſter in. In this caſe the beſt way is to make the patient vomit, either by tickling his throat with a feather, or giving him a vomit. I have frequently known pins which had ſtuck in the gullet for ſeveral days, brought up by ſwallowing a bit of tough meat tied to a ſtrong thread, and drawing it quickly up again.

All hard or ſharp ſubſtances, which might hurt or wound the bowels, ought, if poſſible, to be diſcharged upwards. Subſtances that will diſſolve in the ſtomach, if they cannot be brought up, may be puſhed down. When a mouthful of ſolid food ſtops in the gullet, it may often be forced up by giving the perſon a blow on the back betwixt the ſhoulders. If this ſhould not ſucceed, the throat may be tickled with the finger or a feather. I lately ſaw a halfpenny, which had ſtuck faſt in the gullet of a boy about eight years old, thrown up by only thurſting a finger down his throat.

Persons who have the misfortune to fall into the water are often given up for dead, when it is certain they might, by proper care, be recovered. The great intention which ſhould be kept in view is to reſtore the natural *warmth*, and renew the *circulation* and *breathing*. Tho' cold is by no means the cauſe of the perſon's death, yet it will prove an effectual obſtacle to his recovery. For this reaſon, after ſtripping him of his wet cloaths, if he had any on when the accident happened, his body muſt be ſtrongly ly rubbed for a conſiderable time with coarſe linen cloths as warm as they can be made. As ſoon as a bed can be got ready and well heated, he may be laid in it, and the rubbing ſtill continued. Warm cloths ſhould be laid to his ſtomach and bowels, and hot bricks, or bottles filled with warm water, to the ſoles of his feet. He ſhould likewiſe be bled. The moſt proper part for this operation is in the jugular vein, both becauſe it is moſt likely to bleed, and affords the moſt ſudden relief to the head.

In order to renew the breathing, a ſtrong perſon may blow his own breath into the patient's mouth with all the force he can; or, what will ſucceed better, the ſmoke of tobacco may be blown into the lungs, by means of a pipe or funnel. I have known a pig drowned and reſtored to life, two or three different times ſucceſſively, by blowing air into its mouth with a pair of bellows. It will likewiſe be proper to throw up the ſmoke of tobacco into the inteſtines, in form of a clyſter, by means of a proper pipe. Strong volatile ſalts ought alſo to be applied to the noſe, or ſpirits of hartſhorn, burnt feathers, &c. The noſe ought likewiſe to be tickled with a feather dipped in volatile ſpirits, and warm ſpirits of wine ſhould be rubbed upon the temples, pit of the ſtomach, &c.

If theſe do not ſucceed, the perſon may be put into a warm bath, or laid among warm aſhes. Dr Tiſſot mentions an inſtance of a girl who was

was reſtored to life, after being taken out of the water to all appearance dead, by laying her naked body upon hot or warm aſhes; by covering her with others equally hot; by putting a bonnet round her head, with a ſtocking round her neck ſtuffed with the ſame, and heaping coverings over all.

THE ſame method muſt be purſued for the recovery of perſons ſtrangled as for thoſe who are drowned.——Such as have the misfortune to be ſtunned by a fall, a blow, or the like, muſt alſo be treated nearly upon the ſame principles. Every method muſt be taken to keep up the genial warmth, and to reſtore the vital functions Nor ought we to deſpair too ſoon of ſucceſs. I have been happy enough to recover a perſon who was taken up for dead by a fall from a horſe, after ſix hours endeavours, during the greater part of which time he hardly ſhewed any ſigns of life.

NOTHING is more certain than that life, when ſeemingly loſt, might often be reſtored by perſiſting for a ſufficient time in the uſe of proper means; and that many of thoſe unhappy perſons who periſh by accidents, are really loſt for want of due care. Surely all the laws of religion and humanity call upon us to do every thing in our power to ſave the lives of our fellow men. Who would not chuſe to be the happy inſtrument of preſerving an uſeful member of ſociety, and perhaps of preventing the ruin of an innocent family?

FINIS.

Printed in the United States
By Bookmasters